CELL ACTIVATION AND APOPTOSIS IN HIV INFECTION

Implications for Pathogenesis and Therapy

ADVANCES IN EXPERIMENTAL MEDICINE AND BIOLOGY

Recent Volumes in this Series

CELL ACTIVATION AND APOPTOSIS IN HIV INFECTION

Implications for Pathogenesis and Therapy

Edited by

Jean-Marie Andrieu
Wei Lu
Laennec Hospital
Paris, France

SPRINGER SCIENCE+BUSINESS MEDIA, LLC

Library of Congress Cataloging-in-Publication Data

Cell activation and apoptosis in HIV infection : implications for
   pathogenesis and therapy / edited by Jean-Marie Andrieu and Wei Lu.
        p.   cm. -- (Advances in experimental medicine and biology ; v.
   374)
     Proceedings of the First International Symposium on Cellular
   Aproaches to the Control of HIV Disease, held July 11-12, 1994, in
   Paris, France--T.p. verso.
     Includes bibliographical references and index.
     ISBN 978-0-306-45063-1   ISBN 978-1-4615-1995-9 (eBook)
     DOI 10.1007/978-1-4615-1995-9
     1. HIV infections--Pathophysiology--Congresses. 2. Apoptosis-
   -Congresses. 3. Lymphocyte transformation--Congresses.
   I. Andrieu, Jean-Marie. II. Lu, Wei. III. International Symposium
   on Cellular Approaches to the Control of HIV Disease (1st : 1994 :
   Paris, France) IV. Series.
     [DNLM: 1. HIV Infections--immunology--congresses. 2. HIV
   Infections--therapy--congresses. 3. HIV Infections--immunology-
   -congresses. 4. Apoptosis--immunology--congresses. 5. T
   -Lymphocytes-- immunology--congresses.   W1 AD559 v.374 1995 / WC
   503 C393 1995]
   QR201.A37C45 1995
   616.97'92--dc20
   DNLM/DLC
   for Library of Congress   95-17728
                                                           CIP

Proceedings of the First International Symposium on Cellular Approaches to the Control of HIV Dis
held July 11–12, 1994, in Paris, France

ISBN 978-0-306-45063-1

© 1995 Springer Science+Business Media New York
Originally published by Plenum Press, New York in 1995

10 9 8 7 6 5 4 3 2 1

PREFACE

In the past decade, the global efforts in the control of HIV disease were basically concentrated on the search for anti-retroviral agents. So far, anti-HIV therapies have been shown to be disappointing because of rapid development of drug-resistant mutant variants. Despite this drawback in the therapeutic fight against HIV infection, antiviral research should be actively pursued.

However, failure of antiviral therapy indicates that other avenues of research should be rapidly explored with the same energy. In this setting, striking advances have been recently made in the dissection and understanding of the viro-immunological processes governing the progressive destruction of lymphoid organs associated with AIDS development, and HIV-induced activation and apoptosis have been identified as key phenomena of the immune system destruction.

This book assembles the most recent advances on basic and clinical aspects of T-cell activation/apoptosis in HIV infection and their implications for immunotherapy. These data were presented at an international symposium held on July 11-12, 1994, in Paris. The book is partitioned into 21 chapters covering four comprehensive fields: 1) T-cell/macrophage activation and HIV infection; 2) Apoptosis and viropathogenesis of HIV disease; 3) Apoptosis and immunopathogenesis of HIV disease; 4) Mediators of T-cell activation/apoptosis and therapeutic applications.

We hope that this book will assist the readers in understanding recent advances in the viro-immunopathogenesis of HIV disease as well as the rationales for potential immune-cell-targeted therapeutic interventions.

Jean-Marie Andrieu
Wei Lu

ACKNOWLEDGMENTS

We graciously thank Philippe Even, dean of the Faculty of Medicine Necker, René Descartes University for his continuous encouragement and support; Simon Wain-Hobson (Paris), Sven Britton (Huddinge), Jacques Corbeil (San Diego), and Jean-Claude Ameisen (Lille) for chairing the different sessions of the symposium. The symposium was supported by Agence Nationale de Recherches sur le SIDA (ARNS) and Association de Recherche pour le Traitement des Seropositifs (ARTS).

CONTENTS

T-CELL/MACROPHAGE ACTIVATION AND HIV INFECTION

APOPTOSIS AND VIROPATHOGENESIS OF HIV DISEASE

APOPTOSIS AND IMMUNOPATHOGENESIS OF HIV DISEASE

MEDIATORS OF T-CELL ACTIVATION/APOPTOSIS AND
THERAPEUTIC APPLICATIONS

CD4+ AND CD8+ T LYMPHOCYTE ACTIVATION IN HIV INFECTION
Implications for Immune Pathogenesis and Therapy

Jeffrey Laurence[*]

Laboratory for AIDS Virus Research
Cornell University Medical College
New York, New York

INTRODUCTION

Studies initiated some 30 years ago by Dr. Howard Temin demonstrated that the state of host cell activation at the time of retroviral infection influences greatly reverse transcription and viral expression (1). Similarly, helper/inducer (CD4+) and cytolytic (CD4+ and CD8+) T lymphocyte activation plays a crucial role in the life-cycle of HIV. Indeed, HIV has adopted a transcriptional strategy resembling that used by certain cellular genes that regulate T cell signalling and growth (2), as modulated by viral *cis* and *trans*-acting elements. This enables HIV to establish a persistent infection in T cells from which replication competent virus may be induced through a variety of pathways. Similarly, macrophage-tropic virus, thought responsible for initial infections in humans, establishes a reservoir in monocytes which is susceptible to differentiation and activation signals (3). Such chronicity in either cell lineage may not represent true molecular latency, with absent expression of viral transcripts and protein. Yet latency and viral persistence both involve two essential elements: initial restriction at the level of proviral transcription or initiation, regulated at HIV's long terminal repeat (LTR) and, perhaps, through intragenic enhancers (4); and a second level of control, with the fate of initiated transcripts dependent upon the viral regulatory elements *tat* and *rev* (5). It is also significant that viral replication can be dissociated from cellular growth, with both proliferative and non-mitogenic T cell activation signals sufficient to induce HIV transcription (6). The extraordinarily high turnover of HIV viruses (10^9/day) and rapid death of productively HIV-infected ($t_{1/2}$ = 2-15 days) in the periphery vs. lymph node also attests to the complex regulatory control of HIV replication (7).

Aberrant T cell activation is another factor in the pathophysiology of HIV disease. It can be mediated by HIV infection or indirectly, via: incomplete cross-linking or down-

[*] Requests for reprints to: Jeffrey Laurence, M.D. Cornell University Medical College, 411 E. 69th Street, Room KB-122, New York, NY 10021, USA.

Cell Activation and Apoptosis in HIV Infection
Edited by Jean-Marie Andrieu and Wei Lu, Plenum Press, New York, 1995

modulation of membrane receptors, including the T cell antigen receptor (TCR), CD3,CD4,CD8 & CD28; defects in antigen presenting cells (APC); superantigen (SAg) phenomena; and suppression of T cell co-stimulatory signals and growth factors. Such signals, even if incapable of eliciting an optimal CD4+ T cell response, may still permit induction of HIV replication and cytolytic T lymphocyte (CTL) activity. The latter, if inappropriately directed at autologous lymphocytes or APCs bearing processed HIV Env antigens, may exacerbate the loss of CD4+ cells (8).

This review probes potential mechanisms by which classic and aberrant CD4+ and CD8+ T lymphocyte activation, as initiated by host cellular responses to infectious HIV, HIV Env products and diverse immunogens, APC alterations and other factors contribute to T cell anergy, apoptosis, and ultimately modulation of HIV replication and/or host immune responsivity. These findings may have direct bearing on the course of HIV disease and the likely success of certain modalities of therapy for HIV/AIDS, as well as for the development of protective and therapeutic anti-HIV vaccines.

CELLULAR ACTIVATION AND TRANSCRIPTIONAL CONTROL OF HIV REPLICATION

Viral persistence may be viewed at three distinct levels: persistence in the population as a whole, in the individual host, and within a cell or group of cells (9). In terms of the latter, viruses persist by limited growth in a cell population (carrier state); continuous multiplication without cytopathic effects (steady-state infection); true latency; or cell-to-cell passage without maturation (intracytoplasmic persistence, characteristic of infection of cells which normally remain in G_o, such as monocytes) (9).

Macrophage-tropic virus appears to be responsible for initial infection *in vivo* and, as a persistent fixed reservoir of HIV, may have a central role in transmitting virus to recirculating T cells (3). By combination of endpoint dilution DNA polymerase chain reaction (PCR), *in situ* DNA PCR, and *in situ* RNA hybridization it appears that, *in vivo*, < 1% of CD4+ T cells carrying proviral sequences express viral transcripts, in peripheral blood or lymphoid tissue, at most stages of HIV disease (5). What has not been definitively established is whether the majority of these cells harbor a replication competent virus in a truly latent form, or defective proviruses. *In vitro* models pertinent to such discrimination are incomplete, as they generally rely on chronically infected, transformed cell lines. Preliminary data involving rescue of HIV from peripheral blood mononuclear cells (PBMC) indicate that, in this arguably more physiologic state, reactivation of latent provirus is not simply a function of cellular proliferation. Instead, T cell-monocyte interactions may be required. Evidence for such chronic immune activation *in vivo* comes from high circulating levels of β_2-microglobulin, acid labile α-interferon, neopterin, soluble interleukin-2 receptor (sIL-2R), soluble CD8, and major histocompatibility complex type II (MHC-II)+ lymphocytes. But viral persistence and latency are thus best explored in terms of the relative levels of restriction to viral gene expression at the level of an individual cell.

Starting at such a level, HIV typically integrates into the genome of its target, with reactivation, replication, and dissemination attendant on the level of host cell activation, itself influenced by myriad factors (5, 10). Indeed, while initiation of reverse transcription occurs simultaneously in both activated and quiescent T and B lymphocytes, monocytes, and probably other cell types, it terminates prematurely and proceeds more slowly in quiescent cells. Stimulation of such cells may reinitiate DNA synthesis off of partial reverse transcripts, but this mode of viral rescue is highly inefficient (11). And proviral DNA in quiescent cells is labile, degrading with a $t_{1/2}$ of <24 hrs *in vitro* (12). The molecular biology underlying these events has been exhaustively analyzed *in vitro*, is covered by other authors in these collected reviews, and will be discussed here only as it pertains to immune cell activation and signalling.

In vitro, < 5% of initial infectious doses of HIV-1 can be rescued 15 hrs after infection of a resting T cell (10), a phenomenon dependent upon viral and host products. Such cells, identified by absence of activation markers such as IL-2R and MHC-II antigens, as well as by low DNA synthetic responses, reveal: delayed kinetics for synthesis of LTR U3 DNA and transcription of the regulatory gene *nef*; decreased extension of existing transcripts; and premature termination of reverse transcription (10). Potential mechanisms accounting for these findings include: sequestration of deoxyribonucleotides; production of virion core (Gag) proteins that bind viral RNA; induction of cellular inhibitors of viral RNA transcription; and absence of reverse transcriptase potentiators upregulated in activated lymphocytes (10). Facilitation of HIV replication by TCR cross-linking via anti-CD3 monoclonal antibody can also be augmented by cross-ligation of CD28, a membrane receptor that can substitute for some of the functions of APC (13), as well as by T cell membrane antigen-adhesion molecule interactions such as CD2:LFA3 and CD18:ICAM-1 (5). The role of these accessory cells and accessory molecules in virus-cell activation will be developed later in this review. Transcriptional control of viral replication may be summarized by two basic events: induction of sequence-specific transcriptional factors, and chromatin reorganization to permit effective interaction of the induced factors with their proviral targets (5). The level of viral replication in individual cells may also be modified by the relatively random integration of HIV, with proviral transcription influenced by surrounding genomic DNA (5). This general pathway can account for both the lack of requirement for cell proliferation in viral induction, as well as dissociation of such proliferation from an inevitable enhancement of virion production. For example, NF-κB, a member of the *rel* family of transcriptional enhancers, is found in nearly all eukaryotic cells, coupled to its inhibitor, IκB, in an inactive form. Cellular activation, with or without cell proliferation, leads to upregulation of a variety of protein kinases one of which, in phosphorylating IκB, permits translocation of NFκB to the nucleus its binding to transcriptional enhancer sequences of the HIV LTR, and facilitation of RNA pol II activity.

Infectious Co-Factors for Cell and HIV Activation

Viral co-pathogens may also serve to regulate HIV replication through a variety of cellular activation and transcriptional events. The ability to directly *trans*-activate HIV replication *in vitro* is linked to specific and promiscuous transcriptional factors encoded by all of the herpesviruses—cytomegalovirus (CMV), Epstein-Barr Virus (EBV), herpes simplex viruses (HSV-1,2), and human herpesvirus type 6 (HHV-6)—as well as by hepatitis B (HBV), human T cell lymphotrophic virus (HTLV-I and-II), and papovaviruses (14-16).

In addition, viral co-pathogens may modulate proto-oncogene and tumor suppressor gene transcription, thereby influencing cell activation (through c-*myc*, c-*myb* and c-*fos*) and HIV transcription (e.g., though p53). For example, when T cells are stimulated by protein kinase inducers, mitogens, cytokines or antigen, induction of NF-κB transforms the HIV LTR into a type of housekeeping gene promoter, increasing the assembly of general transcription factors on the LTR to form pre-initiation complexes, and proscribing transcriptional squelching through cellular factors such as wild-type p53. *In vitro*, the wild type p53 tumor suppressor gene product inhibits HIV-LTR-directed transcription through bridging of Sp1 and TFIID sites (17). This is consistent with the finding of high rates of HIV replication in metastatic colon carcinoma cells from an HIV+ individual (18), as such tumors typically contain mutant p53's incapable of complexing with the HIV-LTR. Certain viruses which commonly infect HIV+ individuals also encode proteins which can complex with and inactivate p53 thereby promoting HIV transcription. These include the HBV X protein, E6 of human papillomavirus, and EBNA-V of EBV.

Apart from direct *trans*-activation of the HIV-LTR or suppression of p53 activity, other microorganisms common in HIV infection individuals also enhance HIV replication, at least in *in vitro*. These include: Cryptococcus neoformans, through its capsular polysaccharide (19); EBV, through its latent membrane protein (20); and parvovirus, via an early non-structural (NS) gene product (21). The clinical significance of these latter effects, dependent upon co-infection of single cells with two viruses, is uncertain. However, infection of the host may more broadly influence HIV replication by indirect mechanisms, broad activation of cell proliferation, and cytokine production. Thus, as noted above, HHV-6 can *trans*-activate the HIV-LTR, but it also stimulates the release of cytokines which can activate both cell and virus, as well as induces *de novo* expression of the high-affinity receptor for HIV, CD4, on mature CD8+ T cells, potentially broadening the range of HIV susceptible lymphocytes (16). And the *in vivo* relevance of many of these *in vitro* observations has been corroborated by clinical associations. The extent of peripheral HIV replication is highly correlated with CMV antigenemia (22), as determined by the presence of p24 Gag antigen and the rapidity of CD4+ T cell decline (14,23). Similarly, coinfection of keratinocytes and macrophages by HSV-1 and HIV-1 has been noted within cutaneous HSV lesions, with cyclical enhancement of proliferation of both viruses in single cells (24), and transient but marked increases in HIV viremia may occur during clinically apparent HSV-1 reactivation (25).

Infectious agents may also serve as cellular activators via SAg phenomena (26), or blockade of factors linked to suppression of viral and cell growth, or do both. For example, certain mycoplasmas can enhance viral and retroviral replication by inhibiting production of the antiretroviral product α-interferon (27), and are involved in SAG-mediated TCR cross-linking and cell activation (28).

Immunization and Cell Activation

It is reasonable to speculate that *any* stimulus to the immune system, whether by intercurrent infection, exposure to novel or recall antigens, injury accompanied by inflammation, immunizations, etc. might enhance HIV expression at least transiently. This is consistent with the fact that primary and secondary effector cells and memory cells express a variety of activation antigens and accessory molecules not found on naive lymphocytes (29) (Table 1). Indeed, an elevation in numbers of infected PBMC, ranging from 2- to 25-fold, was seen within 1-2 weeks of administration of inactivated vaccinia or HBV vaccines to HIV-1 infected chimpanzees (30) (Fig 1). This is consistent with the increase in HIV transcripts seen by RNA PCR (>10-fold) and plasma viremia determinations (>5-fold) following influenza immunization of HIV+ individuals (31). A peak in virus replication was again noted at 1-2 weeks after immunization, falling to baseline values only after several months. An identical response obtained in an independent study of a similar influenza immunization program (32). Similarly high-dose IL-2 infusions in HIV-1+ patients, either continuous or intermittent, leads to transient increases in viremia, despite antiretroviral therapy (33).

Pre-activation of uninfected CD4+ T lymphocytes may also lead to enhanced viral replication and accelerated T cell death following viral exposure. This has been demonstrated in animals with PB$_j$-14, an unusual isolate of the simian immunodeficiency virus (SIV) which, in pig-tailed macaques and cynomolgus monkeys, leads to immediate skewing of CD4+ T cells towards the activated CD45^{hi} subset and death of all animals within 6 to 10 days. In contrast, rhesus macaques, with fewer circulating activated T cells pre- and post-viral exposure, have a more prolonged course following PB$_j$-14 inoculation (34). This isolate has a SAg-like effect, *in vitro* and *in vivo*, inducing T cell proliferation in a Vβ-restricted manner. Pre-existing target cell activation has also been linked epidemiologically to enhance susceptibility to *acquisition*

Table 1. T-cell subsets: Phenotype by effector function*

Subset	Naive	Characteristics		
		Primary effectors	Memory	Secondary effectors
Cell cycle	G_o	G_1	$G_o(G_1?)$	G_1
Frequency in periphery	10-5	?	10^{-3}	10^{-2}
Cytokines	IL-2	$T_HO/T_H1/T_H2$	$T_HO(T_H1/T_H2)$	$T_HO/T_H1/T_H2$
Antigen-presenting cells	Dendritic cells	Dendritic cells/B/Mϕ	Dendritic cells/B/Mϕ	Dendritic cells/B/Mϕ
Phenotype				
CD44	low	high	high	high
L-selectin	high	low	low	low
CD45RA	high	high or low	low	low
Integrins	low	high	medium	high
Effector function	−	+	+	+

*Adopted from: Bradley LM, Croft M, Swain SL. Immunol Today 1993; 14:197-201.

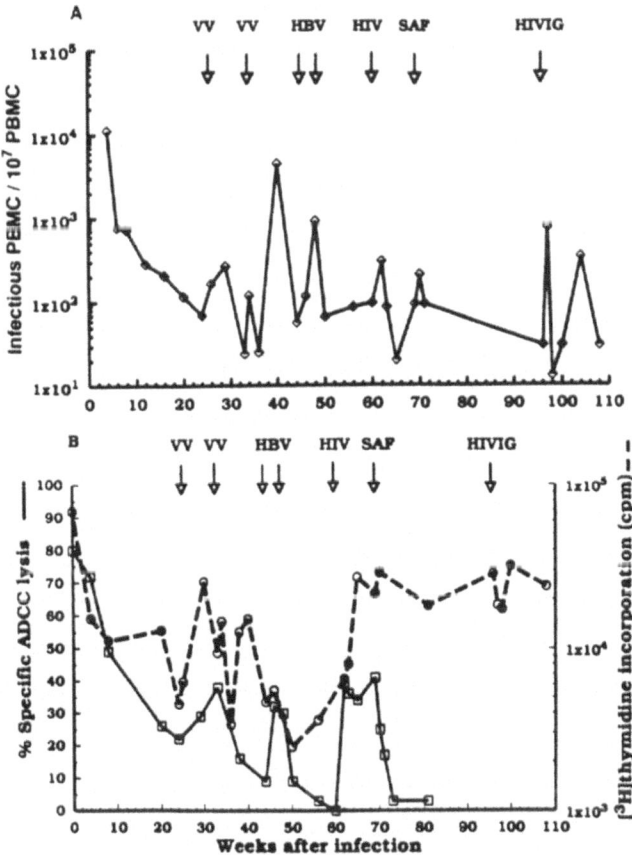

Figure 1. Correlation of virologic and immunologic parameters with immune stimulation in HIV-1 infected chimpanzee C-487. Time 0: inoculatiion with cell-free LAV-1b; VV: inactivated vaccinia virus; HBV: hepatitis B vaccine; HIV: inactivated HIV; HIVIG: purified human immunoglobulin, pooled from HIV-1+ individuals. (Reproduced, with permission, from: Fultz PN, Gluckman J-C, Muchmore E, Girard G. AIDS Res Hum Retroviruses 1992; 8:313-317.)

of an HIV infection (35). This may account, at least in part, for the facility with which HIV appears to be acquired heterosexually in Africa and certain parts of Southeast Asia, where multiple parasitic and venereal infections among HIV at-risk populations are associated with activated T cells, both in the lymphoid network and at mucosal tissues.

CELL ACTIVATION AND VIRAL ESCAPE FROM IMMUNE SURVEILLANCE

In HIV infection there appears to be a continuous production of high levels of virus (7), suggesting that replication and transcription, while extensively regulated, is never abolished. The basis for viral mutation is established early, and erosion of the host's immune response permits further evolution of the infection. Indeed, most models predicting CD4+ T cell decline based upon HIV-mediated cytopathicity demand such an increase in viral diversity. Its rapidity and nature are difficult to quantify, however, as sequence diversity is usually evaluated by DNA PCR, whereas *antigenic* diversity is the most pertinent factor clinically (36). In addition, the infectivity of any established variants, as well as short-lived viral "swarms" or "quasi-species", is usually unknown. The spectrum of variant viral sequences within one host is typically greater than that among primary infectious isolates, with but as few as one in 60,000 virions fully capable of replication and infectivity, requisite for viral propagation (36).

HIV has also evolved diverse mechanisms to counter neutralizing antibody and specific CTL, apart from periodic bursts of variant virus secondary to intermittent cell activation. These include: sequestration in immune privileged sites (e.g., the central nervous system and vitreous humor); alteration in patterns of cytopathicity, growth kinetics and tissue tropism; down-modulation of cellular recognition, adhesion and MHC molecules; induction and encoding of immunosuppressive factors; and alteration of neutralizing and cytolytic epitopes on target cells (37). CTL control, a feature of early HIV disease and probably responsible, in part, for early suppression of viremia following an acute seroconversion reaction, may be evaded through single amino acid substitutions in Env, Gag and Pol, a process not observed in any other natural viral infection (38). Pressures for such mutations include the high turnover rate of virus in the periphery (7), high error rate of the HIV polymerase, the absence of effective editing functions during reverse transcription, the presence of single viral genomes in many cells, and the fact that but a few epitopes dominate the CTL response (38). Emerging variant epitopes capable of complexing with MHC-I may stimulate additional CTL responses. Yet this may be but a pyrrhic victory if such antigenic diversity drives the immune response to exhaustion, as recently proposed by Nowak and associates (39).

This rapidity of development of HIV escape mutants has led some to argue for early initiation of antiretroviral therapy in HIV disease (12). However, AZT has no effect on the induction of HIV from chronically infected cells, at least as assessed *in vitro* (40), and little impact on cell activation. It can retard expression of some markers linked to T lymphocyte and APC stimulation, including CD38 on CD8+ T cells and CD71 on CD20+ B cells, but has no effect on the corresponding CD4+ T cell molecules, such as CD45RA or Leu-8 (41), and may even suppress anti-HIV CTL development.

T CELL ACTIVATION

Optimal stimulation of CD4+ T cells requires engagement not only of the TCR/CD3 complex by antigenic peptides presented in the context of MHC-II, a process often referred to as "signal 1", but additional co-stimulatory or "signal 2" events provided by cross-linking

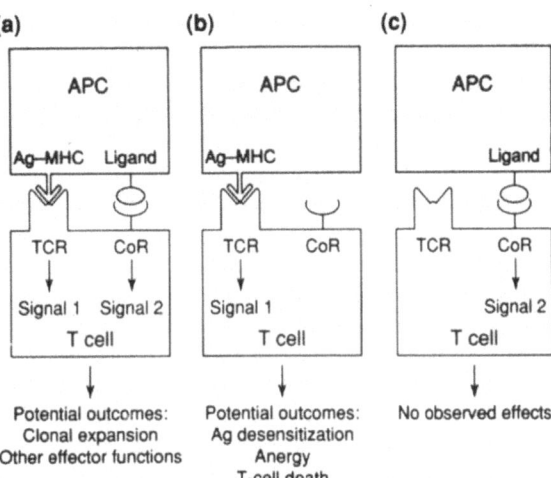

Figure 2. Model of potential outcomes of the interaction between T lymphocytes land antigen presenting cells. While encounter of quiescent T cells expressing CD28 with a B7 ligand in the absence of TCR stimulation does not lead to an obvious change in phenotype, it appears sufficient to upregulate HIV replication if that T cell were infected. (Reproduced, with permission, from: June CH, Bluestone JA, Nadler LM, Thompson CB. Immunol Today 1194; 15:321-331.)

of accessory receptors on the T cell surface with ligands on APCs, including monocyte/macrophages, dendritic cells, B lymphocytes, endothelial cells and possibly CD4+ T cells themselves (42) (Fig. 2). These latter ligands include the β_2 integrin LFA-I (CD 11a), CD2, and CD28. Their engagement leads to increases in $[Ca^{++}]_i$ and translocation of protein kinase C (PKC), required for expression of previously silent cellular and viral genes changes in cell phenotype, and entry of cells into G_1. Cellular consequences of these signals are illustrated in Fig. 3. It should be noted that, while signal 2 alone has no observable effects on APC or T cell phenotype (42), in the form of a B7-CD28 interaction it is sufficient to induce transcription and replication of HIV in naturally infected T cells (44). And alternate signal 1s, including ligation of CD4 by autoantibody or gp120 independently of TCR, may lead to CD4 cell deletion *in vitro* and *in vivo* (45).

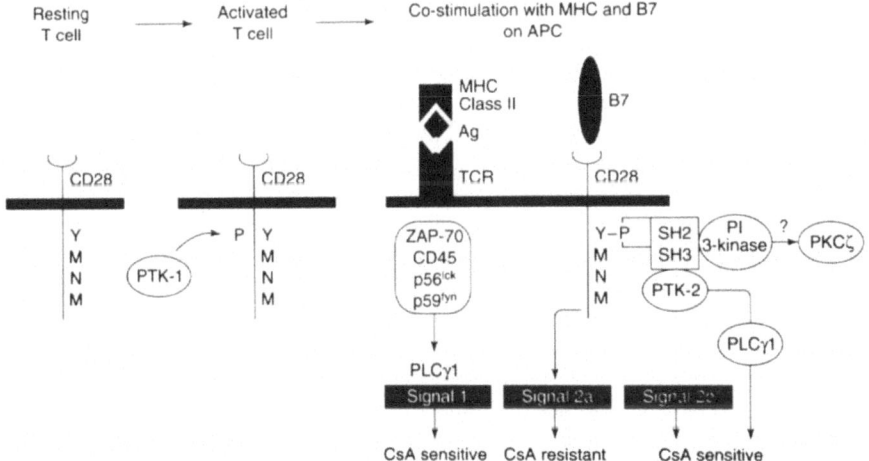

Figure 3. Proposed model of signal transduction events mediated by T cell receptor (TCR)-MHC-antigen (Ag) interactions and CD28-B7 interactions. P: phosphorylation; CsA: cyclosporin A; protein tyrosine kinase (PTK); PLC$_g$1: phospholipase C$_g$1. (Reproduced, with permission, from: June CH, et al. Immunol Today 1994; 15:321-331.)

T cell cycle progression, as opposed to activation, is then dependent upon three main factors: IL-2 concentration, IL-2R density, and the duration of the IL-2/IL-2R interaction. Entry of a T cell from G_0 into G_1 is followed by a lag; semi-synchronous entry into S phase then occurs in the presence of saturating concentrations of IL-2 (100pM) and a normal number of IL-2 receptors per cell (2500). These receptors become saturated within 10-15 minutes, at least *in vitro*, and probably result in an all or non-triggering. T cell proliferation is determined by the presence of high affinity ($k_d=10^{-12}$M) IL-2 binding sites, requiring cooperativity among three intracellular portions of the complete IL-2R receptor: the α (55kd dalton), β (75kd), and γ (65kd) chains. IL-2 dissociates slowly from its ligand complex then is internalized rapidly and completely degraded, not recycled. It appears to be a kinase substrate, and is rapidly phosphorylated by p56[lck] as well as other phosphokinases.

Agents that block cell activation regardless of their impact on cell proliferation, may inhibit induction of HIV (6). And cellular activation with PKC induction is essential for HIV-infected T cells to become fusogenic. Thus cholera toxin, an inhibitor of PKC through its effect on inositol triphosphate and diacylglycerol production, and H7, an isoquinoline and non-competitive inhibitor of PKC, can both prevent unstimulated but not previously stimulated T lymphocytes from forming syncytia (43). This occurs regardless of the mitogenic nature of the initiating signal (13). Indeed, two primary signal-transduction pathways are coupled to CD28, one that is dominant in activated T cells and is sensitive to the immune suppressive drug cyclosporin, and one that occurs in resting T cells and is cyclosporin resistant (Fig.3). This must be kept in mind as strategies are suggested for the use of agents such as cyclosporin to depress cellular activation in HIV+ individuals.

ABERRANT CELL ACTIVATION

HIV infection itself can alter cell signalling. For example, it results in decreased T cell expression of CD28, perhaps mediated by *tat* or SAg, and an increase in the CD28 ligand, B7, on activated APCs. Indeed, B7+, HIV-infected T cells can present MHC alloantigens to CD4+ T cells (46,47). This initiates an unfortunate cascade of virologic and immunologic events. First, it can trigger viral replication. Second, clonal anergy can be induced in the T_H1 CD4+ subset following stimulation via TCR/CD3 in the absence of complete co-stimulation through CD28 or similar receptors (48). T_H1 cells are important to the control of viral replication as they promote CTL and elaborate IL-2. Precursors for T_H1, the T_H0 cells, may then be forced through a differentiation pathway skewing T cell development towards the T_H2 subpopulation, manifest by decreased IL-2 production, decreased antigen specific CTL activity, and enhancement of IL-4, IL-5, and IL-10, which can induce HIV replication and further depress T_H1 growth (48). While helper T cells responses are reduced and immuno-globulin class switching diminished following loss of membrane CD28, CTLs can still be activated, suggesting that alternate co-stimulatory pathways may exist (49).

Cellular, bacterial, viral and HIV-encoded or induced SAgs, apart from contributing to enhanced viral replication by triggering cell proliferation, may also lead to inappropriate T cell activation and anergy. Clonal deletion, characteristic of early thymocytes exposed to low levels of SAg, is not an obligatory consequence of the anergic state, however. Mature anergized T cells, recognized by their inability to produce IL-2 to specific antigen, may persist for extended periods of time *in vitro* and *in vivo* (50). The exact outcome of a SAg exposure thus appears to depend on the ontologic state of the T cell, the level of antigen exposure, and the type of APC involved in assisting SAg-mediated bridging of TCR and MHC on the T cell and APC, respectively (51). Consistent with this hypothesis, HIV appears to selectively replicate to extremely high levels within the Vβ12 subset of CD4+ T cells *in vitro* and, as assessed by quantitative DNA PCR of TCRVβ-selected subsets, *in vivo* (21).

Here, either HIV or an HIV associated product is acting as a classic SAg. In addition HIV can induce, *in vitro*, the expansion of certain TCR Vβ-selected T cells (50). Indeed, upwards of 60% of HIV exposed Vβ8+ T lymphocytes may be so rendered incapable of subsequent antigenic responses (50). This phenomenon may be another means for evading the immune system, with SAgs capable of eliciting anergy in CD4+ and C8+ CTL populations.

The metabolic consequences of such events are numerous. Inositol lipid hydrolysis with formation of diacylglycerol (DAG) and inositol-1,4,5-triphosphate (IP_3) is a critical but not exclusive signal transduction pathway coupled to the TCR-CD3 complex. It appears to be unaffected following initial HIV infection (51), but is depressed in chronic infection. Activation of a group of protein tyrosine kinases, including p56[lck], ZAP-70 and p59[fyn], as well as the CD45 phosphotyrosine phosphokinase, assist in generating signal 1 (Fig 3), and may be affected within hours after HIV infection. Inhibition of certain of these intracellular signals consequent to tyrosine kinase activation by HIV or its Env components can lead to cytopathic effects with prominent syncytium formation (52). While the pathophysiology of this process is yet unclear one such enzyme, p56[lck], when complexed with CD4 in an HIV infected cell, is inappropriately translocated to the cytoplasmic face of the endoplasmic reticulum. This movement appears to directly precede lymphocyte lysis (53).

The kinetics of disruption of these metabolic pathways by HIV may also correlate with the immune defects seen. Lymphokine-mediated signal transduction regularly utilizes a different signaling machinery from the inositol phospholipid pathway used by lymphocyte antigen receptors (54), with the two pathways normally able to thereby synergize to induce the complete cycle of lymphocyte activation and proliferation. The principal type of CD4+ T cell lost in HIV infection is a memory lymphocyte phenotypically characterized as CD44[hi], CD29[hi], and CD45RO+/RA-. This is reflected by the stages of functional defects seen, with an initial decrease in T cell recall responses to specific antigen followed by depressed responses to alloantigen and then mitogen. Only much later is generation of MHC restricted CD8+ CTL affected. This is corroborated *in vitro*. HIV selectively inhibits the proliferative response of clonal CD4+ T lymphocytes to alloantigen at early time points at which other alloantigen-dependent responses were unperturbed. Specifically, impaired blastogenesis could be dissociated from alloantigen-specific induction of the B cell activation molecule CD23, IL-4 release, and inositol lipid hydrolysis (51). Membrane expression of pertinent T cell receptor molecules, including CD2, CD3, and TCR remained intact. Using MHC class II-specific human CD4+ helper T cell clones, the proliferative defect was shown to be an early consequence of HIV infection, occurring within 4 d of viral inoculation and preceding increases in mature virion production. It was generalizable to three distinct methods of T cell activation, all independent of antigen-presenting cells: anti-CD3 mediated cross-linking of the CD3/TCR complex; anti-CD2 and phorbol 12-myristic 13-acetate (PMA); and anti-CD28 plus PMA. These abnormalities were not mitigated by addition of exogenous IL-2, even though expression of IL-2R was unaltered (51).

Lymphocyte Homing

Many immunocyte subsets exhibit preferences, maintained across species barriers, as to the types of lymphoid or other tissues they preferentially interact with. This phenomenon is predicated on associations among membrane adhesion molecules of the selectin, integrin and immunoglobulin supergene families on T cells and specialized high endothelial venules. It has been termed "homing," albeit it generally involves short-range events, with most cells continuing to recirculate. States of cellular activation can influence such homing. For example, trafficking patterns differ between naive and antigen-activated memory T cells, with the former expressing low levels of LFA-3, CD44(H-CAM) and VLA-4, and high levels of LE-CAM-1 and CD45, a situation reversed for memory cells (55) (Table 1). HIV itself, in budding off the plasma membranes of infected CD4+ T cells, may concentrate some of these homing and adhesion molecules on their surface (56), potentially impeding immune recognition.

Activated Cytolytic T Cells: Protective and Pathogenic?

Mice selectively depleted of CD4+ T cells *in vivo* can survive infection with viruses such as CMV that are lethal to mice that lack CD8+ CTL, as production of MHC cell-restricted CTL can proceed in the absence of without CD4+ T cell help (57). Similarly, evidence for a temporal association between development of high levels of activated CD28+, MHC-II+, CD8+ CTL precursors for HIV-1 Gag, Pol and Env and control of viremia in a primary HIV infection has been gathered by several groups (58). These CTLs utilize two specific lytic mechanisms, one involving Ca^{++}-dependent release of granules containing the enzyme perforin, and another which does not require exocytosis and involves Fas-mediated induction of apoptosis (59, 60). Unfortunately, specific effector responses are short-lived. As noted above, activation of HIV-infected CD4+ T lymphocytes with attendant viral replication expands the repertoire of variant viruses and can lead to CTL escape (9). CTL activity itself may be antagonized by natural occurring HIV-Gag variants, as the presence of mutant Gag epitopes *in vitro*, in the form of synthetic peptides, can inhibit normal lysis of cells presenting the original immunogenic CTL target (61). In addition, CD8+ T cells themselves are infectable by HIV *in vitro* and probably *in vivo*, a process inhibited by AZT (62). This susceptibility is enhanced during an attempt to lyse specific infected target cells (63), and may be a consequence of the upregulation, in an epitope-specific and MHC-I restricted manner, of the HIV stimulatory cytokine tumor necrosis factor-α (TNF-α) (64).

The possibility that some of these CTL-mediated effects may directly lead to immunopathology in HIV disease must also be considered. This hypothesis is supported by the finding of extensive visceral CD8+ T lymphocyte infiltrations with attendant tissue destruction in salivary glands, lung, kidneys and the gastrointestinal tract in some HIV+ individuals. This phenomena is antigen driven, MHC-I determined, and associated with specific β_1 and β_2 integrin expression (65). Interestingly, individuals with these diffuse infiltrative lymphocytosis syndromes have a relatively low rate of progression to clinical AIDS, some 0.9% per annum (65), and maintain relatively high absolute numbers of CD4+ T cells, regardless of their level of circulating virus. This further complicates an attempt to correlate extent of CD4+ and CD8+ T cell activation with viral load and rapidity of decline CD4+ T cell decline. For example, Gupta and colleagues plotted degree of HIV replication *in vivo*, measured as number of HIV producing cells per 10^6 CD4+ T cells in an RT PCR analysis of *gag* transcripts, against absolute CD4 count (66). While a clear correlation between extent of viral replication and loss of CD4 cells was noted, there were important outliers, with high levels of virus production in individuals with >1000 CD4 cells/mm^3, and other individuals with <100 CD4+ cells/mm^3 producing very low levels of viral transcripts.

The general trend—high viral load correlated with rapidly declining CD4 count—is consistent with the view of HIV as a direct cytopathic agent leading to cytolysis, syncytium formation, humoral and cellular autoimmunity, and cytokine disregulation. The outliers—healthy carriers with high titers of HIV and high T cell counts, and others with low viral loads but profound CD4 depletion—may support a concept raised by Zinkernagl (9) and others: AIDS as a consequence of immunopathologic mechanisms secondary to a conventional CTL responses against infected CD4+ T cells and APCs, but probably simply represents an immune system exhausted in its ability to replenish rapidly turning-over T cells in the face of continuous viral growth (7). Other indirect mechanisms for T cell depletion in HIV infection, which may arise as a consequence of global but inappropriate T cell activation, including apoptosis, are consistent with this hypothesis. For example, CTL-mediated deletion of APCs can deprive CD4+ T cells of relevant stimuli or growth factors which ordinarily proscribe programmed cell death. It is also consistent with a disturbing new observation concerning administration of a HLA-A3 restricted, CD8+ CTL clone specific for HIV-1 Nef to a 36 year old male with a relatively high ($\geq$ 500/mm^3) CD4 count but high levels of HIV p24 antigenemia. These cells were highly effective at killing HIV+ cells in an MHC-restricted manner. However, their *in vivo* infusion, in the presence or absence of high-dose IL-2, led to dramatic declines in CD4 count and increases in p24 by $\geq$ 4-fold (Dr. Scott Koenig, personal communication). While this is not characteristic of the majority of HIV+ patients who have received *ex vivo* expanded, HIV-specific CTL, it raises the specter of both CD8-mediated cytopathology and cellular activation as important factors for the acceleration of HIV disease.

In addition, CD4+, gp120-specific T cells appear to be able to lyse autologous activated CD4+/MHC-II+ T cells in the presence of soluble gp120 (7). Because most circulating CD4+ T cells are MHC-II negative, it is unclear whether this model can account for a significant decrease of such cells *in vivo*. Such a process may, however, lead to the early loss of recall or anamnestic responses characteristic of HIV disease (51), since these effects depend on previously activated cells that either remain MHC-II+ or rapidly regain MHC products during the restimulation process (67). This mechanism may also account for the inability to prime for new CD4+ responses, as all newly stimulated CD4+ T cells will express MHC-II, and are capable of bindings and processing gp120 (67).

Antigen Presenting Cells in T Cell Activation

Specific antigen and self-MHC are necessary for T cell antigen recognition, but they are not sufficient. Effective antigen presentation, involving the metabolic conversion of intact proteins into a form able to be expressed from the cell membrane in association with MHC, is also required. Antigen entering the cell in endocytic vesicles is typically seen in conjunction with MHC-II by CD4+ T cells, as would sgp120 on an uninfected T cell, and antigen synthesized in the cytoplasm with MHC-I by CD8+ CTL, such as an HIV-infected APCs (67). APC also mediate several important functions in T cell activation, including Fc receptor cross-linking of T cell ligands to form a multimeric complex, and the secretion of cytokines such as IL-1 (54). In terms of APCs, microbial killing may be maintained for prolonged periods while defects in C3R-mediated clearance and IL-1 production occur much earlier. Activation requirements for previously stimulated T cells are less stringent than for virgin quiescent cells, necessitating only this APC cross-linking function. As noted above, cross-linking of TCR/CD3, CD2 or Thy1 in the presence of APCs can provide a primary activation signal to the T cell, facilitating proliferation in the absence of other exogenous signals (54).

Activated APCs themselves can induce viral expression in chronically infected T cells. For example, marked polyclonal activation of B lymphocytes is an early and consistent feature of HIV infection (68); these cells can upregulate HIV in infected T and monocytic cell lines. This phenomenon can be reproduced by supernatants from B cell cultures of HIV+ donors which contain high levels of IL-6 and TNF-α, both capable of inducing HIV at transcriptional and post-transcriptional levels (69). And HIV-LTR activity is highly dependent on cellular transcription factors in undifferentiated monocytes; in differentiated macrophages HIV-1 *tat* facilitates autonomy from absolute control mechanisms (70). This suggests a novel adaptation of LTR enhancers in the replication of HIV within monocytes. In quiescent monocytes, the predominance of transcriptional silencers and relative lack of certain transcription factors such as LBP-1 is manifest.

Table 2. Selective functional loss of antigen specific T cells is due to presentation of antigen by autologous antigen-presenting cells exposed to HIV*

APC	Proliferative response				Phenotype	
	D(A3+)		F(A2+)		CDC with anti-HLA	
TT	−	+	−	+	A3	A2
Co-culture						
A	1-1	21-2	1-0	1-1	5%	95%
B	1-0	1-1	1-0	19-9	95%	5%

*Co-cultures A and B only respond in the presence of antigen presented by syngeneic and not allogeneic APC. T cell activation was measured as IL-2 production, and results indicate thymidine incorporation (ct/min x 10^{-3}) by the IL-2 responsive phytohaemagglutinin (PHA) blasts used as indicator cells. (Reproduced, with permission, from: Manca F, Newell A, Valle M, et al. Clin Exp Immunol 1992; 87:15-19.)

APC function is impaired in PBMC derived from HIV+ donors, or following direct infection *in vitro*. Such defects could enhance susceptibility to opportunistic infections in a host already compromised by T cell depletion (71), and may also interfere with orderly T cell activation. Thus, when antigen-specific T cells are pulsed by monocytes in the presence of HIV, they are functionally deleted following subsequent exposure to APC in the absence of HIV in an MHC-II restricted manner (72) (Table 2). This is consistent with the observation that the defective function of specific T cells precedes generalized loss of CD4+ T cells.

Therapeutic Implications

The phenomena described above have direct bearing on the design and likely success of various forms of therapy for HIV infection, as well as for the development of preventative vaccines. For example, while rsCD4 has been ineffective as a direct antiviral strategy, both in late clinical stages and against "street isolates" of HIV-1 *in vitro*, it may block loss of CD4+ T cells through the MHC-II restricted killing pathway. In contrast, an individual not fully protected by an HIV vaccine containing gp120 may become more susceptible to rapid development of immunodeficiency following infection because of the pre-induction of CD4+ CTL, as well as inappropriate CD4 stimulation with possible induction of anergy (67). Suppression of over-activated or inappropriately activated T lymphocyte and APC populations at any stage of HIV disease, utilizing agents capable of interferring with discrete parts of immunocyte signalling and viral transcription, including cyclosporin, FK-506 rapamycin, glucocorticoids, as well as novel agents such as tamoxifen (74) should be pursued. These observations may also contribute to defining immunologic distinctions among rapid progressors, long-term survivors, and long-term non-progressors of HIV infection, as viral co-factors, T cell activation, and viral load correlate, if yet imperfectly, with advancing disease (73).

ACKNOWLEDGMENTS

This work was supported by National Institutes of Health Grant AI33322; US Army Medical Research and Acquisition Activity Grant DAMD 17-90-Z-0049; and awards from the American Foundation for AIDS Research.

REFERENCES

1. Temin HM. 1967. Studies on carcinogene is by avian sarcoma virus. V. Requirement for new DNA synthesis and for cell division. *J Cell Physiol* 69:53-64.
2. Greene WC, Bohnlein E, Ballard DW. 1989. HIV-1, HTLV-1 and normal T-cell growth:transcriptional strategies and surprises. *Immunol Today* 10:272-278.
3. Mosier D, Sieburg H. 1994. Macrophage-tropic HIV: critical for AIDS pathogenesis? *Immunol Today* 15:332-339.
4. Verdin E, Becker A, Bex F, et al. 1990. Identification and characterization of an enhancer in the coding region of the genome of human immunodeficiency virus type 1. *Proc Natl Acad Sci USA* 87:4874-4878.
5. Laughlin MA, Pomerantz RJ. 1994. Cellular latency in HIV-1 infection. *Clinics Lab Med* 14:2:239-255.
6. Tong-Starksen SE, Luciw PA, Peterlin BM. 1989. Signaling through T lymphocyte surface proteins, TCR/CD3 and CD28, activates the HIV-1 long terminal repeat. *J Immunol* 142:2:702-707.
7. Wei X, Ghosh SK, Taylor ME, et al. 1995. Viral dynamics in human immunodeficiency type 1 infection. *Nature* 373:117-122.
8. Siliciano RF, Lawton IT, Knall C, Karr RW, Berman P, Gregory T, Reinherz EL. 1988. Analysis of host-virus interactions in AIDS with Anti-gp120 T cell clones: Effect of HIV sequence variation and a mechanism for CD4+ cell depletion. *Cell* 54:561-575.
9. Mahy BWJ. 1985. Strategies of virus persistence. *British Med Bull* 41:1:50-55.
10. Zinkernagel RM, Hengartner H. 1994. T-cell-mediated immunopathology *versus* direct cytolysis by virus: implications for HIV and AIDS. *Immunol Today* 15:262-268.
11. Zack JA, Haislip AM, Krogstad P, Chen ISY. 1992. Incompletely reverse-transcribed human immunodeficiency virus type 1 genomes in quiescent cells can function as intermediates in the retroviral life cycle. *J Virol* 66:3:1717-1725.
12. Schnittman SM, Greenhouse JJ, Lane CH, Pierce PF, Fauci AS. 1991. Frequent detection of HIV-1-specific mRNAs in infected individuals suggests ongoing active viral expression in all stages of disease. *AIDS Res Hum Retroviruses* 7:361-367.
13. Gruters RA, Otto SA, Al BJM, Verhoeven AJ, Verweij CL, Van Lier RAW, Miedema F. 1991. Non-mitogen T cell activation signals are sufficient for induction of human immunodeficiency virus transcription. *Eur J Immunol* 21:167 172.
14. Laurence J. 1990. Molecular interactions among herpesviruses and human immunodeficiency viruses. *J Inf Dis* 162:338-346.
15. Laurence J. 1992. Viral cofactors in the pathogenesis of HIV disease. In: Wormser GA, ed., *AIDS and Other Manifestations of HIV Infection* 77-83. (Raven Press, NY)
16. Lusso P, Gallo RC. 1994. Human herpesvirus 6 in AIDS. *Lancet* 343:555-556.
17. Duan L, Ozaki I, Oakes JW, Taylor JP, Khalili K, Pomerantz RJ. 1994 The tumor suppressor protein p53 strongly alters human immunodeficiency virus type 1 replication. *J Virol* 68:4302-4313.
18. Embretson J, Zupancic M, Beneke J, Till M, Wolinsky S, Ribos JL, Burke A, Haase AT. 1993. Analysis of human immunodeficiency virus-infected tissues by amplification and *in situ* hybridization reveals latent and permissive infections at single-cell resolution. *Proc Natl Acad Sci USA* 90:357-361.
19. Pettoello-Mantovani M, Casadevall A, Kollmann TR, Rubinstein A, Goldstein. 1992. Enhancement of HIV-1 infection by the capsular polysaccharide of cryptococcus neoformans. *Lancet* 339:21-23.
20. Hammarskjold ML, Simurda MC. 1992. Epstein-Barr Virus latent membrane protein transactivates and human immunodeficiency virus type 1 long terminal repeat through induction of NFkB activity. *J Virol* 66:6496-6501.
21. Sol N, Morinet F, Alison M, Hazan U. 1993. Trans-activation of the long terminal repeat of human immunodeficiency virus type 1 by the parvovirus B19 NS1 gene product. *J Gen Virol* 74:2011-2014.
22. Lazzarotto T, Campisi B, Re MC, Albertini F, Furlini G, Dalla Casa B, Landini MP. 1994. An *in vivo* study on active cytomegalovirus infection in relation to active HIV replication in HIV-I infected drug addicts. *J Infect* 28:287-291.
23. Webster A, Phillips AN, Lee CA, Janossy G, Kernoff PB, Griffiths PD. 1992. Cytomegalovirus (CMV) infection, CD4+ lymphocyte counts and the development of AIDS in HIV-1-infected hemophiliac patients. *Clin Exp Immunol* 88:6-9.
24. Heng MCY, Heng SY, Allen SG. 1994. Co-infection and synergy of human immunodeficiency virus-1 and herpes simplex virus-1. *Lancet* 343:255-258.
25. Semple M, Loveday C, Weller I, Tedder R. 1991. Direct measurement of Viraemia in patients infected with HIV-1 and its relationship to disease progression and zidovudine therapy. *J Med Virol* 35:38-45.
26. Laurence J, Hodtsev AS, Posnett DN. 1992. Superantigen implicated in dependence of HIV-1 replication in T cells on TCR Vβ expression. *Nature* 358:255-259.

27. Clyde Jr. WA, Chanock RM, Tully JG. 1990. Mycoplasmas. In Davis BD, Dulbecco R, Eisen HV *Microbiology* 707-715.
28. Mycoplasma and SAg
29. Bradley LM, Croft M, Swain SL. 1993. T-Cell memory:new perspectives. *Immunol Today* 14:5:197-199.
30. Fultz PN, Gluckman JC, Muchmore E, Girard M. 1992. Transient increases in numbers of infectious cells in an HIV-infected chimpanzee following immune stimulation. *AIDS Res Hum Retroviruses* 8:313-317.
31. O'Brien WA, Oucak S, Namazie A, Kalhor H, Mao S-H, Zack JA. 1992. HIV-1 replication can be increased in blood from seropositive patients following influenza immunization. *J Cellul Biochem* 16E:Q441.
32. Ho DD. 1992. HIV-1 viraemia and influenza. *Lancet* 339:1549.
33. Kovacs JA, Baseler M, Dewar R, et al. 1993. Sustained increases in CD4+ lymphocytes in HIV-infected patients treated with intermittent interleukin-2 therapy. *1st Intl Conf Hum Retroviruses* Washington DC, Dec 12-16, Abst. 301.
34. Rosenberg YJ, White BD, Papermaster SF, Zack P, Jarling PB, Eddy GA, Burke DS, Lewis MG. 1991. Variation in T-lymphocyte activation and susceptibility to SIV$_{PBj-14}$-induced acute death in macaques. *J Med Primatol* 20:206-210.
35. Kalinkovich A, Manyan S, Weisman Z, Harpaz N, Bentwich Z. 1994 Immune activation, a co-factor for HIV transmission in Thailand? *Lancet* 343:1506-1507.
36. Bangham CRM, McMichael AJ. 1990. Why the long latent period? *Nature* 348:388.
37. Pircher H, Moskophidis D, Rohrer U, Burki K, Hengartner H, Zinkernagel RM. 1990. Viral escape by selection of cytotoxic T cell-resistant virus variants *in vivo*. *Nature* 346:629-633.
38. Phillips RE, Rowland-Jones S, Nixon DF, Gotch FM, Edwards JP, Ogunlesi AO, et al. 1991. Human immunodeficiency virus genetic variation that can escape cytotoxic T cell recognition. *Nature* 354:453-459.
39. Nowak MA, May RM, Anderson RM. 1990. The evolutionary dynamics of HIV-1 quasi-species and the development of immunodeficiency diseaase. *AIDS* 4:1095-1103.
40. Poli G, Orenstein JM, Kinter A, Folks TM, Fauci AS. 1989. Interferon-α but not AZT suppresses HIV expression in chronically infected cell lines. *Science* 244:575-577.
41. Bass HZ, Hardy WD, Mitsuyasu T, Wang YX, Cumberland W, Fahey JL. 1992. Eleven lymphoid phenotypic markers in HIV infection: selective changes induced by zidovudine treatment. *J AIDS* 5:890-897.
42. June CH, Bluestone JA, Nadler LM, Thompson CB. 1994. The B7 and CD28 receptor families. *Immunol Today* 15:321-331.
43. Mohagheghpour N, Chakrabarti R, Stein BS, Gowda SD, Engleman EG. 1991. Early activation events render T cells susceptible to HIV-1 induced syncytia formation. *J Biol Chem* 266:11:7233-7238.
44. Asjo lB, Cefai D, Debre P, Dudoit Y, Autran B. 1993. A novel mode of human immunodeficiency virus type 1 (HIV-1) activation: ligation of CD28 alone induces HIV-1 replication in naturally infected lymphocytes. *J Virol* 67:4395-4398.
45. Wang Z, Orlikowsky T, Dudhane A, et al. 1994. Deletion of T lymphocytes in human CD4 transgenic mice induced by HIV-gp120 and gp120-specific antibodies from AIDS patients. *Eur J Immunol* 24:1553-1557.
46. Haffar OK, Smithgall MD, Bradshaw J, Brady B, Damle NK, Linsley PS. 1993. Costimulation of T-cell activation and virus production by B7 antigen on activated CD4+ T cells from human immunodeficiency virus type 1-infected donors. *Proc Natl Acad Sci* 90:11094-11098.
47. Pichler WJ, Wyss-Loray T. 1994. T cells as antigen-presenting cells. *Immunol Today* 15:312-315.
48. Gajewski TF, Lancki DW, Stack R, Fitch FW. 1994. "Anergy" of T$_H$O helper T lymphocytes induces downregulation of T$_H$1 characteristics and a transition to a T$_H$2-like phenotype. *J Exp Med* 179:481-491.
49. Shahinian A, Pfeffer K, Lee KP, et al. 1993. Differentiated T cells co-stimulatory requirements in CD28-deficient mice. *Science* 261:609-612.
50. Dadaglio G, Garcia S, Montagnier L, Gougeon ML. 1994. Selective Anergy of Vβ8+ T cells in HIV-infected individuals. *J Exp Med* 179:413-424.
51. Laurence J, Friedman SM, Chartash EK, Crow MK, Posnett DN. 1989. Human immunodeficiency virus infection of CD4+ helper T cell clones. Early proliferative defects despite intact antigen-specific recognition and interleukin-4 secretion. *J Clin Invest* 83:1843-1848.
51. Schattner E, Laurence J. 1994. HIV-induced T lymphocyte depletion. *Clinics Lab Med* 14:221-238.
52. Cohen DI, Tani Y, Tian H, Boone E, Samelson LE, Lane HC. 1992. Participation of tyrosine phosphorylation in the cytopathic effect of human immunodeficiency virus-1. *Science* 256:542-545.
53. Crise B, Rose JK. 1992. Human immunodeficiency virus type 1 glycoprotein precursor retains a CD4-p56^{lck} complex in the endoplasmic reticulum. *J Virol* 66:4:2296-2301.

54. Altman A, Coggeshall KM, Mustelin T. 1990. Molecular events mediating T cell activation. *Adv Immunol* 48:227-360.

55. Editorial. 1992. Lymphocyte recirculation: the need for site-specific receptors to dictate T-lymphocyte localization into different tissue sites. *Scand J Immunol* 35:627-632.

56. Meerloo T, Sheikh A, Bloem AC, de Ronde A, Schutten M, van Els CAC, Roholl PJM, Joling P, Goudsmit J, Schuurman HJ. 1993. Host cell membrane proteins on human immunodeficiency virus type 1 after *in vitro* infection of H9 cells and blood mononuclear cells. An immuno-electron microscopic study. *J Gen Virol* 74:129-135.

57. Shearer GM, Singer A, Mizuochi T, Buller M, Hugin A, Morse III HC. 1988. Importance of CD8+ T helper cells function in AIDS. *J Infect Dis* 158:4:893.

58. Koup RA, Safrit JT, Cao Y, Andrews CA, McLeod G, Borkowsky W, Farthing C, Ho DD. 1994. Temporal association of cellular immune responses with the initial control of viremia in primary human immunodeficiency virus type 1 syndrome. *J Virol* 4650-4655.

59. Burrows SR, Fernan A, Argaet V, Suhrbier A. 1993. Bystander apoptosis induced by CD8+ cytotoxic T cell (CTL) clones: implications for CTL lytic mechanisms. *Internat Immunol* 5:9:1049-1058.

60. Landay AL, Mackewicz CE, Levy JA. 1993. An activated CD8+ cell phenotype correlates with anti-HIV activity and asymptomatic clinical status. *Clin Immunol* 69:1:106-116.

61. Klenerman P, Jones-Rowland S, McAdam S, Edwards J, Daenke S, Lalloo D, Koppe B, Rosenberg W, Boyd D, Edwards A, Giangrande P, Phillips RE, McMichael A. 1994. Cytotoxic T-cell activity antagonized by naturally occurring HIV-1 gag variants. *Nature* 369:403-407.

62. Mercure L, Brenner BJ, Phaneuf D, Tsoukas C, Wainberg, MA. 1994. Effect of 3'-azido-3'-deoxythymidine and 2',3'-dideoxyinosine on establishment of human immunodeficiency virus type 1 infection in cultured CD8+ lymphocytes. *Antimicrob Agents Chemo* 38:5:986-990.

63. De Maria A, Colombini S, Schnittman SM, Moretta L. 1994. CD8+ cytolytic T lymphocytes become infected *in vitro* in the process of killing HIV-1 infected target cells. *Eur J Immunol* 531-536.

64. Harrer, T, Jassoy C, Harrer E, Johnson RP, Walker BD. 1993. Induction of HIV-1 replication in a chronically infected T-cell line by cytotoxic T lymphocytes. *J AIDS* 6:865-871.

65. Itescu S, Dalton J, Zhang Z, Winchester R. 1993. Tissue infiltration in a CD8 lymphocytosis syndrome associated with human immunodeficiency virus-1 infection has the phenotypic appearance of an antigenically driven response. *J Clin Invest* 91:2216-2225.

66. Gupta P, Kingsley L, Armstrong J et al. 1993. Enhanced experession of human immunodeficiency virus type 1 correlates with development of AIDS. *Virology* 196:586-595.

67. Germain RN. 1988. Antigen processing and CD4+ T cell depletion in AIDS. *Cell* 54:441-444.

68. Laurence J., Grimison B, Rodriguez-Alfagewe C, Astrin SM. 1993. A model system for regulation of chronic HIV-1 infection in peripheral B lymphocytes. *Virology* 196:433-441.

69. Rieckmann P, Poli G, Kahrl JH, Fauci AS. 1991. Activated B lymphocytes from human immunodeficiency virus-infected individuals induce virus expression in infected T cells and a promonocytic cell line, U1. *J Exp Med* 173:1-5.

70. Moses AV, Ibanez C, Gaynor R, Ghazal P, Nelson JA. 1994. Differential role of long terminal repeat control elements for the regulation of basal and tat-mediated transcription of the human immunodeficiency virus in stimulated and unstimulated primary human macrophages. *J Virol* 68:1:298-307.

71. Schrier RD, McCutchan AJ, Venable JC, Nelson JA, Wiley CA. 1990. T-cell-induced expression of human immunodeficiency virus in macrophages. *J Virol* 64:7:3280-3288.

72. Manca F, Newell A, Valle M, Habeshaw J, Dalgleish AG. 1992. HIV-induced deletion of antigen-specific T cell function is MHC restricted. *Immunol* 87:15-19.

73. Laurence J. 1994. Characteristics of long-term survivors and long-term nonprogressors with HIV infection. *AIDS Updates* 7(3):1-13.

74. Laurence J, Sellars MB, Sikder SK. 1990. Effect of tamoxifen on regulation of chronic HIV-1 infection of HIV LTR-directed transcription. *Blood* 75:696-703.

MARKERS OF IMMUNE CELL ACTIVATION AND DISEASE PROGRESSION

Cell activation in HIV disease

M. Peakman,[1] M. Mahalingam,[1] A. Pozniak,[2] T. J. McManus,[2]
A. N. Phillips,[3] and D. Vergani[1]

[1] Department of Immunology
[2] Department of Genito-Urinary Medicine
King's College School of Medicine
London SE5 9PJ
[3] University Department of Public Health
Royal Free Hospital School of Medicine
Rowland Hill Street
London NW3 2PF, United Kingdom

SUMMARY

Immune cell activation is a feature of infection with the human immunodeficiency virus (HIV). Here we report our studies on a cohort of over 400 patients with HIV infection studied cross-sectionally and longitudinally to examine the relationship between markers of immune cell activation and disease progression. To examine disease progression, 340 patients with HIV infection but without AIDS were followed for a total of 574 patient years, during which 56 developed AIDS.

In our first study, 157 patients in CDC groups II-IV were examined cross-sectionally for in vivo expression of the activation markers HLA-DR and CD25 on CD3, CD4 and CD8 T cells. Levels of CD3+ HLA-DR+ T cells are high in HIV infection and show a significant negative correlation with CD4 counts (r=0.52; p<0.001). The appearance of HLA-DR+ CD3+ T cells is an early feature of asymptomatic HIV+ patients, with a greater proportion (82%) showing abnormally high levels of these than abnormally low levels of CD4 (52%; p<0.001). Examining activation of the CD4 subset specifically is likely to be of greater interest, given that this cell is the viral target. Indeed, we found that in the cross-sectional study, levels of HLA-DR+ and CD25+ CD4 lymphocytes show a step-wise linear increase with increasing disease severity (significant test for linear trend; p<0.001). In our previous studies, only declining CD4 count has shown such a significant linear trend. These data suggest that measuring activated CD4+ T cells in the periphery may be a powerful predictive tool.

In our second study, we examined the expression of other markers acquired (CD45R0) and lost (CD45RA) following activation of naïve T cells. Examining expression of these on CD4 and CD8 cells cross-sectionally in 71 HIV+ patients, we found abnormalities in percentage levels of CD45RA+ and CD45R0+ populations, none of which showed any relationship to disease severity. Intriguingly, however, we noted that the surface density of both CD45RA and CD45R0 molecules on CD4 and CD8 cells was markedly and significantly reduced at all stages of HIV infection (eg relative specific fluorescence reduced by up to 50%; p<0.001). This abnormality was confirmed in studies using antibodies to a common epitope on all CD45 isoforms (pan-CD45) and to the CD45RB isoform.

Finally, returning to the question of immune cell markers of activation and disease progression, we have examined some of the best documented markers in our longitudinal study. The aim of the study was to identify independent predictive markers. Both neopterin and β_2-microglobulin predict progression to AIDS with a relative hazard of up to 7.0 for neopterin and 3.4 for β_2-microglobulin (p<0.0001 for both). Both predict AIDS independently of CD4 count, although neopterin (p<0.0001) performs much better than β_2-microglobulin (p<0.04). Our results suggest that combining markers may be a more powerful approach to prediction.

In summary, immune cell activation is a feature of early HIV infection and some markers may have a powerful predictive value of progression to AIDS. Cross-sectional studies suggest that markers of activation of the CD4 lymphocyte itself could be powerful predictors, while longitudinal studies indicate that combining CD4 count with other independent markers may considerably enhance the power of prediction.

INTRODUCTION

There is in vitro evidence to suggest that activation of cellular immunity may promote the progression of HIV infection. CD4+ T lymphocytes have a greater susceptibility to infection by HIV when activated and both HIV entry and HIV envelope-dependent cell-to-cell fusion require T cell activation (1,2). In turn, activation of T lymphocytes chronically infected with HIV triggers the transition from latency to active viral replication in vitro (3). If these activation-dependent infection-promoting events occur in vivo, the study of T cell activation may provide both pathogenic insights and markers of disease severity in HIV infection.

One approach to assessing T cell activation is the study of surface molecules usually absent or expressed at a very low level on quiescent T cells such as HLA-DR and CD25. HLA-DR is a major histocompatibility complex class II molecule and is expressed on T cells after antigenic or mitogenic stimulation reaching a peak after approximately seven days. On the other hand, CD25, the receptor for the T cell growth and activation factor IL-2, is induced earlier with peak expression occurring at 48-72 hours.

To examine T cell activation and its relationship to disease severity in HIV infection, we measured the expression of HLA-DR and CD25 on T lymphocytes and on the helper/inducer (CD4+) and suppressor cytotoxic (CD8+) subsets in HIV+ patients with disease of varying severity.

CD4+ T lymphocytes can be broadly divided into "naive" and "memory" cell populations, based on expression of different isoforms of CD45 (leucocyte common antigen) on the cell surface. The high molecular weight CD45 isoform (CD45RA) is a marker of the human "naive" subset of T lymphocytes, whilst the low molecular weight isoform (CD45R0) is a marker of the reciprocal "memory" subset (4,5). Transition from naive to memory cell is paralleled by conversion from CD45RA to CD45R0 expression (6-8). In vitro studies have shown that HIV characteristically infects CD4+ memory cells, arguing for a corresponding decline of this population in vivo (9). The accumulated evidence from previous studies performed to date is inconclusive, however. In order to examine alterations in T cell naive and memory cells in vivo in HIV infection more precisely, we measured CD45RA and CD45R0 expression on CD4+ and CD8+ T lymphocytes in peripheral blood from HIV positive patients at different stages of the disease. To examine further the relationship between CD45 and HIV infection, we used a monoclonal antibody which identifies the CD45RB isoform, and one which binds all isoforms (pan-CD45).

To further examine the relationship between these markers of T cell activation and disease severity, activation markers were compared with accepted indices of disease progression namely, CD4 count and β_2-microglobulin and with neopterin, a marker of both disease progression and cellular immune activation. In addition, we report the results of a longitudinal study, examining the ability of markers of cell activation to predict the onset of AIDS in our cohort.

MATERIALS AND METHODS

Activated T Cell Subsets

Subjects. 157 patients with HIV infection (150 males, 7 females; median age 29 years, range 21-42) in whom the diagnosis was made on the basis of positive testing for the presence of anti-p24 antibody (Wellcome Diagnostics, Dartford, UK) and p24 antigen (Abbott Diagnostics, Maidenhead, UK) were studied. When divided according to the Centres for Disease Control (CDC, Atlanta) classification, 66 patients fell in the asymptomatic group (CDC group II), 45 in the persistent generalized lymphadenopathy group (PGL, CDC group III), 10 had acquired immunodeficiency syndrome (AIDS) related complex (ARC, CDC group IVA) and 36 had AIDS (CDC group IVB-E). 53 healthy HIV seronegative blood donors recruited from the South-East Thames Regional Blood Transfusion Service were used as normal control subjects (51 males, 2 females; median age 34 years, range 22-44).

Two-Colour Immunofluorescence and Flow Cytometry. Two-colour immunophenotyping of peripheral blood lymphocytes was performed by flow cytometry using a lysed whole blood technique and a FACScan (Becton Dickinson, Mountain View, California) as previously described (10). The following combinations of monoclonal antibodies were used: PE-conjugated anti-HLA-DR or anti-CD25 in combination with FITC -conjugated anti-CD3, CD4 or CD8 (all Becton Dickinson).

Statistical Analysis. Differences between control subjects and HIV+ patients in different CDC groups were compared using an analysis of variance (ANOVA) method with tests for linearity as previously described (11,12). All variables in each test group had the normality of their distribution tested by the Kolmogorov-Smirnov goodness of fit test, and the distributions were always found to be consistent with the hypothesis of normality. Mean values for each variable in the HIV infected subjects and in controls were compared using the Student's t test. Correlations were studied with Pearson's linear regression analysis.

Frequency distributions were analyzed using the χ^2 or Fisher's exact probability test for small numbers as appropriate.

Naive and Memory T Cell Subsets

Subjects. 71 patients with HIV infection (68 males, 3 females; median age 32 years, range 24-41) were studied. When divided according to the CDC classification, 23 patients were in CDC group II, 20 in CDC group III and 28 in CDC groups IVB-E. Twenty healthy laboratory staff of similar age and sex with no known risk factors for HIV infection served as normal control subjects (all males; median age 29 years, range 28-34).

Three-Colour Immunofluorescence and Flow Cytometry. Monoclonal antibodies conjugated with either fluorescein isothiocyanate (FITC), phycoerythrin (PE), peridinin-chlorophyll-a-protein (PerCP) or biotin were used, in a similar staining technique to that described above, and according to the manufacturer's instructions. The biotin-conjugated monoclonal antibodies were revealed in a second step using saturating amounts of strepta-vidin (AMS Biotechnology, Oxford, UK). The following combinations of antibodies were used: PE-conjugated anti-CD45RA (2H4, Coulterclone, Luton, Bedfordshire, UK), FITC-conjugated anti-CD45R0 (UCHL1, Dako, High Wycombe, Buckinghamshire, UK) and PerCP-conjugated anti-CD4 or anti-CD8 (Becton Dickinson); FITC-conjugated anti-CD45RB (PD7/26; a gift from Dr DY Mason, John Radcliffe Hospital, Oxford, UK) and biotin-conjugated anti-CD4/CD8 (Becton Dickinson); PE-conjugated anti-CD45 (Serotec, Kidlington, Oxford, UK), FITC-conjugated anti-CD8 (Dako, High Wycombe, Buckingham-shire, UK) and biotin-conjugated anti-CD4 (Becton Dickinson).

Results of CD45RA and CD45R0 co-expression are given as a percentage of the main CD4+ and CD8+ populations.

The density of expression of CD45RA, CD45R0, CD45 and CD45RB molecules on the surface of CD4+ and CD8+ lymphocytes is given as the relative specific fluorescence (RSF). Relative specific fluorescence values were expressed as mean arbitrary units (AU) $\pm$ SD and were calculated according to the following formula: [RSF= antilog (mean fluorescence channel number/number of channels per decade)] (13).

Statistical analysis was performed using an identical approach to that described above.

Longitudinal Study of Activation Markers in Prediction

Subjects. 403 patients (335 males (83%)), with HIV infection were recruited into the longitudinal study. Of these 340 did not have AIDS at entry, and these were followed for a total of 574 patient years. Patients were sampled at 3 month intervals during follow-up and CD4 count, neopterin, β_2-microglobulin measured as previously described (11,12).

Statistical Analysis. The Cox proportional hazards model was used to assess the association between potential prognostic markers and risk of AIDS.

RESULTS

Activated T Cell Subsets

Activation of CD3+ T Cells. In HIV+ patients considered as a whole, levels of CD3+HLA-DR+ T lymphocytes were higher compared with the control group (p<0.001) (Table 1). Levels of CD3+HLA-DR+ T lymphocytes were higher in patients in all CDC groups (II, III, IVA and IVB-E) compared with controls (p<0.001) but there were no differences between patients in successive CDC groups.

In contrast, levels of CD3+CD25+ T lymphocytes were significantly lower than the control group in all HIV+ patients considered together (p<0.001) (Table 1). In patients in CDC group III, percentages of CD3+CD25+ T lymphocytes were similar to control, and in

Table 1. Means (SD) and statistical comparison of percentages of activated (HLA-DR+ and CD25+) CD3+, CD4+ and CD8+ T cell subsets in HIV+ subjects and controls

	Controls (n=53)	All HIV+ (n=157)	CDC II (n=66)	CDC III (n=45)	CDC IV (n=46)	Test for linear trend $(F_{4,205})$
% Lymphocytes CD3+HLA-DR+	10.4 (5.3)	46.9† (19.3)	46.8† (19.8)	45.9† (17.3)	49.1† (22.6)	NS
% Lymphocytes CD3+CD25+	14.4 (5.2)	10.2† (10.4)	9.1† (6.5)	13.9 (15.4)	8.4† (8.8)	NS
% Lymphocytes CD4+HLA-DR+	9.7 (4.2)	26.9† (15.4)	21.4† (9.9)	25.0† (15.5)	37.0† (17.7)	52.3*
% Lymphocytes CD4+CD25+	11.0 (4.5)	29.3† (12.0)	24.0† (7.9)	31.7† (10.4)	34.2† (15.8)	71.4*
% Lymphocytes CD8+HLA-DR+	18.7 (9)	55.8† (14.5)	52.5† (13.5)	63.8† (12.0)	51.8† (15.5)	NS
% Lymphocytes CD8+CD25+	5.7 (2.9)	5.8 (5.5)	5.4 (4.7)	6.8 (6.1)	5.3 (6.2)	NS

Note: † $p < 0.001$ (HIV patient groups versus controls).
The $F_{4,205}$ statistics assess the type of trend (linear or non-linear) across the groups. Low values suggest no trend, whereas high values for $F_{4,205}$ suggest that the trend is linear (*$p<0.001$).
Modified from reference 10, with permission.

CDC groups II, IVA and IVB-E significantly lower than control subjects ($p<0.001$ for all). Levels of activated CD3+CD25+ T lymphocytes were higher in patients in CDC group III and lower in CDC group IVA compared with the preceding CDC group.

Activation of Cd4+ T Cells. Levels of CD4+ lymphocytes expressing the activation markers HLA-DR and CD25 were higher in all HIV+ patients considered as a whole and in each CDC group compared with control subjects ($p<0.001$) (Table 1). There was a stepwise increase in levels of CD4+HLA-DR+ lymphocytes with increasing severity of disease, with significantly higher levels in CDC group IV than in the preceding CDC group ($p<0.001$). This progressive activation with disease severity showed a significant test for linear trend ($p<0.001$) without a significant departure from linear trend ($p<0.001$). A similar pattern was seen in levels of activated (CD25+) CD4+ lymphocytes, with stepwise increases with each CDC group and a significantly higher level in CDC group III compared with CDC group II ($p<0.001$) (Table 1). Again, the test for linearity of increasing levels of activated (CD25+) CD4+ lymphocytes with increasing disease severity was significant ($p<0.001$), without significant departure from linearity.

Activation of Cd8+ T Cells. Levels of CD8+HLA-DR+ lymphocytes were higher in all HIV+ patients compared with control subjects ($p<0.001$) (Table 1). Levels of CD8+HLA-DR+ T lymphocytes were higher in patients in CDC groups II, III and IV compared with control subjects ($p<0.001$ for all three). Levels were significantly higher in CDC group III and significantly lower in CDC group IV compared with the preceding CDC group ($p<0.001$ for both).

Levels of CD8+CD25+ lymphocytes were similar in all of the disease groups and control subjects (Table 1).

Frequency of Abnormal Levels of T Cell Activation and Abnormal CD4 Counts in Asymptomatic Patients. The presence of a low CD4 count provides a marker of disease severity and risk of progression to AIDS in asymptomatic patients. In the present study

Table 2. Means (SD) and statistical comparison of percentages
of CD4+ and CD8+ T cell subsets (CD45RA+R0- and
CD45RA-R0+)in HIV+ subjects and controls

	Controls (n=20)	All HIV+ (n=71)
CD45RA+R0-CD4+	39.6	26.5†
	(13.3)	(16.0)
CD45RA-R0+CD4+	50.9	53.8
	(13.6)	(19.0)
CD45RA+R0-CD8+	61.3	37.5†
	(13.8)	(13.1)
CD45RA-R0+CD8+	26.7	46.9†
	(11.9)	(14.5)

Note: † p< 0.001: This symbol refer to comparisons between
HIV patient groups and controls.

abnormally low CD4 counts (less than mean minus 2SD of control subjects) were found in 34/66 (51.5%) of patients in CDC group II. This was compared with the proportion of patients in CDC group II possessing abnormally elevated levels of CD3+, CD4+ and CD8+ lymphocyte activation (greater than mean plus 2SD of control subjects).

In asymptomatic patients with HIV infection high levels of CD3+HLA-DR+ T lymphocytes were found in a greater proportion of patients (54/66, 81.8%) than abnormally low levels of CD4+ lymphocytes (34/66, 51.5%) (p<0.001).

When the same analysis was performed on the smaller group of asymptomatic patients on whom CD4 and CD8 lymphocyte activation studies had been carried out, 18/20 patients (90%) had abnormally high levels of CD8+HLA-DR+ lymphocytes, compared with 12/20 (60%) having low CD4 counts, though this difference failed to reach conventional levels of statistical significance (p= 0.07).

Naive and Memory T Cell Subsets

Expression of CD45RA and CD45R0 on CD4+ T Lymphocytes. Percentage levels of naive CD4+ lymphocytes (i.e CD45RA+R0-) were lower in the HIV positive group compared to controls (p<0.001) (Table 2). Relative specific fluorescence (RSF) of CD45RA on CD4+ T lymphocytes was lower than controls in all HIV positive patients considered as a whole (p<0.001) (Table 3).

Percentages of memory CD4+ T lymphocytes (i.e. CD45RA-R0+) had a reciprocal relationship with CD45RA expression, levels of memory cells tending to be higher in patients although this did not reach statistical significance (Table 2). Relative specific fluorescence of CD45R0 on CD4+ T lymphocytes was lower than controls in all HIV positive patients considered together (p<0.001) (Table 3).

Expression of CD45RA and CD45R0 on CD8+ T Lymphocytes. Percentage levels of naive (CD45RA+R0-) CD8+ T lymphocytes were lower than controls in all HIV positive patients considered as a whole (p<0.001). Relative specific fluorescence of CD45RA on CD8+ T lymphocytes was lower than controls in all HIV positive patients considered as a whole (p<0.001) (Table 3).

Table 3. Relative specific fluorescence of CD45RA and CD45R0 on CD4+ and CD8+ lymphocytes

	Controls (n=20)	All HIV+ (n=71)
CD45RA+ CD4 lymphocytes	3.91 (2.31)	2.30† (1.57)
CD45R0+ CD4 lymphocytes	3.95 (2.89)	2.19† (1.03)
CD45RA+ CD8 lymphocytes	17.92 (16.03)	5.40† (6.99)
CD45R0+ CD8 lymphocytes	3.04 (1.85)	1.99† (0.64)

Note: † $p < 0.001$: This symbol refers to comparisons between HIV patient groups and controls.

Percentage levels of memory (CD45RA-R0+) CD8+ T lymphocytes were higher than controls in all HIV positive patients considered as a whole ($p<0.001$) (Table 2).

Relative specific fluorescence of CD45R0 on CD8+ T lymphocytes was lower than controls in all HIV positive patients considered as a whole (Table 3).

Expression of CD45 and CD45RB on CD4+ and CD8+ T Lymphocytes. Percentage levels of CD4+ and CD8+ T lymphocytes expressing CD45 or CD45RB were similar to controls in all HIV positive patients and were close to 100% (data not shown).

Relative specific fluorescence (RSF) of CD45 and CD45RB on CD4+ and CD8+ T lymphocytes were lower in the HIV positive group compared to controls ($p<0.0001$ for both).

Prediction of Progression to AIDs. Table 4 shows the relative hazards for progression to AIDS in the cohort of non-AIDS HIV+ patients followed prospectively. Only CD4 count, neopterin and ß$_2$-microglobulin levels were independently predictive of progression to AIDS.

Table 4. Relative hazard for progression to AIDS in the longitudinal study of 340 HIV+ patients for a total of 574 patient years

Marker	Range	Person-years at risk	Number with AIDS	Relative hazard
CD4 Lymphocyte count	<50	32.8	26	30.53
(/µl)	50-	153.2	21	5.73
	200-	385.8	9	1.00
				($p<0.0001$)
Neopterin	<15	168.8	7	1.00
(nmol/l)	15-	209.6	20	2.19
	30-	80.5	25	6.98
				($p<0.0001$)
ß$_2$-microglobulin	<4	270.2	4	1.00
(mg/l)	4-	129.2	27	3.35
	6-	63.0	9	2.15
				($p<0.0001$)

DISCUSSION

These studies demonstrate that the decline of CD4 cells in HIV infection is strongly associated with an increase in the levels of activation markers on the CD4 population, supporting the hypothesis of a relationship between activation and death of CD4 cells. The additional observation that the levels of activation of the cytotoxic/suppressor T cell subset increase with the decline of CD4 cells may suggest a mechanism whereby the CD4 cells are eliminated. Finally, we also show that signs of cellular immune activation are present in the majority of asymptomatic HIV infected patients: these may prove useful early markers of disease when other indicators are still silent.

Initially, our findings indicated that HLA-DR+ T cells are persistently increased in HIV infection and are equally high amongst all patients irrespective of CDC group. In contrast, however, when CD25 was used as an indicator of T cell activation, expression was lower in HIV infected individuals. This apparent divergence in the expression of the two activation markers prompted further studies on the expression of HLA-DR and CD25 on the CD4+ and CD8+ T lymphocyte subsets. The results of these additional studies demonstrate important differences in the activation patterns of the two T lymphocyte subsets, which may be both informative of the pathogenesis of the disease and useful clinically.

The fact that this part of the study was cross-sectional in nature, including patients at all stages of infection, enables us only to speculate on the potency of immune markers in predicting progression of HIV-related disease. Of particular value in this respect is the analysis of linearity of immune changes with increasing disease severity (11,12). The absolute number of CD4 lymphocytes is currently the best marker of disease progression in HIV infection (14-16) and in our previous studies on the relationships between immune parameters and disease progression in HIV infection, the CD4 count alone, and not β_2-microglobulin, neopterin or soluble CD4 has shown a linear increase with disease severity (11). It is of interest, therefore, that in the present study activation of the CD4+ subset increases linearly with disease severity and a longitudinal study will be required to confirm that it is indeed a useful predictor of disease progression. Moreover, the close relationship between CD4 activation and CD4 decline suggests that activation of this subset may be a prerequisite for their destruction.

The predictive power of T cell activation in indicating progression to AIDS and its relationship to the pathogenesis of HIV disease remains to be established, and in addition, the underlying activating stimuli are not known as yet. It is possible that cell activation is secondary to the effects of HIV infection, which is known to result in increased circulating levels of cytokines such as IL-1. However, the finding that CD8+ lymphocytes do not upregulate CD25 argues against high levels of CD25 expression on CD4 lymphocytes being solely due to the influence of cytokines. The presence of persistent activation of the CD4+ cells supports the view that cell activation is a key factor in the pathogenesis of the disease through at least two possible mechanisms (17). First, T cell activation involves the induction of factors which bind to specific regulatory factors, known as B, in both the IL-2 and IL-2 receptor genes. Similar binding sites are located in the long terminal repeat sequences of the HIV genome. Activation of T cells and induction of IL-2 and IL-2 receptor production could simultaneously result in upregulation of synthesis of HIV mRNA (18-21). A second possibility is activated CD8+ T cells may represent the cytotoxic T cell response to HIV, hence their relationship with declining CD4 counts. Since the virus is tropic for CD4+ cells this would support the proposal by Levy et al that the prinicipal role of the CD8 cytotoxic/suppressor cell in HIV infection is to target the CD4 lymphocyte and possibly mediate its destruction (23,24).

This study also shows that the frequency of abnormally high levels of activated HLA-DR+ T lymphocytes is a greater discriminator of asymptomatic patients than a low CD4 count. This finding is of importance, since the CD4 count is frequently used to provide diagnostic information in cases of suspected immunodeficiency in which there are reasons for not performing an HIV test or the HIV test is negative. Additional diagnostic information may be gained by also measuring levels of activated T lymphocytes.

Studies on naive and memory CD4+ T lymphocytes in HIV infection have been performed to establish whether either subset has a higher susceptibility to infection and destruction by the virus. Support for the possibility that CD45-mediated functions are defective comes from our finding that the surface density of CD45 molecules, whether of the RA, R0 or RB isoform, is significantly reduced in HIV infection, and by the altered distribution of the CD45RB isoforms. In contrast, surface density of other constitutively expressed surface molecules such as CD4 and CD8, did not change. The reduction in CD45 isoform surface density is present in asymptomatic patients and does not change with disease progression. It thus coincides with the appearance of impaired T cell proliferation to specific antigens and mitogens in vitro, and a lack of response to recall antigens demonstrable in vivo (25,26). Our findings may be of relevance to this anergic state. CD45 is thought to be involved in T cell activation since it possesses tyrosine-specific phosphatase domains, and purified CD45 has phosphotyrosine phosphatase activity (27-28). T cell activation requires such tyrosine kinase activity and reduced expression of CD45 on the cell surface could account for T cell unresponsiveness. Therefore, the dysregulation of CD45 isoform expression could be a key component in the pathogenesis of T cell immunodeficiency in HIV infection.

Our longitudinal study demonstrates that in non-AIDS HIV+ patients in whom the date of seroconversion is not known, CD4 count, β_2-microglobulin and neopterin levels are independent predictors of progression to AIDS. Neopterin is more powerful than β_2-microglobulin in predicting AIDS onset, and future studies will be aimed at determining whether combinations of these independent markers can be used to enhance the predictive power of the single markers used alone.

ACKNOWLEDGMENTS

Meera Mahalingam was supported by the Joint Research Committee of King's College Hospital, which supported these projects in conjunction with the South East Thames Regional Health Authority.

REFERENCES

1. Rosenberg ZF, Fauci AS. Activation of latent HIV infection. *J Natl Inst Hlth* 1990;**2**:41-45.
2. Mohagheghpour N, Chakrabarti R, Stein B, Gowda SD, Englman EG. Early activation events render T cells susceptible to HIV-1 induced syncytia formation. *J Biol Chem* 1991;**266**:7233-7238.
3. Gowda SD, Stein BS, Mohagheghpour N, Benike CJ, Engleman EG. Evidence that T cell activation is required for HIV-1 entry in CD4+ lymphocytes. *J Immunol* 1989;**142**:773-780.
4. Beverley PC. Minireview: Human T cell subsets. *Immunol Lett.* 1987;**14**:263-67.
5. Smith SH, Brown MH, Rowe D, Callard RE, Beverley PC. Functional subsets of human helper-inducer cells defined by a new monoclonal antibody, UCHL1. *Immunology.* 1986;**58**:63-70.
6. Akbar AN, Terry L, Timms A, Beverley PCL, Janossy G. Loss of CD45R and gain of UCHL1 reactivity is a feature of primed T cells. *J Immunol.* 1988;**140**:2171-78.
7. Akbar AN, Salmon M, Janossy G. The synergy between naive and memory T cells during activation. *Immunol Today.* 1991;**12**:184-88.

8. Beverley PCL. Is T cell memory maintained by cross-reactive stimulation? *Immunol Today.* 1990;**12**:189-92.

9. Schnittman SM, Lane HC, Greenhouse J, Justement JS, Baseler M, Fauci AS. Preferential infection of CD4+ memory T cells by human immunodeficiency virus type 1: evidence for a role in the selective T-cell functional defects observed in infected individuals. *Proc Natl Acad Sci* 1990;**87**:6058-62.

10. Mahalingam M, Peakman M, Davies ET, Pozniak A, McManus TJ, Vergani D. T cell activation and disease severity in HIV infection. *Clin Exp Immunol* 1993;**93**:337-43

11. Peakman M, Senaldi G, Foote N, McManus TJ, Vergani D. Naturally occurring soluble CD4 in patients with HIV infection. *J Infect Dis* 1992;**165**:799-804.

12. Senaldi G, Peakman M, McManus TJ, Davies ET, Tee DEH, Vergani D. Activation of the complement system in human immunodeficiency virus infection: relevance of the classical pathway to pathogenesis and disease severity. *J Infect Dis* 1990;**162**:1227-32.

13. Klein NJ, Levin M, Strobel S, Finn A. Degradation of glycosaminoglycans and fibronectin on endotoxin stimulated endothelium by adherent neutrophils: relationship to CD11b/CD18 and L-selectin expression. *J Infect Dis* 1993;**167**:890-898.

14. Phillips AN, Lee CA, Elford J et al. Serial CD4 lymphocyte counts and the development of AIDS. *Lancet* 1991;**337**:389-391.

15. Lange JMA, Dewolfe F, Goudsmit J. Marker for progression in HIV infection. *AIDS* 1989;**3** (Suppl 1):153-160.

16. Philips AN, Lee CA, Elford J et al. The cumulative risk of AIDS as CD4 lymphocyte count declines. *J AIDS* 1992;**5**:148-152.

17. Mcdougal JS, Mawla A, Cort SP et al. Cellular tropism of human retrovirus HTLV-III/LAV. *J Immunol* 1985;**135**:3151-61.

18. Bachelerie F, Alcami F, Arenzana S et al. HIV enhancer activity perpetuated by NF-kB induction on infection of monocytes. *Nature* 1991;**350**:709-712.

19. Nabel GJ. Tampering with transcription. *Nature* 1991; **350**:658.

20. Nabel GJ, Baltimore D. An inducible transcription factor activates transcription of human immunodeficiency virus in T cells. *Nature* 1987;**326**:711-713.

21. Riviere Y, Blank V, Kourilsky P et al. Processing of the precursor of NF-kB by the HIV-1 protease during acute infection. *Nature* 1991;**350**:625-626.

22. Baltimore D, Feinberg MB. HIV revealed : toward a natural history of the infection. *N Engl J Med* 1989;**321**:1673-75.

23. Levy J. Immunological factors involved in long term survival. Presented at the VIIIth International Conference on AIDS, July 22, 1992, Amsterdam.

24. Mackewicz C, Levy J. CD8+ cell anti-HIV activity: Nonlytic suppression of virus replication. *AIDS Res Hum Retr* 1992;**8**:1039-1.

3

THE ROLE OF THE CELL CYCLE IN HIV-1 INFECTION

Jerome A. Zack

Division of Hematology-Oncology
Department of Medicine
UCLA School of Medicine
and Jonsson Comprehensive Cancer Center
Los Angeles, California 90024-1678

SUMMARY

Infection of quiescent lymphocytes with human immunodeficiency virus type 1 (HIV-1) does not result in production of progeny virus. We have previously reported that although HIV-1 can enter quiescent lymphocytes with high efficiency, the reverse transcription process does not go to completion. This results in a viral genome which is composed partly of viral RNA and partly of viral DNA. If a mitogenic signal is applied shortly after infection to a cell harboring such a structure, reverse transcription can go to completion and progeny virus will be produced. However, this partially reverse transcribed structure is extremely labile, and the efficiency of virus rescue decreases rapidly, with increasing times between infection and activation. Our laboratory is using inhibitors of cell activation to identify at which stage of the cell cycle this block to reverse transcription occurs. We have found that agents that arrest the cell in the late G_1 phase of the cell cycle do not alter the ability of the virus to complete reverse transcription. However, agents that inhibit activation of the cell by blocking transition through G_1 prevent completion of reverse transcription. It thus appears that immunosuppression of the target cell may be a means of preventing productive infection of the cell.

We have also been using the severe combined immunodeficient mouse implanted with human tissue (SCID-hu) as an *in vivo* model to study HIV-1 pathogenic properties. When human fetal thymic implants in these animals are infected by HIV-1, profound depletion of CD4-bearing human thymocytes is seen. The depletion appears to initially be more pronounced in the immature CD4/CD8 double-positive thymocyte subset than in the more mature CD4+/CD8- subset. The reason for this preferential cell death is currently under investigation; however, this suggests that factors involved in cell differentiation may play a role in the pathogenic process.

Cell Activation and Apoptosis in HIV Infection
Edited by Jean-Marie Andrieu and Wei Lu, Plenum Press, New York, 1995

INTRODUCTION

Many years ago, Howard Temin noted that fibroblasts rendered quiescent by serum starvation were not susceptible to productive infection by retroviruses.[1] In the case of human immunodeficiency virus type 1 (HIV-1) infection, the vast majority of potential target cells (CD4+ T-lymphocytes) in the peripheral blood are in a resting or G_0 state. Thus, how the virus behaves in these cells may be very important for pathogenesis. Similarly, HIV infection of cells undergoing differentiation as opposed to merely proliferation may play a role in disease progression. Model systems to study how HIV interacts with cells in different stages of replication/differentiation are being explored to better understand how the virus replicates and causes disease.

HIV INFECTION OF QUIESCENT CELLS

Our laboratory and others have shown that *in vitro* infection of quiescent peripheral blood lymphocytes (PBL) with HIV-1 does not result in productive infection.[2-5] However, if a mitogenic stimulus is applied after virus addition, productive infection proceeds and progeny virions are released into the culture medium.[4-6] Furthermore, the longer the time-frame between infection and subsequent mitogenic stimulation is, the less virus production is seen.[4,6] These data suggested that a latent, labile viral intermediate could be formed by HIV-1 in quiescent T-cells. Subsequent molecular analysis by our laboratory, using quantitative polymerase chain reaction (PCR) analysis with primer pairs specific for various stages of HIV-1 reverse transcription, revealed that while HIV-1 could efficiently enter quiescent T-lymphocytes; however, the process was not readily completed.[4] The efficiency of completion of this process was about 1-5%. Stimulation of cells harboring incomplete DNA species resulted in renewed reverse transcription and elongation of these genomes.[7]

Analysis of incomplete reverse transcripts in quiescent cells not stimulated after infection revealed that this partially reverse transcribed intermediate decayed with time, most likely due to the activity of cellular nucleases. This degradation of the viral genome is probably the mechanism for the decrease in progeny virus rescue seen with subsequent stimulation of infected quiescent cells at later timepoints.

Partial reverse transcripts have been found in cell-free HIV-1 virions.[8,9] However, analyses using azidothymidine (AZT) treatment of quiescent cells and detailed kinetic experiments indicated that the incomplete viral genomes found in infected quiescent cells were newly synthesized intracellularly, and not the result of virion-associated partial reverse transcripts.[7] Thus, there appears to be a block to completion of reverse transcription in quiescent cells. This block may be partially due to a smaller nucleotide pool in quiescent versus activated T-lymphocytes. Treatment of activated cells with hydroxyurea, which halts the conversion of ribonucleotides to deoxyribonucleotides by decreasing ribonucleotide reductase activity, decreases the ability of the cell to reverse transcribe viral RNA.[10] However, this does not appear to be the entire story for quiescent cells, as hydroxyurea-treated cells have a lower ability to initiate reverse transcription than that seen in quiescent cells (Zack et al., in preparation). Furthermore, treatment of quiescent cells with high concentrations of extracellular nucleosides did not result in an increased amount of reverse transcription.[7] This latter treatment is effective in partially increasing the slower rate of reverse transcription seen after HIV-1 infection of primary macrophages.[11]

Additional blocks to productive infection occur in quiescent cells at later stages of the viral replication cycle. The laboratory of Mario Stevenson has shown that *in vivo*, quiescent T-lymphocytes harbor fully reverse transcribed yet unintegrated viral genomes.[12] These partial reverse transcripts may be the result of the few viral genomes that proceed past the block to reverse transcription seen in our *in vitro* studies. The lack of integration of these genomes is likely due to the requirement for active transport of viral DNA into the nucleus, a process which is ATP-dependent.[13] These various blocks to productive infection in quiescent cells may be partially responsible for lowering viral load *in vivo*.

THE EFFECT OF CELL-CYCLE INHIBITORS OR HIV-1 REVERSE TRANSCRIPTION

To determine the stage of the cell cycle required for completion of reverse transcription, our laboratory used various inhibitors of the cell cycle added prior to or following stimulation with phytohemmagglutinin (PHA) and subsequent infection. Infected cells were analyzed by quantitative PCR for complete reverse transcripts (Zack et al., in preparation). The effect on the cell cycle was measured by tritiated thymidine incorporation. These studies showed that treatment of cells with aphidicolin, which arrests cells at the G_1/S phase border of the cell cycle, decreased the ability of the cells to proliferate, yet did not affect viral reverse transcription. These results are consistent with those seen by others using drug treatment of T-cell lines,[13] and suggest that the block to reverse transcription occurs prior to S phase.

When cyclohexamide, which abolishes new protein synthesis, was added as early as six hours following stimulation with PHA, although cell proliferation was halted, viral reverse transcription was unaffected. However, if this agent was added prior to stimulation, reverse transcription did not proceed to completion, resulting in a phenotype that resembled infection of quiescent cells. Thus, the block to reverse transcription appears to occur early in the G_1 phase of the cell cycle, and this process requires cellular protein synthesis.

Cyclosporin A, which halts the transcription of certain cellular genes and thus prevents T-cell activation[14] was next assessed for its ability to affect reverse transcription. When added prior to PHA stimulation in concentrations that were not toxic to the cells (25 μg/ml), this agent inhibited the completion of reverse transcription. Thus, it appears that prevention of T-cell activation can influence an early phase of the viral replication cycle. These results suggest that immunosuppressive agents might be useful in halting viral replication *in vivo* under certain circumstances, such as known virus exposure (i.e., contaminated needlestick in a hospital setting or birth of a child to an HIV-infected mother). It is conceivable that a specific immunosuppressive agent could be identified which, when administered immediately following this type of exposure, could prevent reverse transcription. This might subsequently allow endogenous cellular nucleases to degrade the incompletely reverse transcribed viral genome, resulting in prevention of infection.

THE EFFECT OF HIV-1 INFECTION ON DIFFERENTIATING CELLS

During natural HIV-1 infection, cells other than fully differentiated PBL are infected, including cells in various hematolymphoid organs such as lymph nodes[15,16] and the thymus.[17-20] Thus, the virus has the opportunity to infect immature CD4-bearing cells and perturb differentiation. Our laboratory and others have shown that HIV-1 infection of human thymic implants in severe combined immunodeficient (SCID)/human chimeric (SCID-hu) mice[21,22] results in severe depletion of human CD4-bearing thymocytes resembling that seen in humans.[23-26] This depletion appears to initially manifest itself in the immature CD4+/CD8+ thymocyte subset, followed by depletion of the more mature CD4+/CD8- subset. At early timepoints following infection, viral DNA is preferentially found in this double-positive population,[23] and may subsequently be found in various thymocyte subsets.[26]

Why infection and subsequent depletion of the immature CD4+/CD8+ subset is initially seen in human thymic implants in SCID-hu mice is an intriguing question. Flow cytometric analysis indicates that the level of CD4 on the surface of the immature cells is not appreciably higher than on the more mature population, so virus binding and entry is likely not the mechanism resulting in increased infection at early timepoints. Rather, it is likely that this immature population is the more metabolically active population, which allows for increased viral replication in this subset. These cells are actively undergoing differentiation to more mature stages, and this subset appears to have a higher percentage of cells in cell cycle than the more mature subsets, as assessed by propidium iodide staining and flow cytometric analysis (S. Kitchen and J. Zack, unpublished observations). Thus, it appears that infection and depletion of cells at various stages of T-cell differentiation may be very important in viral pathogenesis.

CONCLUSIONS

It is clear that cellular replication and differentiation play important roles in virus replication both *in vitro* and *in vivo*. Infection and replication of HIV-1 requires a multitude of host factors that appear to interact at virtually every stage of the viral life cycle. Further *in vitro* and *in vivo* studies will be required to fully understand the complex interactions between HIV-1 and its target cells in humans. These studies may point the way for the development of novel therapeutics targetted at the interfaces between viral and cellular processes, thereby allowing for successful intervention against disease progression.

ACKNOWLEDGEMENTS

This work was supported by NIH grants AI33259 and AI36059.

REFERENCES

1. Temin HM. 1967. Studies on carcinogenesis by avian sarcoma viruses. V. Requirement for new DNA synthesis and for cell division. *J. Cell. Physiol.* 69:53-64.
2. Folks T, Kelly J, Benn S, Kinter A, Justement J, Gold J, Redfield R, Sell KW, Fauci AS. 1986. Susceptibility of normal human lymphocytes to infection with HTLV-III/LAV. *J. Immunol.* 136:4049-53.
3. Stevenson M, Stanwick TL, Dempsey MP, Lamonica CA. 1990. HIV-1 replication is controlled at the level of T cell activation and proviral integration. *EMBO J.* 9:1551-60.
4. Zack JA, Arrigo SJ, Weitsman SR, Go AS, Haislip A, Chen ISY. 1990. HIV-1 entry into quiescent primary lymphocytes: Molecular analysis reveals a labile, latent viral structure. *Cell* 61:213-2.
5. Zagury D, Bernard J, Leonard R, Cheynier R, Feldman M, Sarin PS, Gallo RC. 1986. Long term cultures of HTLV-III infected cells: A model of cytopathology of T cell depletion in AIDS. *Science* 231:850-3.
6. Zack JA, Cann AJ, Lugo JP, Chen ISY. 1988. AIDS virus production from infected peripheral blood T cells following HTLV-I-induced mitogenic stimulation. *Science* 240:1026-9.
7. Zack JA, Haislip A, Krogstad P, Chen ISY. 1992. Incompletely reverse transcribed human immunodeficiency virus type 1 genomes in quiescent cells can function as intermediates in the retrovirus life cycle. *J. Virol.* 66:1717-25.
8. Gao WY, Cara A, Gallo RC, Lori F. 1993. Low levels of deoxynucleotides in peripheral blood lymphocytes: A strategy to inhibit human immunodeficiency virus type 1 replication. *Proc. Natl. Acad. Sci. USA* 90:8925-8.
9. Trono D. 1992. Partial reverse transcripts in virions from human immunodeficiency and murine leukemia viruses. *J. Virol.* 66:4893-900.
10. Lori F, di Marzo Veronese F, de Vico AL, Lusso P, Reitz MS, Jr, Gallo RC. 1992. Viral DNA carried by human immunodeficiency virus type 1 virions. *J. Virol.* 1992;66:5067-74.

11. O'Brien WA, Namazi A, Kalhor H, Mao S-h, Zack JA, Chen ISY. 1994. Kinetics of human immunodeficiency virus type 1 reverse transcription in blood mononuclear phagocytes are slowed by limitations of nucleotide precursors. *J. Virol.* 68:1258-63.

12. Bukrinsky MI, Stanwick TL, Dempsey MP, Stevenson M. 1991. Quiescent T lymphocytes as an inducible virus reservoir in HIV-1 infection. *Science* 254:423-7.

13. Bukrinsky MI, Sharova N, Dempsey MP, Stanwick TL, Bukrinskaya AG, Haggerty S, Stevenson M. Active nuclear import of human immunodeficiency virus type 1 preintegration complexes. *Proc. Natl. Acad. Sci. USA* 89:6580-4.

14. Schreiber SL. 1992. Immunophilin-sensitive protein phosphatase action in cell signaling pathways. *Cell* 70:365-8.

15. Embretson J, Zupancic M, Ribas JL, Burke A, Racz P, Tenner-Racz K, Haase AT. 1993. Massive covert infection of helper T lymphocytes and macrophages by HIV during the incubation period of AIDS. *Nature* 362:359-62.

16. Pantaleo G, Graziosi C, Demarest JF, Butini L, Montroni M, Fox CH, Orenstein JM, Kotler DP, Fauci AS. 1993. HIV infection is active and progressive in lymphoid tissue during the clinically latent stage of disease. *Nature* 362:355-8.

17. Joshi VV, Oleske JM, Saad S, Gadol C, Conner E, Bobila R, Minnefor AB. 1986. Thymus biopsy in children with acquired immunodeficiency syndrome. *Arch. Pathol. Lab. Med.* 110:837-42.

18. Rosenzweig M, Clark DP, Gaulton GN. 1993. Selective thymocyte depletion in neonatal HIV-1 thymic infection. *AIDS* 7:1601-5.

19. Mano H, Chermann JC. 1991. Fetal human immunodeficiency virus type 1 infection of different organs in the second trimester. *AIDS Res. Human Retroviruses* 7:83-8.

20. Papiernik M, Brossard Y, Mulliez N, Roume J, Brechot C, Barin F, Goudeau A, Bach J-F, Griscelli C, Henrion R, Vazeux R. 1992. Thymic abnormalities in fetuses aborted from human immunodeficiency virus type 1 seropositive women. *Pediatrics* 89:297-301.

21. McCune JM, Namikawa R, Kaneshima H, Shultz LD, Lieberman M, Weissman IL. 1988. The SCID-hu mouse: Murine model for the analysis of human hematolymphoid differentiation and function. *Science* 241:1632-9.

22. Namikawa R, Weilbaecher KN, Kaneshima H, Yee EJ, McCune JM. 1990. Long-term human hematopoiesis in the SCID-hu mouse. *J. Exp. Med.* 172:1055-63.

23. Aldrovandi GM, Feuer G, Gao L, Kristeva M, Chen ISY, Jamieson B, Zack JA. 1993. HIV-1 infection of the SCID-hu mouse: An animal model for virus pathogenesis. *Nature* 363:732-36.

24. Bonyhadi ML, Rabin L, Salimi S, Brown DA, Kosek J, McCune JM, Kaneshima H. 1993. HIV induces thymus depletion *in vivo*. *Nature* 363:728-36.

25. Jamieson BD, Aldrovandi GM, Planelles V, Jowett JBM, Gao L, Bloch LM, Chen ISY, Zack JA. 1994. Requirement of HIV-1 *nef* for *in vivo* replication and pathogenesis. *J. Virol.* 68:3478-85.

26. Stanley SK, McCune JM, Kaneshima H, Justement JS, Sullivan M, Boone E, Baseler M, Adelsberger J, Bonyhadi M, Orenstein J, Fox CH, Fauci AS. 1993. Human immunodeficiency virus infection of the human thymus and disruption of the thymic microenvironment in the SCID-hu mouse. *J. Exp. Med.* 178:1151-63.

4

MOLECULAR BASIS OF CELL CYCLE DEPENDENT HIV-1 REPLICATION
Implications for Control of Virus Burden

M. Stevenson[1,3], B. Brichacek[1], N. Heinzinger[1], S. Swindells[2], S. Pirruccello[1], E. Janoff[4], and M. Emerman[5]

[1] Department of Pathology and Microbiology
[2] Department of Internal Medicine
[3] Eppley Institute for Research in Cancer and Related Diseases
University of Nebraska Medical Center
Omaha, Nebraska 68198-5120
[4] VA Medial Center
Minneapolis, Minnesota 55417
[5] Fred Hutchinson Cancer Research Center
Basic Sciences Division, M774
Seattle, Washington 98194

INTRODUCTION

Retroviruses show a strong cell cycle dependence for productive infection. For example, the onco-retrovirus murine leukaemia virus (MLV) requires proliferating host cells for productive infection (Temin, 1988; Varmus and Brown, 1989). This restriction appears to reflect an inability of viral DNA to localize to the host cell nucleus until the host cell enters mitosis (Roe, et al., 1993; Lewis and Emerman, 1994). This dependence of onco-retroviruses for dividing cells is further illustrated by the poor transduction capacities of onco-retrovirus based retroviral vectors in non-dividing cell systems in vitro (miller, et al., 1990; Springett, et al., 1989).

In contrast to onco-retroviruses such as MLV, the lentivirus HIV does not show a great dependence upon host cell mitosis for establishment of the provirus. Thus, non-dividing cells such as primary macrophages (Gartner, et al., 1986; Nicholson, at al., 1986; Koyanagi, et al., 1988) follicular dendritic cells (Knight, 1990) sustain a productive replication cycle in the absence of cell division as do irradiated monocyte derived macrophages which completely lack cellular DNA synthesis (Weinberg, et al., 1991). In contrast to the permissiveness exhibited by non-dividing metabolically active cells such as macrophages and dendritic cells, non-dividing (quiescent) T lymphocytes which are metabolically inactive, are refractory to productive HIV-1 infection (McDougal, et al., 1985; Zagury, et al., 1986; Zack, et al., 1990; Stevenson, et al., 1990). Quiescent T cells support HIV-1 binding and infection. However, provirus establishment is not observed in these cells (Zack, et al., 1990; Stevenson, 1990). Inefficient provirus establishment by HIV following infection of quiescent T lymphocytes is manifest at several levels. Low levels of ribonucleotide reductase activity limit the nucleotide pool and appear to restrict de novo reverse transcription of in genomic viral RNA (Gao, et al., 1993). Elongation of viral DNA after the first template switch is inefficient (Zack, et al., 1990, 1993) and viral nucleic acids within the context of the preintegration complex access the nuclear compartment of the quiescent host cell very inefficiently (Bukrinsky, et al., 1993a). The latter phenomenon is supported by the predominately extra-chromosomal nature of viral DNA from patient lymphocyte populations enriched for quiescent T cells (Bukrinsky, et al., 1991). Following infection of quiescent T cells by HIV, productive virus infection can be renewed following activation of the infected cells (Zack, et al., 1988; Stevenson, et al., 1990). Thus, HIV infection of quiescent T cells leads to the establishment of a replication intermediate which resumes activity upon subsequent host cell activation. In support of this model, activation of quiescent T cells isolated from HIV-1 seropositive individuals leads to a shift in viral DAN from an extra-chromosomal to an integrated state suggesting hat restricted infection of quiescent T cells, followed by renewed virus replication upon T cell activation in vivo, may provide a mechanism by which virus replication is influenced by the activation state of the host (Zack, et al., 1988, 1990; Stevenson, et al., 1990; Bukrinsky, et al., 1991). From these studies, it is now becoming apparent that permissiveness to HIV-1 replication is strongly influenced by cell cycle parameters. Thus, quiescent (G0) cells are refractory to productive HIV-1 infection while cells arrested at any stage after G0, (G1, S, G2, M) do not appear to profoundly influence provirus establishment.

This paper will provide a synopsis of research aimed at identifying molecular determinants which govern permissiveness of non-dividing cells to HIV-1 infection and, particularly, viral determinants which allow provirus establishment in the absence of mitosis. In addition, research aimed at examining the relationship between T cell activation and, in particular, factors which govern the restriction of quiescent T cells to provirus establishment will be discussed. Recent insight into how the extent of T cell activation may directly impact virus burden in HIV-1 seropositive individuals will be presented in addition to possible implications for the management of HIV-1 infected individuals and the control of virus burden in disease progression.

HOST CELL MITOSIS IS NOT REQUIRED FOR SYNTHESIS OR NUCLEAR IMPORT OF VIRAL NUCLEIC ACIDS

To investigate the relationship between host cell mitosis and nuclear localization of viral DNA we examined the kinetics of circle genome formation following infection of growth arrested cells by HIV-1. Circular forms of the retroviral genome containing 1 and 2 long terminal repeats (LTRs) (Fig. 1) are produced only after synthesis of linear viral DNA and its transport to the nucleus (Varmus and Brown, 1989; Brown, et al., 1987). Thus, PCR using primers directed across the circle junction of the 2 LTR circle or primers which span a single LTR can be used to identify the rate with which nuclear localization of viral DNA occurs under conditions of cell cycle arrest. Cells were arrested in the G1/S phase of the cell cycle using aphidicolin (inhibitor of eucaryotic DNA polymerase alpha [Pedrali-Noy, et al., 1980]). Growth arrested and non-arrested cells were infected with HIV-1 at high multiplicity of infection. The presence of viral DNA and specifically 2 LTR circle forms of viral DNA were measured over the first 24 hours post-infection by PCR (Fig. 2). A state of G1/S arrest neither retarded cell infection and DNA synthesis (as determined by PCR using primers to

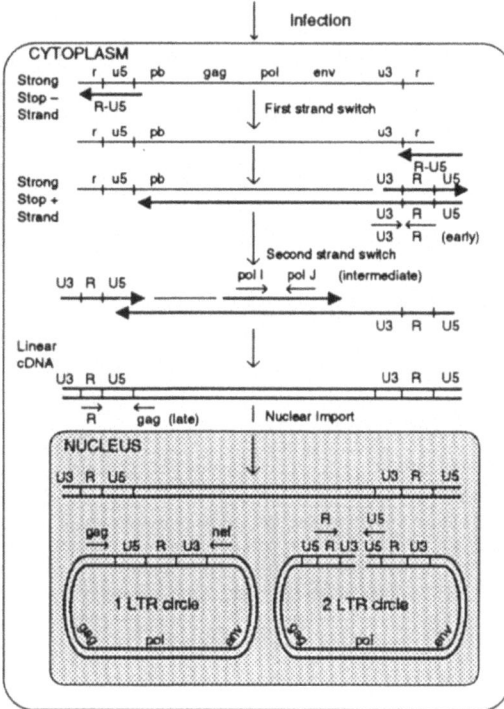

Figure 1. Major reverse transcription in the cytoplasm and nucleus of HIV-1 infected cells. After initiation of reverse transcription, two template switches result in a full length cDNA containing complete plus and minus strand DNA. After transport to the nucleus some linear molecules undergo LTR recombination and intra-molecular ligation resulting in the production of 1 LTR and 2 LTR circles respectively. Primers used for the specific amplification of the various cDNA forms are indicated.

pol gene products) nor accumulation of presence of AZT confirmed de novo viral DNA synthesis. This provided evidence that nuclear localization of viral DNA did not require passage of host cells through mitosis. In agreement with this result, experiments by one of our collaborators (Dr. M. Emerman), using an integration dependent assay (Kimpton and Emerman, 1992) confirmed that under conditions of G2 arrest (gamma irradiation) viral

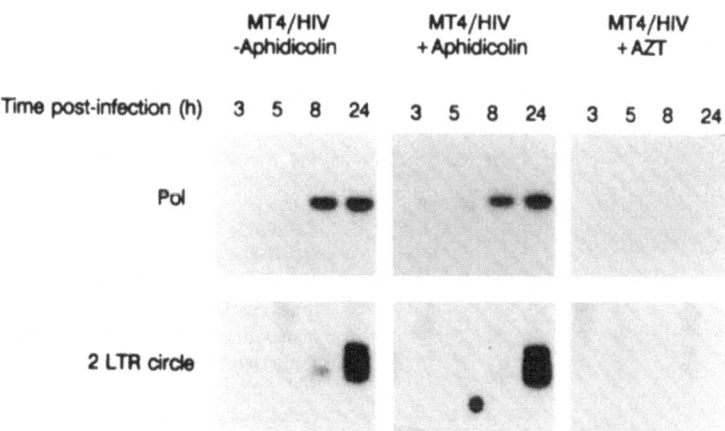

Figure 2. Kinetics of HIV-1 DNA synthesis and nuclear import in proliferating and in G1/S arrested CD4+ T cells. MT4 cell cultures were growth arrested by the action of aphidicolin. Cells were harvested at the indicated intervals and viral DNA synthesis and nuclear import was analyzed by PCR and primers to HIV-1 pol (pol 1/J) and 2 LTR circle products (LTR R.U5) respectively. (Reproduced with permission from Bukrinsky, et al., 1992).

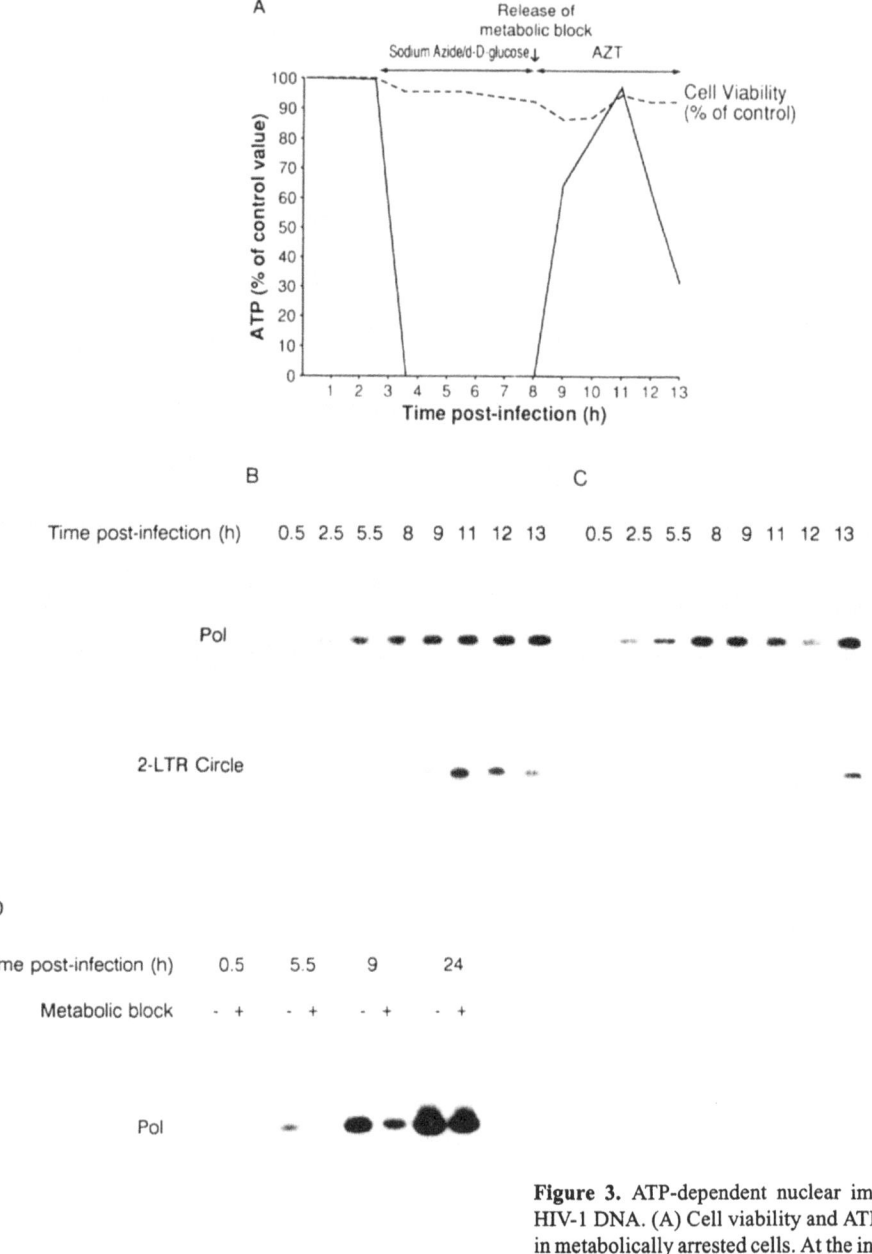

Figure 3. ATP-dependent nuclear import of HIV-1 DNA. (A) Cell viability and ATP levels in metabolically arrested cells. At the indicated times postinfection, samples of control (B) and metabolically arrested (C) cells were removed for measurement of HIV-1 DNA accumulation and intracellular ATP levels by a bioluminescence assay (ATP levels in metabolically arrested cultures are expressed as percentage of ATP levels in HIV-1-infected control MT-4 culture). (D) Nuclear accumulation of HIV-1 DNA in metabolically arrested (lanes +) and control lanes -) MT-4 cells. (Reproduced with permission from Bukrinsky, et al., 1992).

DNA synthesis and provirus establishment was unaffected (Kimpton and Emerman, 1992). Taken together, these studies provide evidence that passage of the host cell through mitosis is not a prerequisite for synthesis of viral DNA, nuclear import viral DNA or integration of viral with host cell DNA.

The experiment outlined above suggests that nuclear localization of viral nucleic acids occurs in the absence of mitosis. In the life cycles of HIV-1, viral nucleic acids remain associated with virion components in the context of a high molecular weight nucleoprotein preintegration complex (Bowerman, et al., 1989). This complex contains all necessary functions for reverse transcription, nuclear import and integration of viral nucleic acids. The association of viral nucleic acids with viral proteins confers upon this complex a high molecular weight property (approximately 160S, Bowerman, et al., 1989). Thus, the rapid nuclear import of high molecular weight nucleoprotein complexes in the absence of mitosis was reminiscent of the active nuclear import processes that govern the nuclear transport of proteins and other macro-molecules larger than 60Kd. In this case, nuclear transport through pores distributed over the nuclear envelope occurs by a process which requires ATP (Newmeyer, et al., 1986) and the presence of a specific nuclear localization signal (NLS) (Dingwall and Laskey, 1992). To investigate the energy requirements of mitosis independent nuclear targeting of viral nucleic acids, intracellular ATP was depleted in T cells by treatment with metabolic inhibitors sodium azide and 2-deoxy-D-gluclose (Richardson, et al., 1988). T cells were infected with HIV to allow viral DNA synthesis to proceed, then ATP was depleted by metabolic arrest. The degree of viral DNA synthesis and nuclear import as evidenced by the lack of 2 LTR circle products in these arrested cultures. The lack of 2 LTR circle formation correlated with an inability to detect viral DNA in the nuclei of metabolically arrested cells (Fig. 3). Upon removal of the metabolic clock, intracellular ATP rapidly returned to control levels which was accompanied by renewed 2 LTR circle formation (Fig. 3). These results suggest an energy dependent mechanism for the transport of HIV-1 DNA to the nucleus to the host cell.

COMPOSITION AND NUCLEOPHILIC PROPERTIES OF THE PREINTEGRATION COMPLEX OF HIV-1

Studies in my laboratory focused on the development of protocols which allow isolation of viral preintegration complexes under conditions which preserve the biological activity of the complex and maintain association of its components. Development of these protocols has been essential since HIV-1 exhibits low particle/infectivity ratios (1 infectious particle per 10^3 to 10^4 virions [Kimpton and Emerman, 1992]) and viral preintegration complexes are present in very small quantities in actual infected cells. In addition , HIV-1 preintegration complexes have short biological half-lives and are very sensitive to detergent. Acutely infected cells are subject to hypotonic lysis followed by fractionation of high molecular weight preintegration complexes intensity gradients (Bukrinsky, et al., 1992, 1993a; Bowerman, et al., 1989). The presence of preintegration complexes within individual gradient fractions was confirmed by the presence of in vitro integration activity (Ellison, et al., 1990; Farnet and Haseltine, 1991). The association of viral proteins with the viral nucleic acids was confirmed by immunoprecipitation of viral proteins using monoclonal or poly-clonal antibodies to HIV-1 specific proteins followed by PCR amplification of viral DNA in immunoprecipitates. Using these approaches, my laboratory has provided evidence for the presence of HIV-1 gag matrix (Bukrinsky, et al., 1993a; Karageorgos, et al., 1993) and the accessory gene product Vpr (Heinzinger, et al., 1994) within preintegration complexes of HIV-1. To date there has been no direct evidence of the presence of HIV-1 gag capsid within

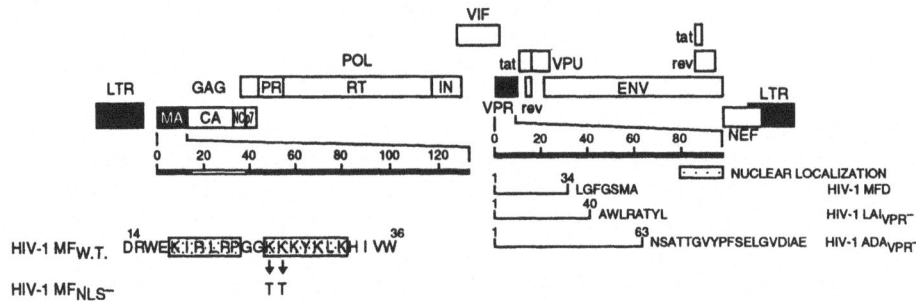

Figure 4. Outline of T cell tropic (MFD, LAI) and monocyte-tropic (ADA) HIV-1 clones which contain single and combined mutations in gag MA NLS and in Vpr. The gag MA NLS shown previously to facilitate nuclear import of viral preintegration complexes in non-dividing cells (Bukrinsky, et al., 1993b) was mutated by gag MA Lys 26, 27 Thr substitutions as described (Bukrinsky, et al., 1993b). The entire MA coding region of HIV-1 MF (Stevenson, et al., 1990) containing the wild type NLS or the double K to T NLS mutations was used to replace MA coding regions of HIV-1 LAI or HIV-1 ADA. Mutation of Vpr in HIV-1 LAI (Peden, et al., 1991) was created by a frame shift at codon 40 of Vpr while mutation of Vpr in HIV-1 ADA was created by a frame shift in codon 63 of Vpr. The putative nuclear localization sequence of Vpr resides in the terminal 17 amino acid of Vpr (Lu, et al., 1993).

preintegration complexes of HIV-1 (Bukrinsky, et al., 1993a; Darageorgos, et al., 1993) which has previously been demonstrated within preintegration complexes of MLV (Bowerman, et al., 1989). Studies from my laboratory now implicate an important role for gag matrix (MA) and Vpr in the nuclear import properties of preintegration complexes of HIV-1 (Bukrinsky, et al., 1993b; Heinzinger, et al., 1994). A series of HIV-1 variants containing mutations within a putative gag MA nuclear Localization signal (NLS) and/or truncations in the Vpr protein were constructed (Fig. 4). Mutations in gag MA were created so as to inactivate a consensus identified between amino acids 8 and 32 of MA while truncations in Vpr were designed to remove a putative NLS at the C terminus of Vpr (which has been reported to reside within the terminal 17 amino acids of Vpr [Lu, et al., 1993]). To examine virus replication in T cells, gag MA and Vpr mutations were introduced into a T cell adapted HIV-1 LAI variant (Peden, et al., 1991) for studies on phenotype in macrophages, these mutations were introduced into HIV-1 ADA, an infectious monocyte-tropic clone of HIV-1 (Westervelt, 1992). HIV-1 LAI virions containing single or combined gag MA NLA and Vpr mutations elicited a spreading infection in dividing CD4+ MT4 cells with kinetics indistinguishable from that of wild type HIV-1 (Fig. 5a). Since terminally differentiated macrophages are natural non-dividing cell targets of HIV-1 in vivo (Shaw, et al., 1985; Koenig, et al., 1986; Wiley, et al., 1986) we examined the phenotype of HIV-1 variants containing single and combined gag MA NLS and Vpr mutations in monocyte-derived macrophages. HIV-1 variants containing either a gag MA NLS mutation or lacking a functional Vpr exhibited an attenuated replication phenotype in monocyte-derived macrophages while a virus variant containing both gag MA NLS and Vpr mutations was greatly attenuated in its ability to elicit a spreading infection in these cells (Fig. 5b). The inefficient replication of combined gag MA NLS/Vpr mutants in macrophages was determined at the level of nuclear localization of viral DNA. Thus, viral DNA synthesis in cells infected with wild type single or combined MA/Vpr mutations was equivalent. However, when macrophages were analyzed for the presence of nuclear forms of viral DNA using primers to 1 LTR circle products (Heinzinger, et al., 1994) or 2 LTR circle products of viral DNA (unpublished), there was a paucity of circle forms of viral DNA in macrophages infected with the combined MA/Vpr mutants suggesting detect in nuclear localization. Since 1 and 2 LTR circle forms of viral DNA are

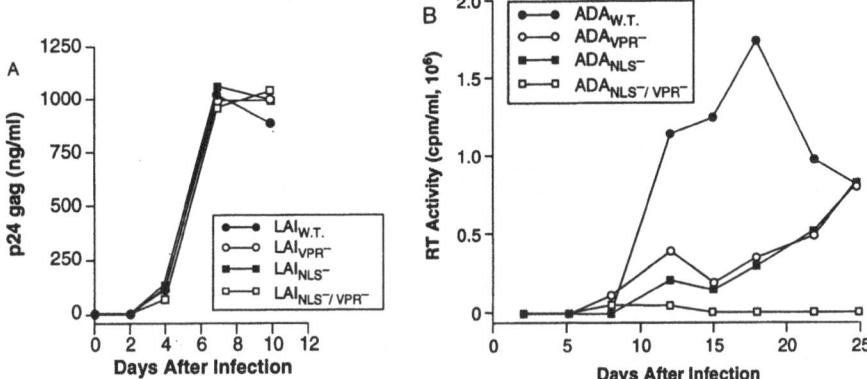

Figure 5. A. HIV-1 variants containing mutations in gag MA NLS and/or in Vpr elicit an efficient spreading infection in proliferating CD4+ MT4 cell cultures. Proliferating MT4 cells were infected with the indicated HIV variants (see Fig. 4) at a multiplicity of infection of 0.1 for 2 hours. Cell were washed twice and resuspended in fresh medium at 1.10^6/ml. Virus production in culture supernatants was determined at 2-3 day intervals by gag p24 ELISA. B. Replication of HIV-1 gag MA NLS and Vpr mutants in monocyte-derived macrophages. Monocytes were isolated by counter-current centrifugal elutriation of mononuclear leukocyte-rich cell preparations obtained from normal HIV-1 and Hepatitis B seronegative donors after leukapheresis. Monocytes were cultured as adherent monolayers in 96 well plates with medium containing 1,000 U/ml monocyte-colony stimulating factor. Macrophages were infected with the indicated HIV-1 variants 7 days after plating. Equal amounts of virus (based on RT activity and gag p24 content) were added to well for 3 hours then cultures were replaced with fresh medium. Reverse transcriptase activity in supernatants (averaged from triplicate wells) was measured at 2-3 day intervals. (Reproduced with permission from Bukrinsky, et al., 1993).

dead-end products of retrovirus replication (Brown, et al., 1987; Lobel, et al., 1989; Ellis and Bernstein, 1989) we confirmed the phenotype of MA/Vpr mutants in an integration dependent assay (Kimpton and Emerman, 1992) which specifically quantitates under single cycle conditions the degree of provirus establishment following HIV infection. On Fig. 6 the ratio of infected non-dividing (G2-arrested) cells to infected proliferating cells by wild type HIV-1 and HIV containing single and combined MA and Vpr mutations is shown. Wild type HIV was able to efficiently infect growth arrested cells which MuLV was unable to efficiently infect G2 arrested cells. The efficiency of infection of non-dividing cells for wild type HIV. In contrast, an HIV-1 variant containing combined MA and Vpr were similar to that observed for wild type HIV. In contrast, an HIV-1 variant containing combined MA and Vpr mutations exhibited a phenotype more representative of the onco-retrovirus MuLV. Taken together, these results indicate that nucleophilic functions associated with either HIV-1 gag MA or with Vpr are sufficient for nuclear localization of viral DNA in the absence of mitosis and for replication of HIV-1 non-dividing cells. As a consequence, mutations in both gag MA and Vpr nucleophilic functions greatly attenuates nuclear localization of viral DNA and replication of HIV-1 in non-dividing cells.

RESTRICTED HIV-1 REPLICATION IN G0 T LYMPHOCYTES

The macrophage represents a natural non-dividing target for HIV-1 infection and the metabolically active state of these cells supplies the energy requirements for the active nuclear import of HIV-1 preintegration complexes. In contrast, the other primary target for HIV infection, the T lymphocytes exists predominantly in a metabolically quiescent G0 state

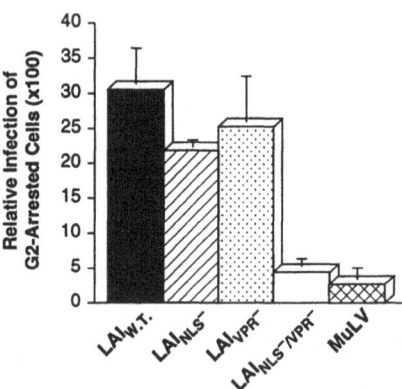

Figure 6. Relative infection of G2-arrested Hela CD4 cells by HIV-1 MA NLS and Vpr mutants. HeLa CD4-LTR/β-gal cells (Kimpton and Emerman, 1992) were arrested in G2 by γ–irradiation and establishment of the provirus was assayed by transactivation of an endogenous LTR-βgalactocidase (β-gal) gene as described previously (Lewis, et al., 1994). In this assay, the HeLa cells have been engineered to express high levels of CD4 and contain a single copy of the bacterial β-gal gene under transcriptional control of the HIV-1 LTR. Upon HIV-1 infection and integration, β-gal is visualized by staining cells in situ with X-gal (BRL). The relative infection of G2-arrested cells is the number of infected cells in the γ-irradiated (non-proliferating) culture divided by the number of infected cells in the proliferating culture from each viral infection. HIV strain designation of the individual clones is as detailed in Figure 4. (Reproduced with permission from Emerman, et al., 1994).

where cellular ATP levels are two logs lower than those observed in activated T cells (M. Stevenson, unpublished observations). Indeed, G0 T cells exhibit a very low density of active nuclear pores when compared with other terminally differentiated cell types (Maul, 1977). Transport of nucleophilic agents to the nuclear pore is energy independent while translocation across the nuclear envelope requires a high energy co-factor (Newmeyer and Forbes, 1988). Thus, as illustrated in Fig. 3 translocation of viral preintegration complexes across the nuclear envelope is rate limiting in G0 cells. In addition to the limited nuclear pore mediated import of HIV-1 DNA in Go T cells, provirus establishment is further limited by inefficient de novo reverse transcription due to low levels of ribonucleotide reductase which limit the nucleotide pool (Gao, et al., 1993) and inefficient elongation of viral DNA after the first template switch (Zack, et al., 1990, 1993). Nucleotide precursor pools have also been proposed to influence rates of reverse transcription following HIV infection of macrophages (O'Brien, et al., 1994; Collin and Gordon, 1994). Using different culture conditions we have observed that rates of viral DNA synthesis and replication following infection of macrophages parallel those observed following infection o activated T cells (Heinzinger, et al., 1994; Baca-Regen, et al., 1994; Heinzinger, et al., submitted). Taken together, it is apparent that the two main targets for HIV-1 infection (T cells and macrophages) provide very different environments for HIV-1 replication depending upon the cell cycle state of the host cell at the point of infection. These issues are summarized on Figure 7.

The restriction to HIV-1 replication in quiescent T lymphocytes can be overcome by subsequent activation of the infected cell (Zack, et al., 1988; Stevenson, et al., 1990) indicating that the extra chromosomal viral DNA within the nucleoprotein preintegration complex serves as a replication intermediate which can lead to provirus establishment when conditions for complete reverse transcription of viral DNA and nuclear import of viral DNA are provided. Clearly, however, T cell activation is an essential pre-requisite for the establishment of the provirus following infection by HIV. This has prompted the suggestion that T cell activation as elicited by exogenous antigen and immune stimulation in non-human

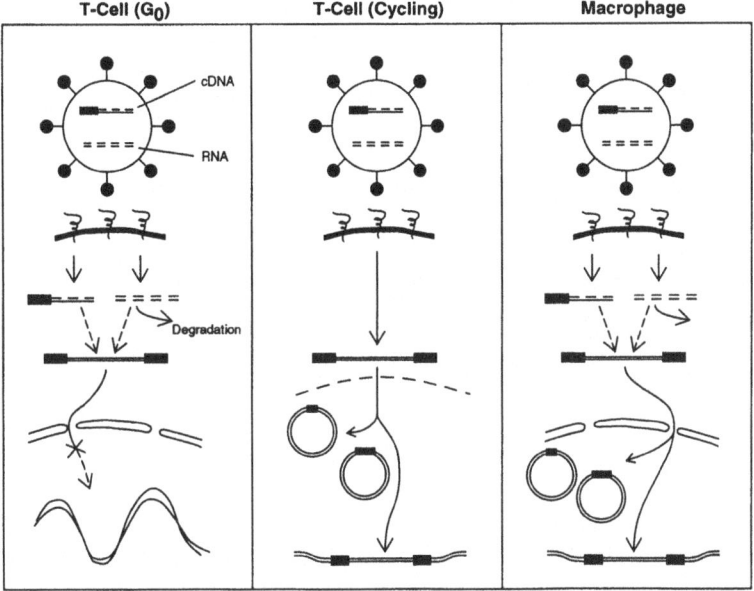

Figure 7. Levels of restriction to HIV-1 infection of non-proliferating host cells. Early events (preceding provirus establishment) in the life cycle of HIV-1 are diagramatically presented together with rate limiting steps that are encountered following infection of non-cycling cells. Following receptor binding and uncoating, viral DNA synthesis in quiescent T cells and macrophages appear inefficient compared to that observed in cycling T cells (Gao, et al., 1993; Zack, et al., 1990; Collin and Gordon, 1994). In some studies, rates of reverse transcription are reduced and as a consequence, incoming genomic viral RNA may be degraded in quiescent T cells (Gao, et al., 1993). In other systems strong stop cDNA synthesis appears unaffected both in G0 T cells and macrophages (O'Brien, et al., 1994). In contrast, quiescent T lymphocytes obtained from HIV-1 seropositive individuals appears to contain predominately full length viral DNA in an extra-chromosomal state (Bukrinsky, et al., 1991). It is possible that the labile nature of viral DNA synthesis in quiescent T cells is a reflection of the limited viability of G0 T cells in culture. Similarly, different systems used for the culture and maintenance of monocyte-derived macrophages may provide very different outcomes in terms of kinetics of viral DNA synthesis in virus spreading infection. Thus, other investigators have observed that viral DNA synthesis in macrophages proceeds at rates exceeding or equal to that observed in activated T cells (Baca-Regen, et al., 1994; Heinzinger, et al., 1994). Since G0 T cells and macrophages are non-dividing, viral nucleic acids must access the nuclear compartment through nuclear pores. This appears to be restricted in G0 T cells but in metabolically active macrophages, is facilitated by active transport mechanisms (Bukrinsky, et al., 1992; 1993b; Heinzinger, et al., 1994). As a consequence, nuclear localization of viral DNA and provirus establishment does not occur in quiescent T cells but is efficient in cycling T cells and monocyte-derived macrophages.

primate models supports the hypothesis that repeated stimulation of the immune system and activation of CD4+ lymphocytes may influence virus burden and progression in AIDS (Rosenberg and Fauci, 1989). A terminal relationship between antigen stimulation and changes in virus burden was demonstrated following exposure of HIV-1 infected chimpanzees to repeated stimulation by various vaccines preparations (Fultz, et al., 1992). Within one to two weeks post inoculation with Hepatitis B virus vaccine, infected PMCs as quantitated by serial endpoint dilution and co-cultivation had increased by over 20 fold and the acute viremic episode subsided after an additional three weeks. A similar dramatic rise in virus burden was observed following inoculation with an activated vaccine virus, Analysis of HIV-1 specified responses indicated that the increased virus burden was accompanied by an activation of the immune system (Fultz, et al., 1992).

Table 1. Increased HIV-1 burden following vaccination of HIV-1
seropositive individuals with Pneumoccal antigens

Time Post-vaccination (Weeks)	1-6	7-17
Fold Increase	x8.3	x6.7
Pneumoccal IgG	(n=7)	(n=6)
Fold Increase	x93.1	x37.8
HIV-1 Virions	(n=9)	(n=7)

Fold increase is calculated as the level of virions or
pneumococcal IgG 1-6 and 7-17 weeks post-vaccination
divided by the levels measured pre-vaccination. HIV-1
virions were quantitated by a modified QC-PCR (Piatak,
et al., 1993) analysis of virus associated genomic RNA.
Pneumococcus-specific IgG was determined by ELISA
(Janoff, et al., 1988).

Future support for the relationship between immune activation and immunopathogenic process was described for SIV infection in rhesus macaques (Popov, et al., 1992).
There is, as yet, a little evidence for a direct relationship between T cell activation and
changes in virus burden in HIV-1 seropositive individuals. Thus, we have attempted to
examine the influence of exogenous antigens (as introduced during vaccination with bacterial antigens) on virus burden. Due to the immunodeficient state, HIV-1 seropositive
individuals are at increased risk of disease such as pnuemococcal bacteremia (Redd, et al.,
1990) and, as a consequence, pneumococcal polysaccharide vaccine is recommended for
adults with asymptomatic or symptomatic HIV-1 infection. A series of asymptomatic HIV-1
seropositive individuals who currently were not on any anti-retroviral therapy were vaccinated with pnuemococcal polysaccharides (Pneumovax). Plasma from vaccinated individuals was collected prior to and at various intervals after vaccination. Extracellular virus
particles were examined in a quantitative competitive PCR (QC-PCR) method as outlined
previously (Piatak, et al., 1993) Pnuemococcus-specific-IgG was measured in order to
evaluate the immune response to the vaccine. Of nine individuals who were examined in
detail, increases in number of extra-cellular virions was observed by one week post
vaccination. Fold increases in HIV-1 virion number and IgG titters at 1-6 and 7-17 weeks
post vaccination are most pronounced in individuals who developed the highest pnuemococcal antigen specific IgG titters. In addition, the degree of virus activation correlated in
most cases with increases in the number of CD4+/CD25+ T lymphocytes following vaccination (B. Brichacek and M. Stevenson, in preparation). Collectively, these preliminary
studies implicate a direct relationship between immune activation and virus burden in HIV-1
seropositive individuals. There are several possible explanations for the increase in virus
burden observed following vaccination with pnuemococcal antigens. The increased number
of activated CD4+ cells following vaccination may provide new targets for de novo
productive infection by HIV-1. Alternatively, activation may reactivate extra-chromosomal
viral DNA residing within quiescent T cells thus leading to renewed virus replication. Studies
are underway to specifically address these issues.

SUMMARY

Research is beginning to yield insight into determinants which govern cell cycle
dependence of provirus establishment by the onco-retroviruses. In the case of HIV-1,

nucleophilic components associated with the viral preintegration complex facilitate mitosis independent nuclear localization of viral DNA and provirus establishment. Differences in the metabolic activity between G0 T cells and macrophages, the two primary targets for HIV-1 infection, lead to significantly different outcomes with regards to provirus establishment following infection of these cells. Thus, macrophages appear fully permissive to productive HIV-1 replication while non-dividing (G0 T cells) restrict virus replication at a step which proceeds nuclear import of viral DNA. The requirement for T cell activation in productive HIV-1 replication has important implications for the relationship between immune activation and virus burden. It remains to be determined whether modulating the immune activation status of the infected individual may provide an opportunity for modulating virus burden and influencing disease course.

REFERENCES

Beca-Regen L, Heinzinger N, Stevenson M, and Gendelman HE. Interferon-alpha induced antiretroviral activities: restriction of viral nuclear acid synthesis and progeny virion production in HIV-1-infected monocytes. J Virol (submitted).

Bowerman B, Brown PO, Bishop JM, and Varmus HE. A nucleoprotein complex mediates the integration of retroviral DNA. Genes Dev, 3:469-478, 1989.

Brown PO, Bowerman B, Varmus HE, and Bishop JM. Correct integration of retroviral DNA in vitro. Cell, 49:347-356, 1987.

Bukrinsky MI, Stanwick TL, Dempsey MP; and Stevenson M. Quiescent T lymphocytes as an inducble virus reservoir in HIV-1 infection. Science, 254:423-427, 1991.

Bukrinsky MI, Sharova N, Dempsey MP, Stanwick TL, and Bukrinskaya AG, Haggerty S, and Stevenson M. Active nuclear import of human immunododeficiency virus type 1 preintegration complexes. Proc Natl Acad Sci USA, 89:6580-6584, 1992.

Bukrinsky MI, Sharova N, McDonald TL, Puohkarakaya T, Tarpley WG, and Stevenson. Association of integase, matrix, and reverse transcriptase antigens of human immunodeficiency virus type 1 with viral nucleic acids following acute infection. Proc Natl Acad Sci USA, 90:6125-6129, 1993a.

Bukrinsky M, Haggerty S, Dempsey MP, Sharova N, Adzhubei A, Spitz L, Lewis P, Goldfarb D, Emerman M, and Stevenson M. A nuclear localization signal within HIV-1 matrix protein that governs infection of non-dividing cells. Nature, 365:666-669, 1993b.

Collin M, and Gordon S. The kinetics of human immunodeficiency virus reverse transcription are slower in primary human macrophages than in a lymphoid cell line. Virology, 200:114-120, 1994.

Dingwall C, and Laskey R. The nuclear membrane. Science, 258:942-947, 19992.

Ellis J, and Bernstein A. Retrovirus vectors containing an internal attachment site: evidence that circles are not intermediates to murine retrovirus integration. J Virol, 63:2844-2846, 1989.

Ellison V, Abrams H, Roe T, Lifson J, and Brown P. Human immunodeficiency virus integration in a cell-free system. J Virol, 64:2711-2715, 1990.

Emerman M, Bukrinsky MI, and Stevenson M. HIV-1 infection of non-dividing cells. (letter) Nature, 369:108, 1994.

Farnet CM, and Hasetine WA. Determination of viral proteins present in the human immunodeficiency virus type 1 preintegration complex. J Virol, 65:1910-1915, 1991.

Fultz PN, Gluckman JC, Muchmore E, and Girard M. Transient increased in numbers of infectious cells in an HIV-infected chimpanzee following immune stimulation. AIDS Res Human Retrov, 8:313-317, 1992.

Gao W, Cara A, Gallo RC, and Lori F. Low levels of deoxynucleotides in peripheral blood lymphocytes: a strategy to inhibit human immunodeficiency virus type 1 replication. Proc Natl Acad Sci USA, 90:8925-8928, 1993.

Gartner S, Markovits P, Markovitz DM, Kaplan MH, Gallo RC, and Popvic M. The role of mononuclear phagocytes in HTLV-III/LAV infection. Science, 233:215-219, 1986.

Heinzinger NK, Bukrinsky MI, Haggerty SA, Ragland AM, Kelwalranami V, Lee MA, Gendelman HE, Ratner L, Stevenson M, and Emerman M. The Vpr protein of HIV-1 influences nuclear localization of viral nucleic acids in non-dividing host cells. Proc Natl Acad Sci USA (in press).

Janoff EN, Douglas JM, Gabriel M, Blaser MJ, Davidson AJ, Kohn DL, and Judson FN. Class-specific antibody response to pneumococcal capsular polysaccharide in men infected with immunodeficiency virus type 1. J Infect Dis, 158:983-990, 1988.

Karageorgos L, Li P, and Burrell C. Characterization of HIV replication complexes early after cell-to-cell infection. AIDS Res Human Retroviruses, 9:817-823, 1993.

Kimpton J, and Emerman M. Detection of replication-competent and pseudotyped human immunodeficiency virus with a sensitive cell line on the basis of activation of an integrated B-galactosidase gene. J Virol, 66:2232-2239, 1992.

Knight SC, and Patterson S. Effect of human immunodeficiency virus on dendritic cells isolated from human peripheral blood. In: Proceedings of Tenth Histocompatibility Workshop, B DuPont (ed.), Springer Verlag, New York, 1990:p378.

Koenig S, Gendelman HE, Orenstein JM, DalCanto MC, Pezeshkpour GH, Yungbluth M, Janotta F, Aksamit A, Martin MA, and Fauci AS. Detection of AIDS virus in macrophages in brain tissue from AIDS patients with encephalopathy. Science, 233:1089-1093, 1986.

Koyanagi Y, O'Brien WA, Zhao JQ, Golde DW, Gasson JC, and IS-Y C. Cytokines after production of HIV-1 from primary mononuclear phagocytes. Science, 241:1673-1675, 1988.

Langhoff E, Terwilliger EF, Bos HJ, Kalland KH, Poznansky MC, Bacon OML, and Haseltine WA. Replication of human immunodeficiency virus type 1 in primary dendritic cell cultures. Proc Natl Acad Sci USA, 88:7998-8002, 1991.

Lewis P, Hensel M, and Emerman M. Human immunodeficiency virus infection of cells arrested in the cell cycle. EMBO J, 11:3053-3058, 1992.

Lewis P, Hensel M. Passage through mitosis is required for oncoretroviruses but not for the human immunodeficiency virus. J Virol, 68:510-516, 1994.

Lobel LI, Murphy JE, and Goff SP. The palindromic LTR-LTR junction of Moloney murine leukemia virus is not an effecient substrate for proviral integration. J Virol, 63:2629-2637, 1989.

Lu YL. Human immunodeficiency virus type 1 viral protein R localization in infected cells and virions. J Virol, 67:6542-6550, 1993.

Maul GG. The nuclear and the cytoplasmic proe complex: Structure, dynamics, distribution and evolution. International Review Cytology Supplement, 6:75-187, 1977.

McDougal JS, Mawle A, Cort SP, Nicholson JKA, Cross GD. Scheppler-Campbell JA, Hicks D, and Sligh J. Cellular tropism of the human retrovirus HTLV-III/LAV I. Role of T cell activation and expression of the T4 antigen. J Immunol, 135:3151-3162, 1985.

Miller DG, Adam MA, and Miller AD. Gene transfer by retrovirus vectors occurs only in cells that are actively replicating at the time of infection. Mol Cell Biol, 10;4239-4242, 1990.

Newmeyer DD, and Forbes DJ. Nuclear import can be separated into distinct steps in vitro: Nuclear pore binding and translocation. Cell, 52:642-653, 1988.

Nicholson JKA, Cross GD, Gallaway CS, and McDougal JS. In vitro infection of human monocytes with human T lymphotropic virus type III/lymphadenopathy-associated virus (HTLV-III/LAV). J Immunol, 137:323-329, 1986.

O'Brien WA, Namazi A, Kalhor H, Mae SH, Zack JA, and Chen IS. Kinetics of human immunodeficiency virus type 1 reverse transcription in blood mononuclear phagocytes are slowed by limitations of nucleotide precursors. J Virol, 68:1258-1263, 1994.

Peden K, Emerman M, and Montagnier L. Changes in growth properties on passage in tissue culture of viruses derived from infectious molecular clones of HIV-1 LAI, HIV-1 MAL, and HIV-1 EL1. Virology, 185:661-672, 1991.

Pedrali-Noy G, Spadari S, Miller-Faures A, Miller AO, Kruppa J, and Koch G. Synchronization of HeLa cell cultures by inhibition of DNA polymerase with aphidicolin. Nuc Acids Res, 8:377-387, 1980.

Piatak M, Saag MS, Yang LC, Clark SJ, Kappes JC, Luk KC, Hahn BH, Shaw GM, and Lifson JD. Hugh levels of HIV-1 in plasma during all stages of infection determined by competitive PCR. Science, 259:1749-1754, 1993.

Popv J, McGrw T, Hofmann B, Vowels B, Shum A, Nishanian P, and Fahey JL. Acute lymphoid changes and ongoing immune activation in SIV infection. J AIDS, 5:391-399, 1992.

Redd SC, Rutherford GW, Sanda MA, Lithson AR, Hadley WK, Facklam RR, and Spika JS. The role of human immunodeficiency virus infection in pneumococcal bacteremia in San Francisco residents. J Infect Dis, 162:1012-1017, 1990.

Richardson WD, Mills AD, Dilworth SM, Laskey RA, and Dingwall C. Nuclear protein migration involves two steps: Rapid binding at the nuclear envelope followed by slower translocation through nuclear pores. Cell, 52:655-664, 1988.

Roe T, Reynolds TC, Yu G, and Brown PO. Integration of murine leukemia virus DNA depends on mitosis. EMBO J, 12:2099-2108, 1993.

Rosenberg ZF, and Fauci AS. The immunophathogenesis of HIV infection. Adv Immunol, 47:377-431, 1989.

Shaw GM, Harper ME, Hahn BH, Epstein LG, Gajdusek DC, Price RW, Navia BA, Petito CD, O'Hara CJ, Groopman JE, Cho ES, Oleske JM, Wong-Staal F, and Gallo RC. HTLV-III infection in brains of children and adults with AIDS encephalopathy. Science, 227:177-182, 1985.

Springett GM, Moen RC, Anderson S, Blaese RM, and Anderson WF. Infection efficiency of T lymphocytes with amphotropic retroviral vectors is cell cycle dependent. J Virol, 63:3865-3869, 1989.

Stevenson M, Haggerty S, Lamonica C, Mann AM, Meier C, and Wasiak A. Cloning and characterization of human immunodeficiency virus type 1 variants diminished in the ability to induce syncytium-independent cytolysis. J Virol, 64:3792-3803, 1990.

Temin HM, Mechanisms of cell killing/cytopathic effects by nonhuman retroviruses. Rev Infect Dis, 10:399-405, 1988.

Varmus H and Brown P. Retroviruses. In: Mobile DNA, DE Berg and MM Howe (Eds), American Society for Microbiology, Washington, DC, 1989:p53-108.

Watkins BA, Dorn HH, Kelly WB, Armstrong RC, Potts BJ, Michaels F, Kufta CV, and Dubois-Dalcq M. Specific tropism of HIV-1 for microglial cells in primary human brain cultures. Science, 249:549-553, 1990.

Weinberg JB, Mathews TJ, Cullen BR, and Malim MH. Productive human immunodeficiency virus type 1 (HIV-1) infection of nonproliferating human monocytes. J Exp Med, 174, 1477-1482, 1991.

Westervelt P, Trowbridge DB, Epstein LG, Blumberg BM, Li Y, Hahn BH, Shaw GM, Price RW, and Ratner L. Macrophage tropism determinants of human immunodeficiency virus type 1 in vivo. J Virol, 66:2577-2582, 1992.

Wiley CA, Schrier RD, Nelson JA, Lampert PW, and Oldstone MBA. Cellular localization of human immunodeficiency virus infection within the brains of acquired immune deficiency syndrome patients. Proc Natl Acad Sci USA, 83:7089-7093, 1986.

Zack JA, Cann AJ, Lugo JP, and Chen ISY. HIV-1 production from infected peripheral blood T cells after HTLV-1 induced mitogenic stimulation. Science, 240:1026-1029, 1988.

Zack JA, Arrigo SJ, Weitsman SR, Go AS, Haislip A, and Chen ISY. HIV-1 entry into quiescent primary lymphocytes: molecular analysis reveals a labile, latent viral structure. Cell, 61:213-222, 1990.

Zack JA, Arrigo SJ, and Chen ISY. Control of expression and cell tropism of human immunodeficiency virus type 1. Adv Vir Res, 38:125-146, 1993.

Zagury D, Bernard J, Leonard R, Cheynier R, Feldman M, Sarin PS, and Gallo RC. Long term cultures of HTLV-III-infected T cells: a model of cyopathology of T-cell depletion in AIDS. Science, 231:850-853, 1986.

5

REGULATION OF MACROPHAGE ACTIVATION AND HIV REPLICATION

Luis J. Montaner,[1] Georges Herbein,[2] and Siamon Gordon[1]

[1] Sir William Dunn School of Pathology
University of Oxford
South Parks Road
Oxford, United Kingdom
[2] Institute of Virology and INSERM U74
Louis Pasteur University
Strasbourg, France

INTRODUCTION

Defining Macrophage Activation

In normal immune responses, macrophages play a key role in the host's defence system combating disease, clearing foreign antigens and protecting against invading microrganisms. The ability of the macrophage (mø) to mediate effective immune responses is associated with its capacity to respond and control its activation upon encountering the appropriate exogenous or endogenous signal. Activation is defined by the stimulus which changes or predisposes to changes in cellular activity, while activation potential is the ability to undergo activation. Since immune activation involves all aspects of immunological responses, we will differentiate between two general types of cytokine-orientated activation when discussing macrophages: pro-inflammatory and immuno-regulatory. Pro-inflammatory activation refers to the state of immunological "alarm" mediated by TNF-α, IL-1β, IL-6 and chemokines, while immuno-regulatory activation refers to responses mediated by IFNs, IL-2, IL-4, IL-10, IL-12, and IL-13. Although discussed separately, these types of activation are not mutually exclusive and seldom occur in isolation.

Macrophages in AIDS: Regulation of HIV

Peripheral blood monocytes/macrophages as well as resident macrophages are susceptible to human immunodeficiency virus (HIV) infection, and their roles during AIDS pathogenesis in immune function and viral spread have been well established [1-4]. Primary infection is correlated with mø-tropic isolates which are maintained in all stages of disease, and HIV-1 causes mø dysfunction (see below). Understanding mø immunological responsiveness (activation potential) after HIV infection and the influencing factors that regulate

Cell Activation and Apoptosis in HIV Infection
Edited by Jean-Marie Andrieu and Wei Lu, Plenum Press, New York, 1995

Table 1. Cytokine and chemokine regulation of HIV growth in acutely
infected primary macrophages. Summary of results observed by
our laboratory, with original references (untested or results different from
thoseobtained by us are shown in parenthesis)

Cytokine	HIV Replication	Reference
TNF-α	↑	5
IL-1β	↑	6
IL-2	↔	Montaner LJ**
IL-3	(↑)	7
IL-4	↓ (↑)	8
IL-7	↑	Montaner LJ**
IL-10	↓	9, 10
IL-12	(↔)	11
IL-13	↓	12
INF-α/β	↓	13
INF-γ	↓(↑)	7
M-CSF	↑	7
GM-CSF	↑	7
RANTES	↔	Herbein G**
MCP-1/3	↔	Herbein G**
MIP-1α	↔	Herbein G**

**unpublished observations

their function is important in characterising the role of infected macrophages in the resulting
virus-induced immune collapse. In addition to infected macrophages' role as immune
effector cells, their responses or dysfunctions must be correlated with their ability to produce
virus. Among known factors that influence mø activation and function are cytokines, which
in addition to being in a state of dysregulation in AIDS, also regulate viral replication in
macrophages (Table 1). Therefore we will review the effect of immune dysregulation by HIV
on the activation potential of macrophages as well as its consequences for HIV infection and
pathogenesis.

PRO-INFLAMMATORY ACTIVATION

Macrophages Fuel a State of Chronic Activation

Normal responses to foreign antigens include an immune activation mediated by
cytokines, such as TNF-α , IL-1β, IL-6, and chemokines, which trigger the immune system
into appropiate action. An effective control of this activation upon achieving immunity to
the antigen is necessary for the renewal of immune function upon re-exposure to new foreign
antigens. AIDS pathogenesis is characterized by a lack of control of immune activation and
a resulting chronically activated state facilitating viral replication in T-cells and increasingly
reducing the host's immunocompetence[14]. Markers of this chronic activation in infected
patients include spontaneous lymphocyte proliferation, lymph node hyperplasia and elevated
serum levels of activation markers (TNF-α, IL-1β, neopterin, β_2–microglobulin, acid-labile
interferon and interleukin-2 receptors).

Table 2. HIV-induced cytokine dysregulation in primary macrophages

		Reference
Gp120 binding studies		
↑	TNF-α, IL-1β	16, 21
↑	INF-β	22
↑	PGE$_2$ and Arachidonic acid metabolites	23
↑	Endothelin-1	24
Productive infection studies		
↑	TNF-α, IL-1β,	15, 25
↑	TNF-α, IL-1β, PGE$_2$	26
↑	INF-α	27
↑	acid labile INF-α	28
↑	INF-β	22
↔	IL-10	11
↓	IL-12	11
↑	MIP-1α (Alveolar mø)	29
↑	GM-CSF (Alveolar mø)	30

Macrophages contribute to immune activation by producing TNF-α and IL-1β upon binding of free (shed) or virion-associated gp120 to mø CD4. This activation occurs irrespective of preferential viral tropism or productive infection [15, 16]. In studying the effects of HIV on production of cytokines by macrophages, both the binding of free gp120 and productive infection have been used to analyse virus-induced changes (Table 2). Therefore, the gp120-induced secretion of pro-inflammatory cytokines results in a positive feedback mechanism for both the continued maintenance of immune activation and virus production [17]. Even though both TNF-α and IL-1β have been shown to upregulate viral replication through an HIV-1 transcriptional activation *via* NF-kβ, only TNF-α decreases LTR proviral synthesis in primary macrophages [18]. The decrease of LTR proviral synthesis has been correlated with a down-modulation of surface CD4[+] by TNF-α although other mechanisms may also be involved. This initial activity upon viral entry by TNF-α suggests a mø-mediated mechanism against superinfection since TNF-α production would be triggered upon gp120 binding, in addition to the described HIV*nef* -induced downregulation of CD4 in lymphocytes. Furthermore, this observation might further explain the decrease of surface CD4[+] expressed on circulating monocytes isolated in AIDS patients with high TNF serum levels[19, 20].

Non-immune Interferons Present but Ineffective

INF-α and IFN-β are also secreted by macrophages upon encountering virus, which have described anti-viral effects[22, 27]. Even though they have both been described to be anti-viral, the ability of virus to productively infect macrophages in vitro shows the ultimate ineffectiveness of the response. Likewise, infection *in vivo* appears to occur in spite of interferons due to the continued viral replication throughout disease and the marked increase of viral load upon end-stage disease. Possible mechanisms by which the virus evades the INF sytem have been reviewed by Lau &William, 1990[31]. However, interferons might play a role in controlling viremia through the asymptomatic stages of AIDS. Symptomatic AIDS is also correlated with an increase of acid-labile INF-α [32, 33]. Although the cell types producing this unusual interferon are still undetermined (it has not been isolated and characterized), there is a report of infected macrophages being able to produce such INF [28].

If confirmed, this would reinforce the notion of a chronically activated mø unable to control viral replication and spread because of ineffective dysregulated mø responses.

Macrophage -induced Activation and Immunosuppresion

Even though a chronic increase of pro-inflammatory cytokines and ineffective interferon responses would indicate a direct mechanism for immune dysfunction in AIDS, infected macrophages secrete higher levels of prostaglandin E_2 (PGE_2) and arachidonic acid metabolites [23]. These products are immunosuppressive. PGE_2 suppresses *in vitro* immune functions of T, B, and NK cells, tumor-cytotoxicity and phagocytosis by macrophages[34]. This mechanism is further supported by a report of decreased cytotoxicity in AIDS patients' infected macrophages in the presence of TNF-α mediated by PGE_2 [35]. In this report the impaired cytotoxicity was partly reversed by a cyclo-oxygenase blocker, indomethacin.

Other mø-mediated immunosuppressive mechanisms include a decrease in IL-12 production [11]. Macrophage IL-12 production has recently been characterized as an important phagocyte product linking natural resistance to adaptive immunity [36, 37]. The consequence of decreased levels of IL-12 would indicate a mø-mediated decrease of T helper cells type I (Th1) responses which are the host's primary mechanism in controlling intracellular pathogens such as HIV.

Impaired Macrophage Activation and Function

The outcome of mø activation upon encountering a foreign antigen or micro-organism, includes cytotoxic mechanisms of cell to cell killing (cytotoxicity) and intracellular clearance (phagocytosis). Alternatively, classical mø activation by the stimulus of T-cell derived INF-γ would increase the activation potential and secretion of IL-12 and TNF-α by macrophages which would act as a positive feedback in augmenting concurrent cell-mediated responses as discussed above.

Following phagocytosis, two mechanisms of intracellular attack can be triggered, an oxygen-dependent (oxidative burst, nitric oxide) and an oxygen-independent (pH, lysosomal enzymes, etc.) pathway [38]. The effects on these mechanisms in infected macrophages have been studied and are summarised in Table 3. Mechanisms mediating these functional effects include the cytokine and PGE_2 dysregulation discussed above. The consequence to the host of having non-functional macrophages is a lack of effective control of opportunistic infections and mø-mediated secondary immune responses due to a decrease in antigen presenting capacity. Therefore, the mø contributes directly to the immunopathology of AIDS by its impaired and ineffective activation potential after HIV infection.

Resident Macrophages as Reservoir of Virus and Macrophage Dysregulation

The body has various resident mø populations in all tissues forming part of the reticuloendothelial system (Brain: microglial cells, Connective tissue: histiocytes, Lung: alveolar macrophages, Liver: Kupffer cells, Kidney: interstitial cells, Lymph node: subcapsular/sinusoidal macrophages, Spleen: marginal zone, red and white pulp macrophages, Bone Marrow: stromal macrophages and promonocytes, Serosa: i.e., peritoneal macrophages, etc.). Concerning HIV-1, the resident populations most widely studied are those in the lung, liver, and brain. Although these are not the only systems in which the mø may contribute to viral replication and pathology they exemplify the active role of mø within tissues in AIDS pathogenesis.

Table 3. HIV-induced phenotypic and functional changes in primary macrophages

		Reference
Gp120 binding studies		
↑	Nitric Oxide (NO)**	39
↓	Chemotaxis and chemotactic receptors	23
↓	Accessory cell function	40
↓	Phagocytosis	41
↓	Anti-fungal (Cryptococcus) activity	42
↓	CD4, Fc receptors (I/II)	40
Productive infection studies		
↔	Oxidative Burst (Macrophages infected *in vitro*)	43
↓	Oxidative Burst (Macrophages infected *in vivo*)	44
↓	Chemotaxis and chemotactic receptors	23
↓	Tumoricidal activity	35
↓	Phagocytosis (opsonized & nonopsonized)	45, 46
↓	Phagocytic degradation	45
↓	Anti-fungal (Aspergillus) activity	46
↓	Anti-fungal (Candida) activity	47
↓	ADCC activity	47
↓	Fc (I/II/III), CR3 receptors	48

** NO presence in human macrophages is presently an area of controversy.[49]

Alveolar Macrophages (Lung). The lung is a site of an alveolar mø population whose activation potential is continually involved in controlling responses to incoming foreign antigens. In AIDS, alveolar macrophages are immunocompromised due to the chronic activation and functional impairment discussed above, resulting in uncontrolled pulmonary infections by opportunistic pathogens such as *Pneumocystis carinii* and fungal infections such as *Cryptococcus neoformans* commonly seen in AIDS patients[50]. The high viral load within alveolar macrophages compared with blood monocytes [51] suggests that the lung contains a viral reservoir of infected macrophages. Two possible mechanisms to explain this preferential site of mø infection are increased chemokine and GM-CSF production by infected alveolar macrophages[29,30]. Chemokine secretion which recruits both monocytes and T-cell subtypes [52, 53] to inflammatory sites is likely to be increased in lung tissue due to increased MIP-1α secretion by infected alveolar macrophages. This effect suggests a higher propensity for uninfected mø recruitment into virus producing areas, probably mediated to some extent by TNF-α and IL-1β action in inducing chemokines such as MCP-1 in primary macrophages[54]. In contrast to TNF-α and IL-1β, chemokines (MCP-1, MCP-3, RANTES, MIP-1α) do not directly affect HIV replication in primary macrophages although increased recruitment could allow for successful infection of T-cells and macrophages. Another characteristic special to infected alveolar macrophages is increased levels of GM-CSF secretion which would support both mø proliferation and virus replication [30]. Both of these effects would contribute to the immunopathogenesis of lung disease and the systemic pro-inflammatory cytokine dysregulation maintaining chronic activation and immune dysfunction.

Kupffer Cells (Liver). While the alveolar macrophages are instrumental in controlling incoming airborne stimuli, the Kupffer cells are the first resident clearance mechanism for incoming stimuli from the intestines except those entering intestinal lymphatics which go to mesenteric lymph nodes. Therefore, Kupffer cell immune dysfunction might render the host susceptible to infections cleared by the Liver. Kupffer cell dysfunction is probable since Kupffer cell pathology has been described in AIDS and these cells have been shown to be latently infected in vivo[55], as well as infectable in vitro [56]

Microglia (CNS). Infiltration of monocyte/macrophages in the brain and subsequent formation of multinucleated cells are characteristic features of neurological HIV disease[3]. In addition to the same effects described above regarding increased TNF-α and IL-1β secretion by infected CNS macrophages[15, 57], increased secretion of endothelins by macrophages after gp120 stimulus has been recently reported [24]. Endothelins, which are strongly positive in AIDS patients' cerebral macrophages, are potent vasoconstrictive peptides which act to maintain smooth muscle contraction. This activity suggests an additional mø activation response in the CNS involved in mediating the cerebral perfusion patterns associated with the AIDS dementia complex.

IMMUNOREGULATORY ACTIVATION

Th1/Th2 Activation

Cytokines have been broadly divided into those supporting cell-mediated responses (IL-2, INFγ, IL-12) and those supporting humoral responses (IL-4, IL-10, IL-13) [36, 58, 59], both of which take place in the context of pro-inflammatory-type cytokines (TNF-α, IL-1β, IL-6) among others. Even though impaired cell-mediated responses are common to AIDS pathogenesis, there are two schools of thought concerning the mechanism mediating this immunopathology:

1. Cell-mediated responses are impaired due to a chronic activation and exhaustion of the immune system leading to decreases in INFγ, IL-2, and IL-12 while increasing TNF-α, IL-1β and IL-6 levels[14].
2. Cell-mediated responses are negatively regulated due to a continued increase of Th-2 type cytokines[60].

Both theories probably have some applicability to AIDS pathogenesis, and both involve an impairment of mø (and T, B, and NK-cell) activation potentials. Recently, evidence supporting the first mechanism has emerged, even though Th2 cytokines are still considered central to T-cell viral replication and immune dysfunction[61, 62].

Immunoregulatory Activation and Macrophage Viral Load

Whereas T-cell activation results in productive infection and enhanced viral production, mø activation does not increase viral replication[65] (Table 4). Both Th1 and Th2-type cytokines control viral replication in macrophages (see Table 1). Therefore, an activated infected mø may not be a target to depletion mechanisms by cytotoxic T cells, NK cells or ADCC mechanisms as are infected T-cells[66-68]. The implications of this difference are a maintained population of activated infected macrophages at either end of the immunoregulatory spectrum which are not induced to produce virus and perhaps supporting the Trojan Horse hypothesis for macrophages in AIDS pathogenesis[3]. Furthermore, infected macrophages stimulated by both LPS or zymozan phagocytosis decrease viral production upon activation[13,69]. However, the concurrent increases of pro-inflammatory cytokines provides

Table 4. Immunoregulatory states of mø activation**

	Interferon-γ Classical	IL-4, IL-13 Alternative	IL-10 Deactivation
MCHII	↑	↑	↓
Antigen presentation	↑	↑	↓
Nitric Oxide	↑	↓	↓
Oxidative Burst	↑	↔	↓
TNF-α, IL-1β, IL-6 induction	↑	↓	↓
Mannose Receptor	↓	↑	↑
HIV replication	↓	↓	↓

**based on discussion by[63,64] dealing mainly with primary murine macrophages.

a competing signal for increase viral production which makes it difficult to characterize broadly the viral replicative consequence of a polarized immunoregulation if present at end-stage disease. More likely, the production of virus in macrophages is determined by both the overall balance after summation of all regulatory signals and the particular cellular site of regulation (i.e., lung. CNS, blood, etc.).

REFERENCES

1. Gartner S, Markovits P, Markovitz DM, et al. The role of mononuclear phagocytes in HTLV III/LAV infection. *Science*. 1986; 233; 215-219.
2. Gendelman HE, Orenstein JM, Martin MA, et al. Efficient isolation and propagation of human immunodeficiency virus on recombinant colony-stimulating factor 1-treated monocytes. *J. Exp. Med.* 1988; 167; 1428-1441.
3. Gendelman HE, Orenstein JM, Baca LM, et al. The macrophage in the persistence and pathogenesis of HIV infection. *AIDS*. 1989; 475-495.
4. Schuitemaker H, Kootstra NA, de Goede REY, et al. Monocytotropic human immunodeficiency virus type 1 (HIV-1) variants detectable at all stages of HIV-1 infection lack T-cell line tropism and syncytium-inducing ability in primary T cell culture. *J. Virol.* 1991; 65; 356-363.
5. Poli G, Bressler P, Kinter A, et al. Interleukin-6 induces human immunodeficiency virus expression in infected monocytic cells alone and in synergy with tumor necrosis factor α by transcriptional and post-transcriptional mechanisms. *J. Exp. Med.* 1990; 172; 151-158.
6. von Briessen H, von Mallinckrodt C, Esser R, et al. Effects of cytokines and lipopolysaccharides on HIV infection of human macrophages. *Res. Virol.* 1991; 142; 197-204.
7. Koyanagi Y, O'Brien WA, Qi Zhao J, et al. Cytokines alter production of HIV-1 from primary mononuclear phagocytes. *Science*. 1988; 241; 1673-1675.
8. Kazazi F, Mathijs JM, Chang J, et al. Recombinant interleukin 4 stimulates human immunodeficiency virus production by infected monocytes and macrophages. *J. Gen. Virol.* 1992; 73; 941-949.
9. Montaner LJ, Griffin P , Gordon S. Interleukin-10 (IL-10) inhibits initial reverse transcription of HIV-1 and mediates a virostatic latent state in primary blood-derived human macrophages in vitro. *J. Gen. Virol.* 1994; In press.
10. Saville MW, Paga K, Foli A, et al. Interlukin-10 suppresses human immunodeficiency virus-1 replication in vitro in cells of the monocyte/macrophage lineage. *Blood*. 1994; 83; 3591-3599.
11. Chehimi J, Starr SE, Frank I, et al. Impaired interleukin 12 production in human immunodeficiency virus-infected patients. *J. Exp. Med.* 1994; 179; 1361-1366.
12. Montaner LJ, Doyle AG, Collin M, et al. Interleukin 13 inhibits human immunodeficiency virus type 1 production in primary blood-derived human macrophages in vitro. *J. Exp. Med.* 1993; 178; 743-747.
13. Kornbluth RS, Oh PS, Munis JR, et al. Interferons and bacterial liposaccharide protect macrophages from productive infection by human immunodeficiency virus in vitro. *J. Exp. Med.* 1989; 169; 1137-1151.

14. Fauci AS. Multifactorial nature of human immunodeficiency virus disease: implications for therapy. *Science.* 1993; 262; 1011-1018.

15. Merrill JE, Koyanagi Y, Zack J, et al. Induction of interleukin-1 and tumor necrosis factor alpha in brain cultures by human ummunodeficiency virus type 1. *J. Virol.* 1992; 66; 2217-2225.

16. Herbein G, Keshav S, Collin M, et al. HIV-1 induces tumour necrosis factor and IL-1 gene expression in primary human macrophages independent of productive infection. *Clin. Exp. Immunol.* 1994; 95; 442-449.

17. Vyakarnam A, McKeating J, Meager A, Beverly PC. Tumour necrosis factors (alpha, beta) induced by HIV-1 in peripheral blood mononuclear cells potentiate virus replication. *AIDS.* 1990; 4; 21-27.

18. Herbein G, Montaner LJ, Gordon S. Tumor necrosis factor displays a bifunctional action on HIV-1 replication in human primary macrophages. *"MRC AIDS Workshop".* 1994; Manchester, UK; Abstr. 26.

19. Rieder P, Riethmuller G. Loss of circulating T4+ monocytes in patients infected with HTLV-III. *Lancet.* 1986; 270.

20. Lahdevirta J, Maury CPJ, Teppo AM, Repo H. Elevated levels of circulating cachectin/tumor necrosis factor in patients with acquired immunodeficiency syndrome. *Am. J. Med.* 1988; 85; 289-291.

21. Merrill JE, Koyanagi Y, Chen ISY. Interleukin-1 and tumor necrosis factor alpha can be induced from mononuclear phagocytes by human immunodeficiency virus type 1 to the CD4 receptor. *J. Virol.* 1989; 63; 4404-4408.

22. Gessani S, Puddu P, Varano B, et al. Induction of beta interferon by human immunodeficiency virus type 1 and its gp-120 protein in human monocytes-macrophages. Role of beta interferon in the restriction of virus replication. *J. Virol.* 1994; 68; 1983-1986.

23. Wahl SM, Allen JB, Gartner S, et al. HIV-1 and its envelope glycoprotein down-regulate chemotactic ligand receptors and chemotactic function of peripheral blood monocytes. *J. Immunol.* 1989; 142; 3553-3559.

24. Ehrenreich H, Rieckmann P, Sinowatz F, et al. Potent stimulation of monocytic endothelin-1 production by HIV-1 glycoprotein 120. *J. Immunol.* 1993; 150; 4601-4609.

25. Lathey JL, Kanangat S, Rouse BT. Differential expression of tumor necrosis factor α and interleukin 1β compared with interleukin 6 in monocytes from human immunodeficiency virus-positive individuals measured by polymerase chain reaction. *AIDS.* 1994; 7; 109-115.

26. Longo N, Zabay JM, Sempere JM, et al. Altered production of PGE-2, IL-1β and TNF-α by peripheral blood monocytes from HIV-positive individuals at early stages of HIV infection. *AIDS.* 1993; 6; 1017-1023.

27. Francis ML, Meltzer MS. Induction of IFN-α by HIV-1 in monocyte-enriched PBMC requires gp120-CD4 interaction but not virus replication. *J. Immunol.* 1993; 151; 2208-2216.

28. Szebeni J, Dieffenbatch C, Wahl SM, et al. Induction of alpha interferon by HIV type 1 in human monocyte-macrophage cultures. *J. Virol.* 1991; 65; 6362-6364.

29. Denis M, Ghadirian E. Alveolar macrophages from subjects infected with HIV-1 express macrophage inflammatory protein-1α : contribution to the CD8+ alveolitis. *Clin. Exp. Immunol.* 1994; 96; 187-192.

30. Agostini C, Trentin L, Zambello R, et al. Release of granulocyte-macrophage colony-stymulating factor by alveolar macrophages in the lung of HIV-1-infected patients. *J. Immunol.* 1992; 149; 3379-3385.

31. Lau AS, Williams BRG. Interferon and tumor necrosis factor in the pathogenesis of HIV infection. *J. Exp. Pathology.* 1990; 5; 111-122.

32. DeStefano E, Friedman RM, Friedman-Kien AE, et al. Acid-Labile human leukocyte interferon in homosexual men with Kaposi's sarcoma and lymphadenopathy. *J. Infect. Dis.* 1982; 146; 451-455.

33. Lau AS, Read SE, William BRG. Down regulation of interferon alpha but not γ receptor expression in vivo in the acquired immunodeficiency syndrome. *J. Clin. Invest.* 1988; 82; 1415-1421.

34. Goodwin JS, Ceuppens J. Regulation of the immune response by prostaglandins. *J. Clin. Immunol.* 1983; 3; 295-315.

35. Rossol S, Gianni G, Rossol-Voth R, et al. Cytokine-mediated regulation of monocyte/macrophage cytotoxicity in human immunodeficiency virus-1 infection. *Med. Microbiol. Immunol.* 1992; 181; 267-281.

36. Trinchieri G. Interleukin-12 and its role in the generation of Th1 cells. *Immunol. Today.* 1993; 14; 335-337.

37. Brunda MJ. Interleukin-12. *J. Leukoc. Biol.* 1994; 55; 280-288.

38. Reiner NE. Altered cell signaling and mononuclear phagocyte deactivation during intracellular infection. *Immunol. Today.* 1994; 15; 374-381.

39. Pietraforte D, Tritarelli E, Testa U, Minetti M. gp120 HIV envelope glycoprotein increases the production of nitric oxide in human monocyte-derived macrophages. *J. Leukoc. Biol.* 1994; 55; 175-182.

40. Durrbaum-Landmann I, Kaltenhauser E, Hans-Dieter F, Ernst M. HIV-1 envelope protein gp120 affects phenotype and function of monocytes in vitro. *J. Leukoc. Biol.* 1994; 55; 545-551.

41. Shiratsuchi H, Johnson JL, Toossi Z, Ellner JJ. Modulation of the effector function of the human monocytes for Mycobacterium avium by human immunodeficiency virus-1 envelope glycoprotein gp120. *J. Clin. Invest.* 1994; 93; 885-891.

42. Wagner RP, Levitz SM, Tabuni A, Kornfield H. HIV-1 envelope protein (gp120) inhibits the activity of human bronchoalveolar macrophages against Cryptococcus neoformans. *Am Rev. Respir. Dis.* 1992; 146; 1434-1438.

43. Dukes CS, Matthews TJ, Weinberg JB. Human immunodeficiency virus type 1 infection of human monocytes and macrophages does not alter their ability to generate an oxidative burst. *J. Infect. Dis.* 1993; 168; 459-462.

44. Chen TP, Roberts RL, Wu KG, et al. Decreased superoxide anion and hydrogen peroxide production by neutrophils and monocytes in human immunodeficiency virus-infected children and adults. *Pediatr. Res.* 1993; 34; 544-550.

45. Wehle K, Schirmer M, Dunnebacke-Hinz J, et al. Quantitative differences in phagocitosis and degradation of Pneumocystis carinii by alveolar macrophages in AIDS and non-HIV patients in vivo. *Cytopathology.* 1993; 4; 231-236.

46. Roilides E, Holmes A, Blake C, et al. Defective antifungal activity of monocyte-derived macrophages from human immunodeficiency virus-infected children against Aspergillus fumigatus. *J. Infect. Dis.* 1993; 168; 1562-1565.

47. Baldwin GC, Fleischmann J, Chung Y, et al. Human immunodeficiency virus causes mononuclear phagocyte dysfunction. *Proc. Natl. Acad. Sci. USA.* 1990; 87; 3933-3937.

48. Kent SJ, Stent G, Sonza S, et al. HIV-1 infection of monocyte-derived macrophages reduces Fc and complement receptor expression. *Clin. Exp. Immunol.* 1994; 95; 450-454.

49. Denis M. Human monocyte/macrophages: NO or no NO? *J. Leukoc. Biol.* 1994; 55; 682-684.

50. Murray JF, Mills J. Pulmonary infectious complications of human immunodeficiency virus infection. Part I and Part II. *Am. Rev. Respir. Dis.* 1990; 141; 1356-1372, 1582-1598.

51. Sierra-Madero JG, Toossi Z, Hom DL, et al. Relationship between load of virus in alveolar macrophages from human immunodeficiency virus type 1-infected persons, production of cytokines, and clinical status. *J. Infect. Dis.* 1994, 169, 18-27.

52. Shall TJ, Bacon K, Toy KJ, Goeddel DV. Selective attraction of monocytes and T lymphocytes of the memory phenotype by cytokine RANTES. *Nature.* 1990; 347; 669-671.

53. Taub D, Conlon K, Lloyd A, et al. Preferential migration of activated CD4+ and CD8+ cells in response to MIP-1α and MIP-1β. *Science.* 1993; 260; 355-358.

54. Matsushima K, Larsen CG, Dubois G, Oppenheim JJ. Purification and characterization of a novel chemotactic and activating factor produced by a human myelomonocytic cell line. *J. Exp. Med.* 1989; 169; 1485-1490.

55. Hufert FT, Schmitz J, Schreiber M, et al. Human Kupffer cells infected with HIV-1 in vivo. *J. Aquir. Immune Def. Syndr.* 1993; 6; 772-777.

56. Schmitt MP, Gendrault JL, Schweitzer C, et al. Permissivity of primary cultures of human Kupffer cells for HIV-1. *AIDS Res. Human Retroviruses.* 1990; 6; 987-991.

57. Tyor WR, Glass JD, Baumrind N, et al. Cytokine expression of macrophages in HIV-1-associated vacuolar myelopathy. *Neurology.* 1993, 43, 1002-1009.

58. Mosmann TR, Coffman RL. Th1 and Th2 cells: Different patterns of lymphokine secretion lead to different functional properties. *Ann. Rev. Immunol.* 1989; 7; 145-173.

59. Zurawski G, de Vries JE. Interleukin-13, an interleukin 4-like cytokine that acts on monocytes and B cells, but not on T cells. *Immunol. Today.* 1994; 15; 19-26.

60. Clerici M, Shearer G. A Th1-> Th2 switch is critical step in the etiology of HIV infection. *Immunol. Today.* 1993; 14; 107-110.

61. Maggi E, Mazzetti M, Ravina A, et al. Ability of HIV to promote a Th1 to Th0 shift and to replicate preferentially in Th2 and Th0 cells. *Science.* 1994; 265; 244-248.

62. Graziosi C, Pantaleo G, Gantt KR, et al. Lack of Evidence for the dichotomy of Th1 and Th2 predominance in HIV-infected individuals. *Science.* 1994; 265; 248-252.

63. Stein M, Keshav S, Harris N, Gordon S. Interleukin 4 potently enhances murine macrophage mannose receptor activity: A marker of alternative immunologic macrophage activation. *J. Exp. Med.* 1992; 176; 287-292.

64. Doyle AG, Herbein G, Montaner LJ, et al. Interleukin-13 alters the activation state of murine macrophages in vitro: comparison with interleukin-4 and interferon-γ. *Eur. J. Immunol.* 1994; 24; 1441-1445.

65. Zack JA, Arrigo SJ, Weitsman SR, et al. HIV-1 entry into quiescent primary lymphocytes:molecular analysis reveals a labile, latent viral structure. *Cell.* 1990; 61; 213-222.

66. Zarling JM, Ledbetter JA, Sias J, et al. HIV-infected humans, but not chimpanzees, have circulating cytotoxic T lymphocytes that lyse uninfected CD4+ cells. *J. Immunol.* 1990; 144; 2992-2998.

67. Brenner BG, Dascal A, Margolese RG , Wainberg MA. Natural killer cell function in patients with acquired immunodeficiency syndrome and related diseases. *J. Leukoc. Biol.* 1989; 46; 75-83.

68. Tanneau F, McChesney M, Lopez O, et al. Primary cytotoxicity against the envelope glycoprotein of human immunodeficiency virus-1: evidence for antibody-dependent cellular cytotoxicity in vivo. *J. Infect. Dis.* 1990; 162; 837-843.

69. Nottet HSLM, de Graff L, de Vos NM, et al. Down-regulation of human immunodeficiency virus type 1 (HIV-1) production after stimulation of monocyte-derived macrophages infected with HIV-1. *J. Infect. Dis.* 1993; 167; 810-817.

6

INVESTIGATIONS ON AUTOLOGOUS T-CELLS FOR ADOPTIVE IMMUNOTHERAPY OF AIDS

Jan van Lunzen, Jörn Schmitz, Kathrin Dengler, Claudia Kuhlmann, Herbert Schmitz, and Manfred Dietrich

Clinical Medicine Section and Department of Virology
Bernhard-Nocht-Institute for Tropical Medicine
Bernhard-Nocht-Str. 74
20359 Hamburg
Germany

ABSTRACT

We report on the preclinical results of an immunotherapeutic approach of AIDS mediated by ex vivo propagated CD4+ and CD8+ T-cells. A mean yield of 6.23×10^9 lymphocytes, containing 1.82×10^9 CD4+, 3.23×10^9 CD8+ T-lymphocytes and 8.39×10^6 CD34+ peripheral blood progenitor cells (PBPC) were be obtained by continuous flow cytapheresis (CFC) in 15 asymptomatic HIV infected patients (CD4-count >350/mm^3). The CD4/CD8 ratio (mean: 0.53, SD: ±0.15) in the cell concentrates reflected the distribution of the circulating lymphocyte subsets in vivo. Absolute lymphocyte counts decreased at a mean of 404/µl (25%) immediately after CFC but were replaced from the extravascular pool within one hour. Neither the CD4/CD8 ratio nor p24-antigen and neopterin levels did change significantly after cell separation. No alteration of the number of proviral DNA copies ($1/10^3$ - $1/10^6$) could be detected in peripheral T-helper cells by semiquantitative PCR after lymphapheresis. Cells were cryopreserved in liquid nitrogen without substantial loss of viability or function. Ex vivo propagation of T-cells in a strictly autologous manner in the presence of PHA+IL-2 for 14d resulted in a 50-fold expansion rate (140-fold in healthy controls, p<0.001). Viral replication could be controlled but not completely eliminated by cocultivation with autologous CD8+ T-lymphocytes as measured by limiting dilution nested PCR (NPCR). The expanded cells showed the typical phenotype of highly activated memory type T-lymphocytes (CD3+ CD45RO+ CD25+ HLA-DR+). The distribution of CD4+ and CD8+ T-cells did not reveal significant changes before and after culture indicating that both subsets were equally expanded. Functionally important membrane or intracellular epitopes which were found to be decreased in HIV infected subjects (CD7, CD55, CD59) before culture were reconstituted after ex vivo propagation of T-cells. The functional importance of the up-regulation of complement regulating epitopes (CD55, CD59) after culture could be proven by a significant inhibition of cytolysis of T-cells in the presence of autologous complement. The majority (75%) of expanded CD8+ T-cells stained positive with mAb TIA-1 which is directed to intracellular granules within cytotoxic T-cells. Furthermore, programmed cell death of expanded T-cells could be prevented by cocultivation with fibroblasts which are believed to secrete a cytokine pattern preventing activated T-cells from apoptosis after withdrawal of IL-2 and other stimuli. Our preclinical data support the idea of reconstituting the immune response of HIV infected patients by adoptive cell mediated immunotherapy in order to an improve prevention and treatment of opportunistic diseases. The methods of cell separation, cryopreservation and ex vivo propagation are established and safe. However, before clinical application and evaluation additional studies are necessary.

INTRODUCTION

The acquired immune deficiency syndrome (AIDS) is characterized by the development of HIV induced immunedefect and subsequent opportunistic infections and malignancies (1). The human immune deficiency virus (HIV) as the causative agent, preferentially infects CD4-receptor expressing cells (e.g., T-helper lymphocytes and monocytes/macrophages)(2-4). Subsequently the depletion of T-helper lymphocytes and severe impairment of the function of T-lymphocytes as well as monocytes/macrophages develop (5,6). The resulting lack of immune regulation by T-helper cells and accessory cells, finally leads to a complete loss of immunological surveillance. The mechanisms of T-cell depletion and malfunction are as yet not completely understood but there are definitely several different factors involved in this process. Direct cytopathic effects of the virus, apoptosis, lysis by cytotoxic T-lymphocytes and the dysregulation of the cytokine pattern in concert, may contribute to the observed immunological abnormalities in AIDS (7-12). Next to the decrease of the absolute number of T-helper cells an impaired response to mitogen and recall antigen stimulation of T-cells frequently occurs during HIV-infection (13). Thus the final state of immune deficiency is caused by a complex deterioration of the normal human immune response as the consequence of the depletion and malfunction of T-cells. Previous studies indicate, that a significant reduction of proliferative capacity can be detected in PBMC of HIV infected patients after exposure to mitogens or recall-antigens compared to healthy controls. The magnitude of this proliferative defect seems to depend on the stage of the disease and may be associated with a numeric depletion of T-helper cells. Thus, we found in a large cohort study which was started in 1985, that those patients who were initially asymptomatic but progressed to ARC or AIDS showed the most pronounced decrease in proliferative capacity of lymphocytes in vitro (German Multicenter Cohort Study, unpublished). This correlated with impaired DTH reaction in vivo, increase of serum neopterin levels and up-regulation of HLA-DR molecules on T-cells. Based on these findings and on the current literature, we summarize that progressive HIV-infection leads to severe functional impairment of T-cells in response to non-specific activation and recall antigens (13, 14). This (partial) anergy results in the loss of immunological surveillance and subsequent development of opportunistic diseases. Both, the depletion of the absolute amount of T-helper cells in the course of the disease and the malfunction of T-cells on the single cell level in concert, seem to contribute to the immunopathogenesis of AIDS. The progressive loss of T-helper cells during the course of HIV-infection cannot solely be explained by direct cytopathic effects of the virus itself, since only a part of T-helper cells have integrated proviral genome, depending on the stage of the disease (15). We have demonstrated earlier that the number of infected T-cells in the peripheral blood is increasing over time and the highest viral load can be found in patients with full blown AIDS (16,17). Furthermore, we could also show that the number of lymphatic tissue T-helper cells integrating proviral genome is 5 to 150-fold higher compared to the peripheral blood in asymptomatic stages of infection. These T-helper cells seem to be latently infected at the transcriptional level rather than productive infection can be observed (18,19). Thus, viral latency might at least partially be explained by antigen trapping and viral persistence in the lymphatic tissue (20). Also it has been described that viral replication is controlled to some extent by cytotoxic HIV-specific CD8+ T-lymphocytes and that this inhibitory capacity is declining over time (21). These data gave raise to the development of immunotherapeutic approaches by retransfusing ex vivo activated CD8+ T-cells into symptomatic patients (22-24). In summary, the treatment of symptomatic HIV infection is momentarily based on three major principles: 1. antiretroviral therapy, 2. prophylaxis and early treatment of opportunistic infections (OI) and 3. reconstitution of immunological responses. Despite intensive research effort, drug therapy offers only limited beneficial effects concerning overall survival and prevention or treatment of OI. Therefore, we concentrate on the scientific evaluation of immunotherapeutic approaches of AIDS mediated by ex vivo propagated autologous CD4+ and CD8+ T-cells. T-cells recovered in early stages of the disease shall be recovered by lymphapheresis, cryopreserved and autologously retransfused after ex vivo propagation when patients have deteriorated to more advanced stages of immunedeficiency. As outlined, both T-cell subsets (CD4+ and CD8+) might contribute to achieve the goal to control viral replication and to restore immunological responses.

PATIENTS AND METHODS

Study Population

Fifteen asymptomatic patients (CDC stage II/III, CD4 count >350/mm^3) with confirmed HIV-1 infection were included in this study. One to four continuous flow cell separations (CFC) were performed on each patient using an IBM-2997 device allowing for half automatic cell sampling. A minimal free interval of two weeks was placed between repeated lymphaphereses. The patient's blood was processed at an anticoagulant citrat dextrose formula A (ACD-A): whole blood ratio of 1:10 over a two to three hour period. Separated cell fractions were directly collected into sterile containers (Cryocyte 500 ml freezing bag, Baxter, Unterschleißheim, Germany) suitable for cryopreservation and storage in liquid nitrogen. Aliquots of fractionated cell samples were separately frozen and later used for phenotypic analysis (CD4$^+$ and CD8$^+$ T-lymphocytes, granulocytes, monocytes, B-lymphocytes, NK-cells, CD34$^+$ peripheral progenitor cells) by flowcytometry and ex vivo propagation. Ficoll-separated PBMC of healthy volunteers served as controls. For estimation of CD34$^+$ peripheral progenitor cells, separated cells were stained with PE-conjugated mAb HPCA-2 and counterstained with FITC-conjugated mAb directed to CD7, CD19 or HLA-DR. These analyses were performed on a minimum count of 1x10^5 cells. Serial estimations of hematological parameters (WBC, RBC, platelets), blood chemistry and coagulation tests were carried out immediately before and after lymphapheresis and after 1h, 3h, 24h and 7d after completed procedure. At the same time phenotyping of circulating lymphocytes was performed after staining with various directly FITC- or PE-conjugated monoclonal antibodies (mAb) directed to several of the cluster of differentiation antigens.

Ex vivo Propagation of PBMC

The Ficoll separated PBMC as well as PBMC obtained by CFC were resuspended at 0.5 x 10^6 cells/ml in AIM-V containing 15% heat inactivated human AB-serum after washing twice in PBS. Cells were referred to 25 cm^2 culture flasks (Nunc, Wiesbaden, Germany) at a final volume of 10 ml cell suspension and preincubated with PHA 1 μg/ml for 48 hours at 37° C in 5% CO_2. After preincubation, human IL-2 (gift from H. Mohr, Blutbank Springe, Germany) was added at a concentration of 25 U/ml. IL-2 and medium was refreshed every third day and total cell number adjusted to 1 x 10^6 cells/ml. Cultures were referred to 175 cm^2 culture flasks (Nunc, Wiesbaden, Germany) when the total volume of cell suspension exceeded 20 ml and kept for 14 days at 37° C in 5% CO_2. Blastogenesis and morphology of cells was assessed every third day by light microscopy. At termination of culture the total cell numbers were measured on a Coulter-type counter after centrifugation of the whole cell suspension at 2000 x g for 10 min to form a pellet and after resuspension in PBS. Viability was estimated using the trypan blue dye exclusion test and propidium iodide staining. Additionally, ex vivo propagated cells were cocultivated with human fibroblasts for 48 hours to allow cultured PBMC a "resting phase" after withdrawal of IL-2.

Flowcytometrical Phenotype Analysis

Phenotype analysis of PBMC was performed as described previously. Briefly, 1 x 106 cells were stained with various directly FITC-, PE- or PerCP conjugated mAb directed to several of the cluster of differentiation antigens. Apart from surface marker expression intracellular staining with the mAb TIA-1 (gift from Coulter, Krefeld, Germany) was performed after permeabilization of the cell membrane to determine cytotoxic T-cells (25). Two and three colour flowcytometric analysis of lymphocyte subsets was performed on a FACScan flowcytometer using Simulset^R and Lysis II^R software (Becton Dickinson, Heidelberg, Germany). Stained cells were gated on live lymphocytes and each analysis was performed on a total number of 1 x 10^4 cells except the analysis of CD34+ progenitor cells where 1 x 10^5 cells were used. Cells were phenotyped before and after culture and in vivo following lymphapheresis as indicated above.

Proliferative Responses of PBMC

The proliferative capacity of PBMC in response to unspecific (PHA, PWM, ConA, Il-2) and specific (recall antigens) stimulation was tested in proliferation assays. PBMC were cultured in triplicate in 96-well flat bottomed microtiter plates at a concentration of 1 x 10^5 cells/ml in AIM-V for 72h at 37° C in 5% CO_2. Mitogens (PHA, PWM, ConA) and Il-2 were added to each well to a final volume of 200μl/well. Specific stimulation with recall antigens was performed by incubating cells with Ag (Candida, PPD, tetanus toxoid, diphteria, proteus) after addition of freshly isolated autologous monocytes/macrophages as antigen presenting cells (APC) for 7 days at 37° C at 5% CO_2. Cultures were pulsed with 1 μCi/well tritiated thymidine (Amersham, Braunschweig, Germany) for six hours and cells were collected onto fibre glass filters using a cell harvestor (Skatron, Lier, Norway). Tritiated thymidine incorporation was determined by liquid scintillation spectroscopy and either expressed as absolute counts per minute (cpm) or stimulation indeces (SI); unstimulated PBMC served as negative controls.

Viral Load

To test the hypothesis that replacement of peripheral T-lymphocytes from lymphatic tissue might increase the rate of infected peripheral T-cells, the number of CD4$^+$ T-lymphocytes with integrated proviral DNA was determined by a semi-quantitative, nested PCR technique before and 3h after lymphapheresis . Ficoll separated PBMC drawn before and after three hours of lymphapheresis were serially diluted (in 0.25 log stages) so that different quantities of cells (1×10^6 - 1×10^1) were used for amplification. Viral load before and after culture of PBMC was determined using the same PCR-assay. In a first step, the samples were amplified using the V3-Not primer as published elsewhere (26). Amplification was carried out within 30 cycles with denaturation at 94° C for 1.5 min, annealing at 50° C for 1.5 min and elongation at 72° C for 3 min. In a second step, 1µl of the specific amplified DNA fragment was reamplified in a nested primer reaction using PCR 1/2 primer (17). The amplification was carried out within 30 cycles with denaturation at 94° C for 1.5 min, annealing at 58° C for 1 min and elongation at 72° C for 2 min. DNA from 10^3 infected (HIVIIIb) and noninfected H9 cells were used as positive and negative controls. Furthermore, the nested PCR reaction was performed on limiting dilutions of ACH-2 cells, a cell line harbouring one viral copy per cell (26). PCR products were analysed by agarose gel electrophoresis. The number of cells integrating proviral genome was finally adjusted to the number of CD4+ cells. Semi-quantitative analysis was performed by comparing the results to the quantities obtained in the PCR of ACH-2 cell dilutions. Thus, ACH-2 cell dilutions served as the standard for quantitation of viral copies (Table 2). These experiments were all done in triplicate. Production of viral antigen in supernatants or antigenemia in serum was determined by a sandwich-type p24 ELISA (Abott, Wiesbaden, Germany). Antigen levels were measured at day 0 and 14 of PBMC culture and on day 0 and 7 after lymphapheresis. Serum neopterin levels as an indicator of macrophage activation was determined at the same time after lymphapheresis by a RIA.

RESULTS

Lymphapheresis

A total of 35 lymphaphereses were performed on the 13 eligible patients. The mean total blood volume processed was 5494 ml (±1615 ml) over a period of 2-3 hours. A mean yield of 6.23×10^9 (±2.65×10^9) lymphocytes could be obtained in a mean volume of 273 ml (±90 ml). The cells were collected into sterile freezing containers, including a mean of 1.82×10^9 (±1.02×10^9) CD4+ and 3.23×10^9 (±1.53×10^9) CD8+ T- lymphocytes (Table 1). Thus, the distribution of helper- and supressor/cytotoxic T-cells in the fractionated cell samples (0.53±0.15) reflected the ratio of circulating subsets in vivo (0.53±0.17). The purity of the lymphocytes was 80-95% (5-10% contaminating monocytes/macrophages) . A substantial amount of CD34+ peripheral progenitor cells (mean: 8.39×10^6) could be detected in the cell samples without prior conditioning of patients with growth factors (e.g. G-CSF, stem cell factor). The separated absolute number of these cells revealed considerable interindividual differences (SD:±7.55×10^6) depending on the absolute amount of PBMC collected and the CD4/CD8 ratio ex vivo. There was a trend towards decreased numbers of separated CD34+ progenitor cells in patients with CD4/CD8 ratios <0.5 ex vivo (data summarized in Table 1, pts. D, E, G). These progenitors coexpressed CD7 and HLA-DR molecules; no expression of CD19 could be detected.

The number of circulating lymphocytes decreased at a mean of 404/mm³ (25%) immediately after lymphapheresis, but cells were fully replaced one hour after the procedure was completed. No changes of the CD4/CD8 ratio *in vivo* could be detected immediately after lymphapheresis or after 1h, 3h, 24h and 7 days. The absolute number of redistributed CD4+ and CD8+ T-lymphocytes showed a slight rebound effect exceeding the initial counts after 1h, 3h and 24h and returned to baseline after 7 days (Figure 1 a-c). Platelets significantly decreased after lymphapheresis but did not fall below the normal range (<120.000/mm³) and were fully replaced after 7 days. Also CFC did not lead to a relevant decrease of total leukocytes and erythrocytes. No coagulation disorders occured. Lymphapheresis was toler-

Table 1. Absolute numbers and distribution of PBMC obtained by leukapheresis of HIV$^+$ patients (mean values ± SD)

Pat.	No.*	Processed Volume (ml)	Collected Volume (ml)	CD4/CD8 In Vivo	CD4$^+$ Cells x 10^9	CD8$^+$ Cells x 10^9	CD4/CD8 Ex Vivo	CD34$^+$ Cells x 10^6	Total No. PBMC x 10^9
A	3	4430	220	0.54	1.62±0.41	3.11±1.00	0.55	n.d.	6.08±1.88
B	3	5556	280	0.66	2.30±0.86	3.16±1.05	0.72	10.35±13.5	7.51±1.21
C	3	5553	240	0.50	1.72±0.22	3.73±0.67	0.45	8.58±5.10	6.50±1.54
D	3	4710	200	0.26	0.62±0.40	2.03±1.55	0.32	0.78±0.94	3.18±2.01
E	3	5050	260	0.53	1.78±1.24	3.80±1.80	0.45	1.59±1.61	7.61±2.65
F	3	6303	340	0.64	1.59±0.61	2.30±0.78	0.68	6.18±3.40	5.39±1.77
G	3	3220	170	0.50	0.91±0.65	1.86±1.47	0.51	1.60±0.39	2.98±2.10
H	1	5330	240	0.20	1.20	5.78	0.20	n.d.	8.03
I	3	5500	300	0.73	2.88±0.64	3.94±0.54	0.71	17.94±1.61	7.52±0.67
J	1	2500	120	0.53	0.74	1.40	0.53	n.d.	2.55
K	3	7266	400	0.73	1.67±0.34	2.41±0.37	0.69	9.02±3.02	5.28±0.95
L	2	6950	330	0.32	1.34±0.09	3.52±0.25	0.38	8.83±0.11	6.15±0.82
M	4	6967	325	0.48	3.45±1.10	4.91±2.43	0.54	17.63±9.10	9.79±3.41
mean: ±SD	35	5494±1615	273±90	0.53±0.17	1.82±1.02	3.23±1.53	0.53±0.15	8.39±7.55	6.23±2.65

* number of lymphaphereses per patient

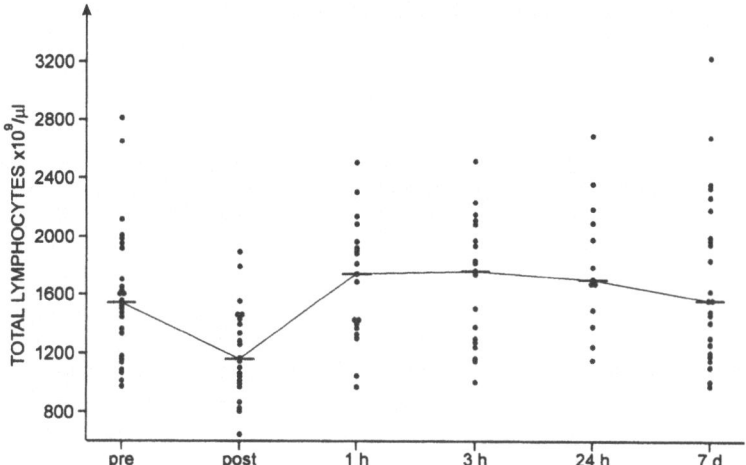

Figure 1. Absolute number of circulating lymphocytes before, immediately after and 1h, 3h, 24h and 7d after lymphapheresis. Counts determined by flowcytometry and given as median values/mm³.

ated well in all patients and did not result in clinical side effects during or following lymphapheresis.

Activation of the immune system or enhancement of viral replication was evaluated by serum neopterin (a product of activated macrophages), HLA-DR expression, p24 antigenemia and by nested PCR. Neither a difference in serum neopterin levels nor a rise in HLA-DR expression or p24-antigenemia could be detected over time (data not shown). The number of PBMC integrating proviral genome adjusted to absolute CD4-count ranged from $1/10^3$ to $1/10^6$ before lymphapheresis and did not increase after the replacement of lymphocytes from extravascular pools (e.g. lymphoid tissue) even after small dilution steps were titrated (0.25×10^3-1.0×10^6 in 0.25 log stages) (Table 2). As little as two viral copies could be detected in serial dilutions of ACH-2 cells, indicating the applicability of our semi-quantitative PCR protocol.

Table 2. Minimal nunmber of PCR-positive cells before and
after lymphapheresis in eight representative patients*

Pt.	before	after 3h
1	1:130	1:130
2	1:290	1:200
3	1:300	1:320
4	1:260	1:310
5	1:400	1:430
6	1:250	1:260
7	1:2900	1:2700
8	1:3400	1:3600
mean	1:990	1:990

*number of positive cells adjusted to CD4 counts,
semi-quantitative PCR analysis was performed
according to the ptotocol as described in the 'Patients
and Methods' section. PCR on dilutions of ACH-2
cells served as standards for quantitation.

Ex vivo Propagation of Autologous T-Cells

A 50-fold expansion rate could be achieved after 14d of bulk lymphocyte culture in HIV infected subject, whereas lymphocytes of healthy donors expanded 140-fold under the same conditions (p<0.001). No alterations of immunological phenotype or function could be observed in cryopreserved PBMC over time. The recovery rate for cryopreserved cells was 85% with a viability of 90%. The expanded PBMC displayed the typical phenotype of highly activated memory-type T-cells (CD3+ CD25+ HLA-DR+ CD45RO+). The results of the phenotype analyses before and after culture for HIV+ and healthy control lymphocytes are summarized in Tables 3a and b. The distribution of CD4+ and CD8+ T-cells of HIV-infected individuals did not reveal significant differences before and after culture (CD4/CD8 ratio: 0.62 vs. 0.59) indicating that both subsets were equally expanded. The majority of CD8+ T-cells stained positive with mAb TIA-1 which is directed to intracellular granules within cytotoxic T-cells. Furthermore, functionally important membrane epitopes (CD7, CD55, CD59) were up-regulated after culture as measured by fluorescence intensity (FI) (Figure 2). The functional significance of this finding was reflected by the inhibition of cytolysis after reconstitution of complement regulating epitopes (CD55, CD59) on T-cells after culture in the presence of autologous complement in propidium iodide uptake assays (data not shown).

Proliferative Responses of Expanded T-Cells

Adoptive immunotherapy of AIDS by retransfusion of ex vivo propagated T-cells will critically depend on the ability of those T-cells generate a proper immune response. The proliferative capacity of expanded T-cells to respond to mitogenic and antigenic stimulation in vitro was tested using lymphocyte proliferation assays. It could be demonstrated that PBMC of asymptomatic HIV-infected patients have a significantly decreased proliferative capacity when compared to healthy controls (mean: 47% response; range: 36%-54%) before culture. We could rule out that this is a HIV-specific effect since PBMC of patients with acute lymphotropic viral infections other than HIV (CMV, EBV) did even show a more pronounced proliferative defect in response to mitogenic and antigenic stimulation (data not shown). Moreover, expanded T-cells of HIV-infected patients are driven into a state of complete anergy after activation in vitro. This loss of proliferative capacity after ex vivo propagation could not be reversed by the addition of autologous APC, whereas responses to Il-2 were fully preserved exceeding the initial counts considerably due to the up- regulation of Il-2 receptors after in vitro activation (Figure 3).

Since in vitro activated T-cells rapidly undergo apoptosis after withdrawal of Il-2, we used human fibroblast cocultures to avoid this detrimental effect and to overcome the "state of anergy" of activated T-cells. Apoptosis of expanded T-cells could be prevented by a "resting-phase" of 24-48h on fibroblasts. This was also observed when the supernatant of fibroblast cultures (fibroblast conditioned medium) was used.

Viral Replication in Vitro

The use of expanded T-cells for immunotherapy will be restricted by enhanced viral replication after in vitro activation. However, we could not detect an increase of the proportion of CD4+ T-cells harboring proviral genome after ex vivo propagation. The proportion of infected T-helper cells decreased by one to two log stages in two thirds of the cases (7/10) and remained stable in the remaining cases after culture as measured by our semi-quantitative PCR protocol (Figure 4). Thus, viral replication could be controlled but obviously not completely eradicated in vitro by cocultivation with autologous CD8+

Table 3a. Phenotype of PBMC of HIV infected donors and healthy controls before and after ex vivo propagation (mean values in %, ±SD, n=20).

	HIV-positive PBMC		HIV-negative PBMC	
	before	after	before	after
CD3+	72.2	89.1*	74.5	94.0*
	±12.5	±7.8	±7.7	±2.5
CD19+	4.6	0.0	6.9	0.0
		±2.5	±1.3	
CD3+CD4+	24.8	31.2	40.0**	42.6
	±10.3	±10.2	±9.7	±7.5
CD3+CD8+	40.1	53.3	28.7**	51.1*
	±12.8	±13.6	±7.5	±8.5
CD3+CD25+	2.8	16.0*	n.d.	n.d.
	±0.8	±4.1		
CD3-CD16/56+	15.0	3.5*	6.9	1.6*
	±10.5	±4.2	±1.3	±0.7

* p<0.05 between before and after ex vivo propagation.
** p<0.05 between HIV-positive donors and healthy controls.

Table 3b. Additional phenotype analysis of ex vivo propagated CD4+ and CD8+ T-cells (mean values in %, ±SD, n=20)

		HIV-positive PBMC		HIV-negative PBMC	
		before	after	before	after
	CD7+	68.0	70.5	89.6**	90.5**
		±9.1	±20.9	±4.3	±6.1
	CD45RO+	44.4	99.1*	41.9	96.0*
		±11.9	±2.2	±4.1	±2.6
CD4+	HLA-DR+	12.0	70.8*	2.0**	45.8*
		±1.9	±7.4	±0.9	±12.5
	TIA-1+	15.7	22.7	2.7**	8.0**
		±9.3	±9.4	±0.6	±1.0
	CD11b+	2.9	11.9*	n.d.	n.d.
		±1.8	±5.5		
	CD7+	58.0	88.0*	86.8**	90.5**
		±15.3	±6.0	±4.3	±6.1
	CD45RO+	41.8	96.0*	41.6	95.3*
		±6.4	±4.1	±11.5	±2.5
CD8+	HLA-DR+	15.6	86.0*	3.2**	46.4*
		±10.1	±2.8	±1.9	±20.7
	TIA-1+	77.2	78.0	49.0**	66.3*
		±8.8	±11.8	±10.4	±11.1
	CD11b+	8.1	21.1*	n.d.	n.d.
		±2.8	±5.9		

* p<0.05 between before and after ex vivo propagation.
** p<0.05 between HIV-positive donors and healthy controls.

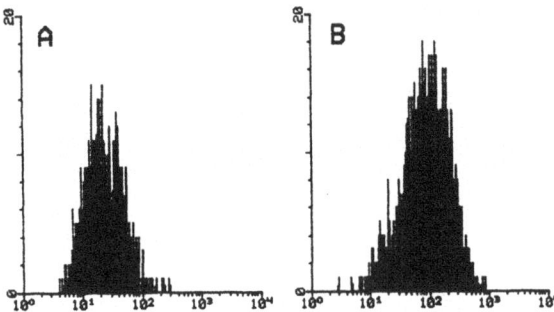

Figure 2. Up-regulation of CD59 molecules on CD8+ T-cells after ex vivo propagation as measured by fluorescence intensity (mean FI before culture (A): 39, after culture (B): 114, p<0.05).

T-lymphocytes. This finding was also reflected by decreasing p24 antigen levels in supernatants after culture as a measure for productive infection.

DISCUSSION

In this study we could show that high yields of T-cells can be safely obtained by lymphapheresis of asymptomatic HIV infected patients, that long term cryopreservation of these cells does not impair phenotype or function and that ex vivo propagation leads to the generation of large numbers of functionally competent T-cells which might be used for autologous adoptive immunotherapy of AIDS. Cell separation did not result in alterations of virological, immunological or clinical parameters (28). The initial decrease of circulating lymphocytes immediately after lymphapheresis was followed by a rapid replacement (within 1h) of cells from marginal pools. This is not a surprising finding since only approximately 2% of the total body lymphocytes can be found in the peripheral blood whereas the remaining 98% are located in lymphoid organs (29). It is noteworthy, however, that the redistribution of lymphocytes from lymphatic tissue did not result in an increase of infected circulating helper cells despite the fact that the proportion of infected T-helper cells in the lymph nodes exceeds the numbers in the peripheral blood by far (18,19). It is also interesting that a relatively high number of peripheral blood progenitor cells was separated without prior preconditioning of patients with growth factors (e.g. G-CSF). The yield of peripheral blood progenitor cells (PBPC) might even be enhanced by the application of growth factors to

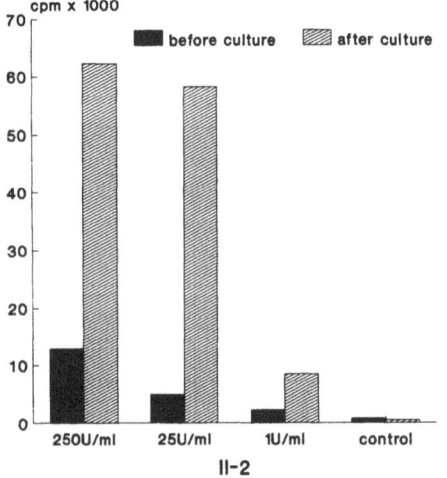

Figure 3. Responses of ex vivo propagated PBMC to different concentrations of Il-2 in proliferation assays after culture.

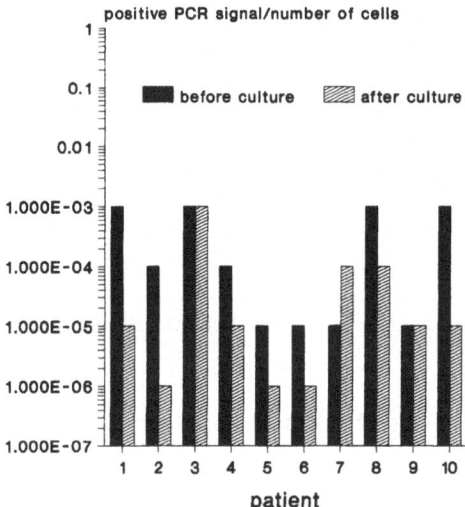

Figure 4. Proportion of CD4+ T-cells integrating proviral genome before and after ex vivo propagation as measured by limiting dilution PCR.

asymptomatic HIV-infected individuals in analogy with the findings in HIV-negative donors (30). These peripheral progenitors might potentially be used in future gene therapy protocols. One important issue of our study was to investigate the feasibility of ex vivo propagation protocols to obtain a sufficient number of T-cells for cell mediated immunotherapy of AIDS. We could demonstrate that a mean expansion rate of a 50-fold increase in total cell number can be achieved by our protocol. Given a total number of 500×10^9 T-cells in the human organism (29) and a mean number of 6×10^9 T-cells obtained by a single cytapheresis it could be possible to replace approximately half $(250-300 \times 10^9)$ of the total body T-cells after in vitro expansion of one cell separation product. One of the major constraints associated with such an approach might be the lack of functional immunological properties of ex vivo propagated T-cells. It is known that PHA and IL-2 driven lymphocytes enter a state of anergy when exposed to antigenic stimulation after in vitro culture and rapidly undergo apoptosis once exogenous IL-2 is withdrawn. However, recent findings indicate that these functional properties are regained after cocultivation of in vitro activated T-cells with fibroblasts or fibroblast conditioned medium (FCM)(31-33). Our preliminary results suggest that activation induced apoptosis following IL-2 starvation can partially be prevented by fibroblasts or FCM. Thus fibroblasts are thought to secrete a pattern of cytokines which is essential for the survival of activated T-cells. The question whether expanded T-cells retain specific immunological function is difficult to assess and as yet widely unanswered. In vitro systems like stimulation of T-cells with recall antigens are associated with a number of inherent limitations and do not necessarily reflect the situation in vivo. Another interesting finding of our study in this context is the reexpression of complement regulating epitopes (CD55, CD59) after ex vivo propagation. This phenotypic appearance can be translated into biological importance since the reexpression of CD55 and CD59 lead to a significant reduction antibody mediated specific lysis of T-cells in the presence of human complement. In this regard activation of the complement cascade in HIV infection might play an important pathogenetic role in T-cell depletion. Concerning the immunological phenotype of the expanded cells we could demonstrate that CD4+ and CD8+ T-cells can equally be expanded expressing activation markers (HLA-DR, CD25, CD45RO) and intracellular molecules associated with cytotoxic T-cells (TIA-1). Viral replication could be controlled but not completely eradicated by cocultivation with autologous cytotoxic CD8+ T-lymphocytes. Viral load of T-helper cells decreased 1-2 log fold after culture in the majority (7/10) of patients. This is in accordance with the findings of Levy and Walker who first described the suppressive effect of CD8+ T-cells on viral replication in vitro (21). Since only a limited number of T-helper cells are found to be infected in these asymptomatic patients ex vivo propagation of T-cells does not lead to a significant enhancement of viral replication when kept in bulk cultures. Whether this in vitro control of viral replication by CD8+ T-cells might be translated into therapeutic approaches in vivo are under study by different groups (22). Recent clinical trials suggest a potentially beneficial effect of ex vivo propagated CD8+ T-cells in vivo but await further confirmation (23,24). In conclusion we feel that our preclinical data support the idea of reconstituting the immune system of patients in advanced stages of HIV infection with autologous ex vivo propagated T-cells which have been obtained earlier in the course of the disease. However, additional research has to be performed before such an approach should be evaluated in clinical trials.

ACKNOWLEDGMENTS

The excellent technical assistance of Anne Bildhauer and Claudia Jülch is gratefully acknowledged. The presented data are part of the medical dissertation of K. Dengler. This research project was supported to a great part by a donation of Ms. G. Bruhn, Hamburg, Germany.

REFERENCES

1. Phillips AN, Lee CA, Elford J, Janossy G, Timms A, Bofill M, Kernoff PB: Serial CD4 lymphocyte count and development of AIDS. Lancet 337:389-392, 1991
2. Barre-Sinoussi F, Chermann JC, Rey F., Nugeyre MT, Chamaret S, Gruest J, Dauguet C, Axler-Blin C, Vezinet-Brun F, Rouzioux C, Rozenbaum W, Montagnier L: Isolation of a T-lymphotropic from a patient at risk for acquired immune deficiency syndrome (AIDS). Science 220: 868-871, 1983
3. Gallo RC, Salahuddin SZ, Popovic M, Shearer GM, Kaplan M, Haynes BF, Palker TJ, Redfield R, Oleske J, Safai B: Frequent detection and isolation of cytopathic retroviruses (HTLV-III) from patients with AIDS and at risk for AIDS. Science 224: 500-503
4. Schnittman SM, Psallidopoulos MC, Lane HC, Thompson L, Baseler M, Massari F, Fox CH, Salzman NP, Fauci AS: The reservoir for HIV-1 in human peripheral blood is a T-cell that maintains expression of CD4. Science 245: 305-308, 1989
5. Miedema F, Petit AJC, Terpstra FG, Eeftinck Schattenkerk JKM, de Wolf F, Al BJM, Roos M, Lange JMA, Danner SA, Goudsmit J, Schellenkens PTA: Immunological abnormalities in HIV-infected asymptomatic homosexual men. J. Clin. Invest. 82: 1908-1914, 1988
6. Schnittman SM, Lane HC, Greenhouse J, Justement JS, Baseler M, Fauci AS: Preferential infection of CD4+ memory T cells by human immunodeficiency virus type 1: evidence for a role in the selective T-cell functional defects observed in infected individuals. Proc Natl Acad Sci 97: 6058-62, 1990
7. Ameisen JC, Capron A: Cell dysfunction and depletion in AIDS: The programmed cell death hypothesis. Immunol Today 12: 102-105, 1991
8. Groux H, Torpier G, Monte D, Mouton Y, Capron A, Ameisen JC: Activation-induced Death by apoptosis in CD4+ T cells from human immunodeficiency virus-infected asymptomatic individuals. J Exp Med 175: 331-340, 1992
9. Tyler DS, Stanley SD, Nastala CA, Austin AA, Bartlett JA, Stine KC, Lyerly HK, Bolognesi DP, Weinhold KJ: Allterations in antibody-dependant cellular cytotoxicity during the course of HIV-1 infection. J Immunol 144: 3375-84, 1990
10. Walker BD, Flexner C, Birch-Limberger K, Fisher L, Paradis TJ, Aldovini A, Young R, Moss B, Schooley RT: Long-term culture and fine specifity of human cytotoxic T-lymphocyte clones reactive with human immunodeficiency virus type 1. Proc. Natl. Acad. Sci. USA, 86: 9514-9518, 1989
11. Clerici M, Shearer GM: A TH1-TH2 switch is a critical step in the etiology of HIV infection. Immunology Today, 14: 107-111, 1993

12. Scott-Algara D, Vuillier F, Marasescu M, de Saint Martin J, Dighiero G: Serum levels of Il-2, Il-1 alpha, TNF-alpha, and soluble receptor of Il-2 in HIV-1 infected patients. AIDS Res. Hum. Retroviruses, 7: 381-386, 1991

13. Gluckman JC, Klatzmann D, Cavaille-Coll M, Brisson E, Messiah A, Lachiver D, Rozenbaum W: Is there correlation of T-cell proliferative functions and surface marker phenotypes in patients with AIDS or LAS? Clin. Exp. Immunology, 60: 8-16, 1985

14. Clerici M, Stocks NI, Zajac RA, Boswell RN, Lucey DR, Via CS, Shearer GM: Detection of three distinct patterns of T-helper cell dysfunction in asymptomatic, human immunodeficiency virus-seropositive patients. J. Clin. Invest. 84: 1892-1899, 1989

15. Hufert FT, v. Laer MD, Schramm C, Tarnok A, Schmitz H: Detection of HIV-1 DNA in different subsets of human peripheral blood mononuclear cells using the polymerase chain reaction. Arch Virol 106: 341-345, 1989

16. Schnittman SM, Greenhouse JJ, Psallidopoulos MC, Baseler M, Salzman NP, Fauci AS, Lane HC: Increasing viral burden in CD4+ T-cells from patients with HIV-infection reflects rapidly progressive immunosuppression and clinical disease. Ann. Intern. Med. 113: 438-443, 1990

17. Hufert FT, v. Laer D, Fenner TE, Schwander S, Kern P, Schmitz H: Progression of HIV-1 infection. Monitoring of HIV-1 DNA in peripheral blood mononuclear cells by PCR. Arch Virol 120: 233 -240, 1991

18. Schmitz J, van Lunzen J, Tenner-Racz K, Großschupff G, Racz P, Schmitz H, Dietrich M, Hufert FT: Follicular dendritic cells retain HIV-1 on their plasma membrane but are not productively infected in asymptomatic patients with follicular hyperplasia. J. Immunol. 153: 1352-1359, 1994

19. Embretson J, Zupancic M, Ribas JL, Burke A, Racz P, Tenner-Racz K, Haase AT: Massive covert infection of helper T-lymphocytes and macrophages by HIV during the incubation period of AIDS. Nature 362: 359-362, 1993

20. Pantaleo G, Graziosi C, Demarest JF, Butini L, Montroni M, Fox CH, Orenstein JM, Kotler DP, Fauci AS: HIV infection is active and progressive in lymphoid tissue during the clinical latent stage of disease. Nature 362: 355-359, 1993

21. Walker CM, Moody DJ, Stites DP, Levy JA: CD8+ lymphocytes can control HIV infection in vitro by supressing virus replication. Science 234: 1563-1566, 1986

22. Whiteside TL, Elder EM, Moody D, Armstrong J, Ho M, Rinaldo C, Huang X, Torpey D, Gupta P, McMahon D, Okarma T, Herberman RB: Generation and characterization of ex vivo propagated autologous CD8+ cells used for adoptive immunotherapy of patients infected with human immunodeficiency virus. Blood 81: 2085-2092, 1993

23. Ho M, Armstrong J, MacMahon D, Pazin G, Huang X, Rinaldo C, Whiteside TL, Tripoli C, Levine G, Moody D, Okarma T, Elder E, Gupta P, Tauxe N, Torpey D, Herberman RB: A phase 1 study of adoptive transfer of autologous CD8+ T lymphocytes in patients with AIDS-related complex or AIDS. Blood 81: 2093-2101, 1993

24. Klimas N, Patarca R, Walling J, Garcia R, Mayer V, Moody D, Okarma T, Fletcher MA: Clinical and immunological changes in AIDS patients following adoptive therapy with activated autologous CD8 T cells and interleukin-2 infusion. AIDS 8: 1073-1081, 1994

25. Tenner-Racz K, Racz P, Thome C, Meyer CG, Anderson PJ, Schlossman SF, Letvin NL: Cytotoxic effector cell granules recognized by the monoclonal antibody TIA-1 are prsent in CD8+ lymphocytes in lymph nodes of HIV-1 infected patients. Am J Pathol 124: 1750-1758, 1993

26. Wolfs TFW, Zwart G, Bakker M, Valk M, Kuiken CL, Goudsmit J: Naturally occorring mutations within HIV-1 V3 genomic RNA lead to antigenic variation dependant on a single amino acid substitution. Virology 185: 195-205, 1991

27. Folks TM, Clouse KA, Justement J, Rabson A, Duh E, Kehrl JA, Fauci AS: Tumor necrosis factor alpha induces expression of HIV in a chronically infected T cell clone. Proc Natl Acad Sci (USA) 86: 2365-2368, 1989

28. van Lunzen J, Schmitz J, Dengler K, Schmidt l, Schmitz H, Dietrich M: Recovery of T-lymphocytes for adoptive immunotherapy by lympapheresis of HIV-infected patients without alterations of virological, immunological or clinical parameters. Br J Hematol 88: 46-51, 1994

29. Westermann J, Pabst R: Lymphocyte subsets in the blood: A diagnostic window of the lymphoid system? Immunology Today 11: 406-410, 1990

30. Dreger P, Haferlach T, Eckstein V, Jacobs S, Suttorp M, Löffler H, Müller-Ruchholtz W, Schmitz N: G-CSF mobilized peripheral blood progenitor cells for allogeneic transplantation: safety, kinetics of mobilization, and composition of the graft. Br J Haematol 87: 609-613, 1994

31. Akbar AN, Borthwick N, Salmon M, Gombert W, Bofill M, Shamsadeen N, Pilling D, Pett S, Grundy JE, Janossy G: The significance of low bcl-2 expression by CD45RO T cells in normal individuals and

patients with acute viral infections. The role of apoptosis in T cell memory. J. Exp. Med. 178: 427-438, 1993

32. Scott S, Pandolfi F, Kurnick JT: Fibroblasts mediate T cell survival: A proposed mechanism for retention of primed T cells. J. Exp. Med. 172: 1873-1876, 1990

33. Pandolfi F, Oliva A, Sacco G, Polidori V, Liberatore D, Mezzaroma I, Giovanetti A, Kurnick JT, Aiuti F: Fibroblast-derived factors preserve viability in vitro of mononuclear cells isolated from subjects with HIV-1 infection. AIDS 7: 323-330, 1993

7

RATIONAL PROBLEMS ASSOCIATED WITH THE DEVELOPMENT OF CELLULAR APPROACHES IN CONTROLLING HIV SPREAD

Aldar S. Bourinbaiar and Sylvia Lee-Huang

Department of Biochemistry
New York University Medical Center
New York, New York 10016

INTRODUCTION

The priority in elucidation of the problems associated with HIV infection has been mainly determined by experimental feasibility rather than by its importance. Molecular biologists have rapidly produced an impressive body of knowledge about the structure of HIV, but this understanding is not sufficient to explain complex biological effects accompanying viral pathogenesis. Physicians, fourteen years into the epidemic have been left with a confused mixture of AZT, CD4 counts, false promises of vaccines, morbidity charts and nothing else. Immunologists, in their turn, disappointed by the results of their own narrow scope of inquiries for a direct explanation of the pathological effect of the virus, started to look for alternative concepts such as self-inflicted immunopathology mediated through the capacity of HIV to mimic host antigens and to trigger autoimmune responses. Although this idea was proposed even before HIV was implicated as a cause of AIDS, mainstream research has been oriented toward goals that were easier to grasp. As a result, little progress has been made to adopt the viral 'kamikaze' phenomenon to the development of a meaningful therapeutic strategy.

HIV infection in humans is commonly associated with the decrease in CD4+ T lymphocytes, an increase in HIV concentration, and impairment in the function of CTL. Although it seems to be clear that the course of the disease is set by initial HIV infection we have very little understanding of the process since the clinical picture is congested with unexplained variables. Recent trends in AIDS research have begun to imply that vaccines and effective antiviral drugs will be not available in the foreseeable future. Accordingly the attention has shifted to cell-mediated immunity, i.e., the induction of HIV-specific CTL. However, the general mechanism by which CTL eliminate viruses remains largely obscure. Even less is known about the relationship between CTL and HIV-infected cells. In this paper we present evidence that questions the necessity of raising CTL responses against HIV.

Cell Activation and Apoptosis in HIV Infection
Edited by Jean-Marie Andrieu and Wei Lu, Plenum Press, New York, 1995

CLOSE ENCOUNTERS OF THE FIRST KIND: CELL-CELL CONTACT

Cellular communication is an essential requirement for triggering CTL activity. The importance of the adhesion of effector cell to the target surface was first pointed out in 1961 by Rosenau and Moon (1). Conditions that favor effector-target contact increase killing, whereas conditions that minimize direct contact, e.g., the presence of dextran sulfate in the medium, abolish killing (2). Contrary to common belief, the initiation of the contact, i.e. binding of CTL to the surface of the target cell, is nonspecific and does not require antigen-bearing MHC molecules. The presence of MHC-antigen complex may enhance the killing ability of CTL but it is not an absolute requirement (3). The envelope proteins of HIV adsorbed to the surface of CD+ lymphocytes appear to induce cytolytic responses without MHC restriction (4). Furthermore, the antibodies against various nonspecific adhesion molecules such as CD8, LFA-1, and ICAM-1 were found to inhibit both adhesion and killing (5).

The process of adhesion results in reorientation of the cytoplasmic components such as the cytoskeleton, Golgi apparatus and centrosomes. Within a few minutes of cell-cell contact they are concentrated in a small area adjacent to the region of contact. This precedes the release of cytolytic granules in a highly polarized manner toward the conjugated target cell (6). The lytic process is, thus, strictly focused and this possibly contributes to the bystander-sparing phenomenon in CTL killing.

The vectorial secretion of the contents of highly specialized cytoplasmic granules is of critical importance to the killing action by CTL and NK cells (7,8). Investigations of the content of secretory granules released by CTL reveal chemically defined mediators of cell-mediated killing (9). The enzymatic activity of serine proteases or granzymes identified in CTL granules (10) appear to be required for the activation of cytolysin, the inactive precursor of perforin, present in the same compartment. The main function of perforin is to facilitate granzyme penetration into the target cell. Serine protease alone, but not perforin, could generate DNA fragmentation - the landmark of the initiation of apoptosis (11,12).

Thus, the encounter of CTL with the target cell leads to a cascade of events that can be divided into four successive stages: first, the cell-cell adhesion; second, the reorientation of cytoplasmic organelles; third, polarized exocytosis of cytolytic granules containing serine proteases and perforin; fourth, initiation of DNA fragmentation and apoptosis.

THE MACHINERY OF HIV SPREAD BY CELL-CELL CONTACT IS A COPYCAT VERSION OF CTL INTERACTION WITH TARGET CELLS

The conditions that favor efficient HIV spread are strikingly similar to the conditions optimizing the activity of CTL. Cell-cell contact is an essential requirement for the initiation of HIV expansion. Physical contact between latent HIV-infected donor cells and the target recipient cells triggers the release of viral particles into a space formed by adjacent cellular membranes, resulting in virus uptake by target cells (13,14). In this manner, CD4-negative cells that were otherwise resistant to cell-free virus infection became susceptible to HIV-1 infection. Furthermore, HIV-carrying cells with impaired adhesion capacity were not capable of infecting cocultured target cells (15). Accordingly, cell-cell contact plays an important role in upregulation of viral expression and enhances the spread of HIV-1. The presence of dextran sulfate in the culture of infected cells with uninfected targets prevented the spread of HIV (16) and this effect was associated with the deterrence of cell-cell adhesion (17).

Classical dogma entertains the notion that transmission of HIV requires the interaction of the cell-surface CD4 receptor and the viral envelope glycoprotein. However, the presence of CD4+ is not an absolute requirement in cell-mediated HIV infection. Several studies have indicated that integrins and other cell adhesion molecules (CAM), e.g., CD8, CD2, LFA-1, ICAM-1, can regulate cell-mediated viral spread. The antibodies directed against CAM or peptide analogues of CAM were found to be effective in preventing cell-to-cell spread of HIV (18-20).

Within a few minutes following the adhesion both types of HIV-harboring vectors, monocytic and lymphocytic cells, were shown to reorient their cytoplasmic components toward the target cell. This event is followed by the exocytosis of virus particles into a confined space formed by adjoining cell membranes of donor-target cells in a fashion that is strikingly similar to the directional release of cytoplasmic granules from CTL (14-15). The viral spread occurring in this preferential manner within the enclosed *claustra* was referred to as claustrophilic transmission. This type of transmission may explain why neutralizing antibodies against HIV were not capable of preventing cell-to-cell transfer of HIV (14). Similarly, antibodies against cytolytic enzymes were not able to enter the enclosed intercellular space formed by effector-target conjugates and thus inhibit CTL activity. Hence, the principles of cell-to-cell HIV spread appear to be a mirror image of the four conditions necessary for CTL function, i.e., adhesion, polarization of the cell, directional discharge of viral particles, and apoptosis.

HAHNEMANN VS. JENNER

Homeopathy was founded in 1796 by Samuel Hahnemann. This theory is considered a nonscientific form of therapy involving treatment with natural remedies. Incidentally, in the same year Edward Jenner introduced a "new" therapy "of the cow" *vaccinae* — well known as a folk remedy for smallpox. Although John Baker, the first official victim of experimental immunology has died as a result of immunization, Jenner's proposal was praised as the basis of modern scientific therapy, whereas homeopathy has been outlawed and ridiculed. However, the basic principles of homeopathic medicine, *similia similibus curentur, experimenta in homine sano, doses minimae and unitas remedii*, reflect the essential requirements of vaccinology. Hahnemann offered the theory of therapy without convincing data, while Jenner, who was not a thinker, started applying the therapy without knowing its principles.

Tremendous effort has been put forward to accommodate the classic immunological paradigm of humoral immunity to the ever-elusive issue of HIV containment. Although in vitro studies have demonstrated convincingly the obedience of HIV to the neutralizing action of virus-specific antibodies, it is not clear whether the humoral immune response will succeed in controlling HIV spread in real life situations. Occurrence of de novo infection has been reported recently in recipients of several experimental vaccines (21). No clinical response was observed in any of the 15 clinical trials of therapeutic vaccines completed to date (22). None of the experimental vaccines in chimpanzees have shown protection against the HIV challenge (23-25). Thus, there are indications that a natural or vaccine-induced immunity will be not able to cope with retroviral infection, but the current state of the art regarding the efficacy of humoral immunity against HIV is such that the interpretation of available data allows two opposite opinions to co-exist, albeit in antagonistic fashion.

However, publicly expressed opinions of scientists doubting the usefulness of vaccination as a means of providing protection against HIV have been rare (26-28) and they apparently have not reversed the mind of the predominantly Jennerian scientific community, since clinical trials of anti-HIV vaccines are actively pursued.

The observation that seropositive individuals progress to AIDS despite circulating anti-HIV Abs has created a predictable rush to explore the possibility that viremia may have persisted due to mutants arising during infection. Longitudinal studies of patients infected with HIV reveal temporal changes in the number of genetically distinct strains of the virus throughout the incubation period, with a slow but steady rise in diversity during the progression to disease. Structure-function studies analyzing site substitution of the HIV envelope have shown that neutralizing Abs recognizing gp120 of susceptible strains of HIV cannot abrogate the infectivity of mutant viruses. Moreover, a single amino acid change in the V3 loop of a mutant can transform a neutralizing V3 antibody into an antibody with virus-enhancing property (29). Although antigenic variation may help to evade normal immunity, in the case of AIDS selective pressure imposed by the decaying immune system will decrease with time. Thus, the increase or decrease in diversity of HIV variants, i.e, variation in antigenic noise, with feedback of positive or negative antibody response, might be of little consequence for the evolution of virulence.

In addition, these studies concentrated on one facet of the problem since in almost all functional, i.e., neutralization assays, the target cells for HIV were invariably CD4+ lymphocytes. However, practically every major type of human cells can be susceptible to HIV infection (30). Unfortunately, very little is known regarding the effect of neutralizing Abs in protecting tissues outside of the blood compartment. It is obvious that the success of an anti-HIV vaccine will be determined by its ability to confer protection to all types of human tissues.

In the past few years we have assessed the neutralizing activity of HIV antisera and HIV MAbs in blocking viral infection of CD4-negative cells, e.g., epithelial cells and placental trophoblasts. These in vitro studies were designed to examine the role of neutralizing antibodies in preventing horizontal and vertical transmission of HIV. It was found that neutralizing antibodies, highly efficient in protecting CD4+ lymphocytes, failed to prevent the infection of CD4-negative cells. This could not be attributed to the variability of virus since we have used the identical IIIB strain of HIV. Furthermore, neutralizing antibodies were incapable of blocking cell-to-cell transfer of HIV (14). Thus, it appears that humoral immunity has limited capacity in controlling HIV infection, particularly when virus is spread by cell-to-cell contact. Future research will reveal whether Hahnemann-Jenner's theory can withstand the HIV challenge.

CTL AS HEROES

The efforts to generate a vaccine against HIV have been focused on inducing neutralizing antibodies. Although these efforts have not succeeded in providing adequate protection it has been observed that vaccination can provoke CTL responses (31). Accordingly, the focus has shifted to induction of cell-mediated immunity — considered essential for recovery from many types of viral infections.

In spite of the fact that there is no single documented recovery from HIV infection the idea that killing of infected cells by CD8+ cells is important in preventing the development of disease has become prevalent in the AIDS field (32,33). This has been supported by clinical observations associating selective impairment of HIV-specific CTL response with disease progression (34,35). Recent findings suggest that the CTL of noninfected sexual partners of HIV-infected individuals or seronegative health care workers exposed to contaminated blood may be responsible for rapid and effective clearance of the virus after exposure (36-37).

Other studies have shown that CTL can control HIV spread by a non-lytic mechanism, corroborating earlier investigations with unrelated viruses showing that activated CD8+ T cells secrete a soluble inhibitor of viral replication (38). The nature of this factor is not known. The inhibitory effect was not dependent on direct cell-cell contact: it was exerted by CD8+ T cells across a semipermeable membrane, and an inhibitory activity was also exerted by the cell-free supernatants from activated CD8+ T cells (39-41). Thus, the issue of whether and how CTL contribute to control of HIV deserves further investigation.

CTL AS VILLAINS

The current dogma entertains the notion that the development of CD8+ cytotoxic T cell responses to viral pathogens is crucial for the prompt resolution of acute infections and for the control of persistent viruses. Although this concept may be true in the case of a "regular" virus it may not apply to HIV. Recent studies have provided evidence that can be interpreted as refuting the original assumption that HIV-specific CTL provide protection to the host.

A major symptom of infection with HIV — the virus known formerly as LAV — is lymphadenopathy. Sections of lymph nodes of HIV patients display follicular hyperplasia and lymphocyte depletion with massive infiltration of effector cells recognized by TIA-1 antibody against 15-kd granule-associated protein of CTL and NK cells or by expression of mRNA for serine esterase B, a protein contained in cytoplasmic granules (42,43). These observations suggest that cytotoxic cells are activated in follicles of HIV lymph nodes and are actively involved in the lysis of immunocompetent cells (44). Development of follicle destruction observed in otherwise asymptomatic patients is likely to represent a major pathway leading to AIDS.

In addition the activation of CTL in situ results in production of TNF-alpha and other lymphokines that could enhance viral replication and thus contribute to viral dissemination and disease pathogenesis (45-47). The ability of HIV to infect CD8+ NK cells was related to TNF production by these cells and may also explain selective depletion of this subset that begins in early stages of HIV infection (48).

CTL AND "ROACH MOTELS"

It is important that the concept of cell-mediated killing of HIV-infected cells should take into account the fact that cell-cell contact triggers not only the release of cytoplasmic serine proteases destined to kill target cells but the release of virions from the target cells as well. These two processes are reciprocal and occur within minutes following cell-to-cell interaction (6,13-14). Incidentally, the functional activation of HIV, i.e., the capacity to infect the host cell, requires cleavage of envelope glycoproteins mediated by the same type of proteolytic enzymes — serine proteases (49,50).

There is no evidence that cytolytic serine proteases released by CTL are capable of directly inactivating HIV. In contrast, Martz et al. have provided compelling evidence showing that reovirus was not inactivated when CTL lysed the host cell (38). Instead the virus was released into supernatant as infectious virions. It cannot be excluded that serine proteases secreted by CD8+ CTL or NK cells can actually activate the infectious capacity of HIV released from the dying target cell. As a result virus-specific killer cells expose themselves to the infectious virus and can be either depleted or chronically infected without undergoing apoptosis. These two possibilities are not merely speculation. There are several well-documented reports in the literature demonstrating that CTL and NK cells containing cytolytic granules are progressively depleted in the course of the disease (51,52). This depletion appears to be specific since the frequency of CTL precursors against other microorganisms such as EBV was maintained at levels observed in healthy controls (53).

Alternatively, CD8+ CTL can be infected with HIV without being killed and can serve as chronic virus carriers. The minimal requirement for in vitro infection of CD8+ lymphocytes is physical contact with infected CD4+ cells. Infected CD8+ T lymphocytes can then spread the infection to CD4+ naive cells. Coculture of HIV+ CTL with uninfected CD4+ cells showed that chronically infected CD8+ cells could transmit the virus to uninfected targets (54,55). Thus, CTL in infected individuals may inadvertently function with the purpose of spreading the virus further in the body by communicating with as-yet-uninfected cells (by analogy with the principle of "roach-motels" made famous in American TV commercials).

In view of these possibilities it is questionable whether current strategies designed to reconstitute or augment CD8+ cytotoxic T cell responses will realize success in preventing the disease.

CTL ARE NEITHER HEROES NOR VILLAINS

Two dissenting opinions appear to coexist in the AIDS field regarding the role of CTL in controlling HIV spread. Some researchers have eventually made conciliatory overtures by showing that depending on the stage of disease CTL can cause either upregulation or suppression of HIV-1 expression (56). They have suggested that the subpopulations of CD8+ T cells that predominate at different stages of HIV-induced disease have different functional properties, including the ability to modulate HIV-specific cell-mediated immunity. However, the phenotype of CTL responsible for either of the effects has not been identified.

Despite the progressive loss of HIV-specific cytolytic activity in the advanced stages of the disease, the cytolytic machinery of CD8+ cells against unrelated pathogens is still functioning even in patients with AIDS (57). The reason for the specific decrease in anti-HIV activity is not known and it has been suggested that it could be due either to a progressive decrease in the pool of HIV-specific CTL or to a functional impairment in their ability to kill or proliferate. NK cells from AIDS patients are able to bind but not to lyse the target cells. This has been attributed to an inability to rearrange the microtubular system of the cytoskeleton and to release the cytotoxic factor (58). However, the mechanism of the impairment in CTL is not known. Direct killing of CD8+ cells may be responsible for the decreased activity of CTL (59). Others have implied that the decrease in activity was associated with a reduced ability of HIV-specific CTL to expand. Most researchers believe that although the progression to disease is associated with overall loss of absolute CD8+ T cells, the percentages of CD8+ cells remain unchanged. These conflicting explanations are due to confusion over the genuine markers of cytotoxic cells. Although our knowledge in this area has been considerably advanced lately, no complete information is yet available concerning the nature and phenotype of cytotoxic lymphocytes.

The above chapters describe both positive and negative roles of CTL in regulation of HIV. It is important to determine whether these roles are played by the same subsets or are executed by separate types of cells.

AIDS AS A GROTESQUE GVHD

Chronic viral, bacterial, and parasitic infections serve as a trigger factor in the breakdown of self-tolerance and the appearance of self-reactivity that is remarkably similar to the symptoms of graft-versus-host-disease (GVHD). Host encoded viral antigens expressed as self antigens post-thymically are immunogenic and are recognized as foreign by activated effector T cells. Such an immune response may cause a disease resembling an autoimmune syndrome characterized by polyclonal B-cell activation, molecular mimicry between viral and host antigens, abnormal expression of immunoregulatory molecules, and cytolytic anti-idiotypic network with alloreactive CTL (60,61). Numerous studies have demonstrated a high degree of homology between HIV proteins and various human antigens, such as the heavy chain of HLA class I and beta chain of HLA class II molecules, platelet GPIIb/IIIa glycoproteins, LFA-3 adhesion molecule, C1q complement, the proteins of the immunoglobulin superfamily, ill-defined nuclear and surface proteins of monocytes and so on. HIV can also mimic the components of the microorganisms that represent etiological agents of most opportunistic infections in AIDS. In addition, the HIV particle appears to borrow intrinsic cellular components of the host cells as it exits through the cell membrane (30). In most HIV-unrelated situations, the appearance of self-reactivity in the sera of patients with chronic infections is not associated with clinical manifestations. However, individuals with HIV develop autoimmune degeneration. In spite of the extensive knowledge that has been accumulated, the specific relationship between HIV infection and autoimmunity is still obscure.

The results of experimental transplantation studies, murine autoimmunity models such as type I diabetes, and LCMV infection models can be relevant to the pathogenesis of chronic HIV infection. The survival of the kidney allograft, pancreatic islet cells, and LCMV-infected mice determined by the tolerance of the host either to self- or foreign immunogens was achieved by antibody treatment either to CD4 or CD3 (62-64). Furthermore, self-tolerance was restored in adult mice once autoimmunity was fully established and was obtained without overt depletion of T cells (65). These studies support the notion that autoimmune conditions could be managed by induction of tolerance to foreign antigens, i.e., by inducing anergy of T cell function.

AIDS AS A HIGH ZONE TOLERANCE

Two types of cellular response are possible that may allow the foreign antigen, i.e., virus to evade immune surveillance. During the initial incubation period HIV is present in low concentrations. The antigenic dose of the virus may be low enough that the virus induces a low zone tolerance to itself (66,67).

However, studies carried out with murine lymphocytic choriomeningitis virus (LCMV) have shown that a confrontation with a low dose of the virus caused death in mice, whereas inoculation with a high dose of the virus resulted in asymptomatic disease (68). Zinkernagel et al., have shown in a similar LCMV model that persistence of the virus in an immunocompetent host can be achieved by inducing high zone tolerance or 'complete exhaustion' of immune T cells (69).

Early stages of HIV infection in humans are characterized by vigorous cellular immune responses of CD8+ subset (70). Several activation markers, including CD38, HLA-DR, and CD69, increase significantly after HIV seroconversion. This activation has been associated with increased T cell death (71). As overt AIDS is characterized by depletion of both CD4+ cells and HIV-specific CD8+ CTL this suggests that HIV infection causes high zone tolerance.

THE MONKEY'S WISDOM: TOLERANCE AS A KEY TO SURVIVAL

Chimpanzees, despite being infected with HIV, do not develop the symptoms of AIDS. The hypothesis that autoimmune phenomena might contribute to the depletion of CD4+ T cells and the development of AIDS in HIV-1 infected humans is supported by the observation of the lack of CTL activation and low levels of anti-HIV, i.e., self antibodies in infected chimpanzees. Infected chimpanzees do not present significant alterations in the percentage of CD4+ subsets -a key determinant in HIV-induced progressive pathogenesis. This might be explained by the fact that CTL from HIV-infected chimpanzees lack detectable lytic activity for uninfected CD4+ cells (72-74). The course of the disease in humans accompanied by the depletion of reactive T cells resembles that of SIV-infected macaques but not of HIV-resistant chimpanzees (75). The chimpanzees producing antibodies to major HIV proteins developed marked lymphadenopathy whereas animals without HIV antibodies had no evidence of disease (76). With the exception of one HIV Ig-treated chimpanzee all immunized and control animals that were challenged were not protected from infection, i.e. HIV could be isolated and/or seroconversion was documented (77). Obviously this does not mean chimpanzees are not able to control HIV replication (78). The CD3+CD8+ T cell population of chimpanzees had the capacity to control the growth of HIV in a non-lytic manner (79). In spite of a number of unanswered questions these well-documented observations deliver a clear message that the immunity of the chimpanzees has adopted highly-selective ignorance tactics as a means of preventing self-destruction triggered by HIV infection.

MUSHROOM SAGA: CYCLOSPORIN

Cyclosporin A (CSA) is certainly one of the most controversial substances proposed as an anti-HIV agent. The rationale for its therapeutic use in AIDS patients is based on the hypothesis of the autoimmune nature of HIV disease and was first conceived and tested in clinics by Andrieu et al (80).

Several *in vitro* studies aimed at elucidating the anti-HIV mechanism(s) of CSA action have been reported. Klatzmann et al., who first investigated this drug *in vitro*, proposed that CSA acts by preventing virus binding to its receptor (81). A similar opinion was shared by Wainberg et al., who in addition suggested that CSA may act indirectly by inducing an antiviral state in treated cells (82). Sawada et al., attributed the effect of CSA to the downregulation of CD4 (83). A French group led by Ameisen linked the action of CSA to the induction of anergy and inhibition of HIV-caused apoptosis in lymphocytes (84). Amendola et al., have reported that prevention of apoptosis by CSA was due to the inhibition of transglutaminase expression (85). Karpas et al., associated the antiviral effect of CSA with the selective growth inhibition of infected cells (86). Bell et al., in their study of eradication of HIV+ cells by virus-specific immunotoxins complemented by CSA treatment, concluded that the anti-HIV effect was due to the prevention of T cell activation required for productive viral replication (87). Luban et al., have proposed that CSA prevents proper assembly of HIV gag protein (88). CSA has been also implicated in blocking the formation of complete viral DNA induced in activated T cells (89).

Since there is already a lack of consensus among researchers regarding the interpretations of experimental data on CSA activity in vitro, we have also attempted to provide additional clutter to this issue. Our approach was based on comparing CSA to 3'-azido-3'-deoxythymidine (AZT), which belongs to the same class of nucleoside immunosuppressants as azathioprine. Both drugs were tested side by side for the effect on immune function of lymphocytes and anti-HIV activity. The assays included monitoring proliferative responses to soluble antigens, i.e., lectins of plant origin PHA and Con A and microbial antigens Diphtheria toxin, Tetanus toxoid, and Candida albicans. Cell-mediated allogeneic immune reaction has been tested in mixed lymphocyte reaction. The least significant effect was observed with cells stimulated with pokeweed lectin: presumably this was due to the fact that PWM does not have a direct mitogenic effect on T lymphocytes. Both drugs displayed a smaller but still appreciable effect when tested for growth inhibition of T cell lines. In contrast to the observation by Karpas et al., no significant difference was observed when HIV+ or HIV- cell lines derived from the same parental line were compared for the dose-response to CSA.

Our results indicate AZT appears to act as CSA, i.e. as an immunosuppressor. This conclusion agrees well with publications suggesting the negative immunosuppressive aspect of AZT (90-92) but disagrees with the report indicating a 100-fold increase in CTL activity after AZT administration (93).

In agreement with earlier studies, both CSA and AZT were effective against *de novo* infection with cell-free virus, providing nearly complete protection at approximately 10^{-7} M. Cell-to-cell HIV transmission has been also prevented, albeit at higher doses. Based on end-point cytotoxic doses, 10^{-3} M and 10^{-5} M for AZT and CSA respectively, it can be concluded that in antiviral assays AZT has higher selective index against HIV.

Since AZT inhibits viral reverse transcription, a step preceding integration, the analysis of integrated HIV DNA formed 4 h postinfection has been carried out. The size and intensity of gag-specific bands has been reduced in CSA-treated cells indicating that this drug prevents proviral DNA formation. Results of the functional assay with viral polymerase enzyme suggest that CSA appears to act as an inhibitor of RT and the effect is comparable to that of AZT. Although CSA has been shown earlier to inhibit DNA and RNA polymerase activities (94,95), no reports describing specifically the anti-RT activity of CSA were found in the literature, and this observation should be confirmed in further studies.

Both drugs, CSA and AZT, demonstrated low efficacy in suppressing viral production in persistently infected T cell lines. When present the effect was correlated with the negative influence on cell growth. The differences between proliferative responses of peripheral lymphocytes and immortalized T lymphocytes were substantial. These results suggest that pharmacological doses of drugs required for controlling HIV RT might also suppress host DNA polymerase involved in the initiation of cell replication (96,97). Thus, the previously reported higher specificity of AZT against viral enzyme observed in infection assays using T cell lines may not hold true in the case of PBMC. It appears that *in vitro* the antiviral effect of both drugs, CSA and AZT, cannot be totally differentiated from the immunosuppressive and/or antiproliferative actions.

The results of our study add a new perception to the problems in the future. However, a major dilemma, revealed by earlier investigators in regard to the action of CSA, remains to be solved. What is more crucial: suppression of autoimmunity via anergy induction (98) or an antiviral effect? The evidence from HIV-positive patients who received organ transplants and were treated with CSA has been controversial. While some investigators warned that CSA therapy had worsened the status of patients, others suggested a better outcome. A third group of investigators cautiously alluded that no effect was observed. These conclusions, as legitimate as they can be, were biased either by small number of subjects in each study or by personal opinions regarding the controversial nature of CSA in immunocompromised patients. The follow-up study by Andrieu et al., published two years after the original study, imploring the autoimmune nature of HIV infection, was also inconclusive (99).

Clinical trials of CSA may provide an answer to the question of whether this mushroom-derived peptide may be of any worth. Based on unfortunate experiences with AZT, though, it is anticipated that CSA, a compound with very similar properties, will not provide a satisfactory solution. This notion is supported by follow-up studies on the low therapeutic benefit of CSA and AZT in the treatment of acquired immunodeficiency syndrome in mice infected with murine retrovirus (100).

FALLOUT OF APOPTOSIS

The first reference to apoptosis in relation to AIDS was made in 1986 by Kotler et al., (101). The last few years have witnessed an explosion of interest in apoptosis as a key to unlocking the mystery of depletion of CD4+ cells during HIV infection. Recent reports have suggested that activation-induced apoptosis of antigen-specific CD4+ T cells may lead ultimately to depletion of this T cell subset during HIV infection (reviewed in 102). Lymphocytes become activated when antigen receptors on the cell surface are cross-linked, or when they are exposed to agents that mimic this signal. Although such activation is usually associated with the production of immune mediators (e.g. antibodies, cytokines) and entry into the cell cycle, it can alternatively lead to death via apoptosis. This activation-induced apoptosis was first observed in developing thymocytes and has been proposed as a mechanism for negative selection, by which immature cells with potential for autoreactivity are eliminated. Activation-induced apoptosis has also been observed in normal, mature lymphocytes under some conditions, and this may account for the phenomena of peripheral depletion, in which mature T cells are eliminated upon exposure to high doses of antigen. This is supported by observations that apoptosis can be induced in the absence of viral infection by a simple cross-linking of CD4 with the viral envelope alone (103). It has been suggested that this can also be an important mechanism whereby CD4+ T cells are depleted in HIV+ individuals (104,105).

The wholesale tendency to replace the old-fashioned concept of the direct cytopathic effect of HIV with a trendy up-to-date explanation such as programmed cell death (which is presumably programmed by that same cytopathic virus) cannot withstand any serious critical scrutiny. There are several incongruities that appear to have no straightforward explanation in either of the opinions. Many, if not all, viral infections can cause some degree of death in lymphocytes of the host. Thus, it is not clear whether HIV-associated PCD is specific to this virus or it is a general phenomenon that always occurs in some proportion of lymphocytes upon any type of viral infection. It has been also noted that despite the occurrence of apoptosis among T cells of mice with MAIDS, their CD4+ T cells are not depleted during the course of disease. Thus, while apoptosis is a characteristic of both MAIDS and AIDS, CD4+ lymphocyte depletion is associated only with the progression of HIV infection (106). In humans the death of T cells was not quantitatively correlated with CD4+ T cell numbers or appearance of more cytopathic, syncytium-inducing HIV variants. Furthermore, the analysis of the phenotype of cells undergoing apoptosis revealed that cell death was not confined to a specific T cell subset nor correlated with expression of certain T cell activation markers. The extent of programmed cell death of T cells in HIV infection was not correlated with progression to disease. Higher incidence of apoptotic cells has been recorded in earlier stages of HIV infection before any decline in CD4+ cell numbers (107-109). On a purely intuitive basis one may infer that the dynamics of apoptosis, similar to what is observed in experimental studies in vitro, would correspond to an acute disease that will eliminate CD4 lymphocytes of the host within a week of time rather than years. However, the high incidence of apoptotic cells does not correlate with the slow depletion of CD4 cells that occurs over a period of <10 years. Taken together these discrepancies seem to indicate that despite the occurrence of HIV-related apoptosis this 'newly'-discovered phenomenon alone may not explain completely the progressive depletion of the CD4 helper T cell population and consequently the impairment of the immune system. In contrast, the slow cell death rate in AIDS fits better a model in which apoptosis is caused by cell-mediated killing carried out by autoreactive CTL.

IMMUNOPHARMACOLOGICAL MODULATION OF HIV-HOST COMPETITION

The evolution of HIV infection, i.e., the increase in viral burden is reciprocal to CD4+ lymphocyte depletion and reflects the failure of limiting virus growth by the CTL deprived of the helper effect of CD4+ lymphocytes. This mathematically simple population model, consisting of three basic elements, allows up to nine mutually non-exclusive outcomes that can cause an imbalance either of quantitative or qualitative nature. This relationship can become even more complex after inclusion of HIV-specific antibodies that can either enhance or neutralize the virus. However, in relation to the host or the virus the possible outcomes can be only positive (survival) or negative (death). Given the fact that infected humans die along with the virus one may assume that this imbalance is negative for both host and parasite. However, as HIV propagates faster than the slow-replicating host the virus has a definite advantage that allows exponential expansion and spread in the host population. An example of positive outcome for the host - which is, in essence, stabilizing Kimura-type selection - is what we observe in chimpanzees (110).

Multicellular metazoan structures such as humans are unified by cell-cell communications and will collapse if individual cells with abnormal expression are not promptly eliminated. This can be achieved either by necrosis or apoptosis (111). However, cell death is only the second stage of a two-step process. CTL are responsible for the initial stage. Given the fact that CTL activity is initiated and determined by the encounter of the first kind, i.e., cellular contact, one must find means that could prevent cell-cell interaction and the resulting disruption of the equilibrium caused by the self/non-self turmoil triggered by HIV. In the contrary case Darwinian laws will determine the fate of the metazoan host in the favor of the 'kamikaze' retrovirus.

Several drugs, mostly known in the past as immunomodulators, are capable to suppress CTL activity. Of particular interest are of course those that are clinically acceptable and can inhibit apoptosis and HIV infection. During the last few years we have identified few 'novel' pharmacological substances that seemed to satisfy these requirements and can be of potential interest in restoring and maintaining the immune homeostasis while serving as anti-HIV agents (see Table 1). These substances are not structurally related and they were not investigated before as inhibitors of HIV. The fact that these compounds manifested antiviral activity might have surprised us, if we did not know that they were related to each other by a common property in regard to down-modulation of CTL and consequently apoptotic events. For example, it is not a coincidence that indefinite allograft survival allowed by CSA treatment was correlated to the reduction of CTL in cellular infiltrates surrounding grafted tissue and inhibition of granzyme degranulation (112,113).

The inhibitors of proteases were known to be involved in regulation of CTL activity by suppressing the action of granzymes and ensuing DNA fragmentation (114). However, serine protease inhibitors can also inhibit HIV since binding capacity and infectivity of

Table 1. Immunopharmacological substances with multiple effects

Name	Action	CTL	PCD	HIV
AZT	DNA polymerase	↑↓	?	↓
Cyclosporin	immunosuppressor	↓	↓	↓
TLCK	serine protease	↓	↓	↓
Coumarins	protease	↓	↓	↓
Bestatin	aminopeptidase	↓	↓	↓
Progesterone	steroid hormone	↓	↓	↓
Estrogen	steroid hormone	↓	↓	↓
hCG	pregnancy hormone	↓	↓	↓

retroviruses depends on the cleavage of envelope glycoproteins believed to assure functional activation of viral fusion proteins (49,50). Without exception, all of the recently-reported 'alternative' HIV receptors are proteolytic enzymes located on the membrane of target cells. Among them are TL2 tryptase, subtilisin-type human endoprotease (furin), dipeptidyl peptidase IV (CD26), leucine aminopeptidase (CD13), thrombin-like protease, etc (115-120). At present, they are not fully characterized and we do not know which one is the most crucial for viral infectivity though one cannot exclude the possibility that HIV is a promiscuous virus. The latest evidence also suggests that even CD4, considered the main HIV receptor, appears to function as a protease since it cleaves gp120 (121). It is thus not surprising that various protease inhibitors that inhibit cell-mediated immunity and apoptosis can also inactivate HIV. Among those multifunctional molecules with demonstrated anti-HIV activity are peptidyl-chloromethylketones (TLCK) — irreversible inhibitors of serine proteases and CTL activity (122,123). Suicide substrates of serine proteases and poly-(ADP-ribose) polymerase belonging to the coumarin family are another example of agents with anti-HIV, anti-CTL, and anti-PCD activities (124-127).

In contrast to TLCK, coumarins are routinely used in clinics. For example, one of the coumarins with anti-HIV activity is warfarin, known as a potent thrombin inhibitor and thus used widely in treating coagulation disorders. Other coumarins have been used as potent immunomodulators in adjuvant therapy of malignancies. Clinical trials of some of these compounds are underway and the results will show whether such drugs are effective in treating HIV infection.

A similar but not identical mechanism has been shown for the antiviral action of sulfated and carboxylated polysaccharides such as dextran sulfate and aurintricarboxylic acid — potent inhibitors of virus-cell adsorption, cell-cell adhesion, CTL activity and known in clinics as anticoagulants (128-130). However, clinical trials of dextran sulfate with AIDS patients have been disappointing and had to be terminated due to an increase in viremia.

Bestatin, a small dipeptide derived from *Streptomyces olivoreticuli* and known as an inhibitor of aminopeptidases, is another anti-HIV substance with multiple effects. Our recent observations indicate that pharmacological levels of bestatin can inhibit cell-free and cell-mediated HIV spread (119). The administration of bestatin was associated with depression of NK and T cell-mediated responses. Oral formulations of bestatin have been employed in clinics as immunomodulating agents useful in cancer and AIDS therapy (131). Therapeutic application of bestatin in treating AIDS as a direct antiviral compound certainly deserves further exploration. Another category of immunomodulating molecules with known inhibitory effects on cell-mediated immunity and apoptosis are female steroid hormones, progesterone and estrogen (132). We have recently shown that physiological concentrations of these hormones can inhibit HIV replication (133). Corticosteroids have been successfully used by Andrieu et al. (personal communication) in treating HIV-infected patients. Thus, steroid-based therapy opens a new perspective in regarding and treating AIDS as an autoimmune disease caused by autoreactive CTL.

Human chorionic gonadotropin (hCG) is another pregnancy-associated hormone of interest. This immunomodulating glycoprotein is composed of two non-covalently bound α and β subunits. The amino acid sequence of α subunits of related gonadotropic hormones of the pituitary gland - follicle-stimulating hormone, luteinizing hormone, and thyrotropin - is identical, while the β chain is hormone-specific (134). The β monomer alone has no reproductive activity and can be found beyond pregnancy. The presence of βhCG-like substances is quite common among microorganisms, indicating that hCG may have been conserved throughout evolutionary history. Virulent strains of *Mycobacterium tuberculosis* species produce hCG-like molecules — an observation suggesting that they may act as natural immunosuppressors (135). βhCG is produced ectopically by various tumors affecting the testicles, stomach, liver, bladder, and kidney — possibly to prevent CTL-mediated tumor recognition. Although it is not well understood how hCG may regulate CTL reactivity and allogeneic reactions against cellular antigens in MLR or fetal transplant, there is a general consensus that hCG can modulate the function of immunocompetent cells and control apoptotic cell death (136,137). hCG is a ubiquitous molecule. Normal human lymphocytes can release hCG when in contact with lymphocytes from an HLA mismatched individual (138). Interestingly, hCG has been also reported to inhibit proteolytic activity of serine proteases (139).

We have investigated whether hCG can suppress viral production and viral transmission resulting from cell-cell contact between virus-carrying lymphocytes and target cells (140,141). It was found that inhibition of viral replication can been achieved at low physiological levels of hCG. Further investigations revealed that the β monomer, considered a physiologically inactive molecule, exhibits anti-HIV activity that is identical to the effect of the dimer (142). These results suggest that β hCG may represent an important, new class of natural antiviral substances free of hormonal side-effects. So far, the only other known antiviral glycoprotein produced in the human body is interferon, which in certain aspects appears to be related to the family of gonadotropins (F. Dianzani, personal communication). Based on the fact that hCG can be produced by normal lymphocytes it cannot be excluded that this veto molecule is indeed that same elusive molecule responsible for CTL-mediated non-lytic suppression of HIV replication reported earlier (39-41).

These quasi-serendipitous coincidences leading to the discovery of a series of anti-HIV substances across the whole range of seemingly unrelated compounds suggested to us that our approach, based on stressing the pivotal importance of cell-to-cell communication as a means of spreading virus as well as harnessing viral spread, may hold the key to the control of HIV disease. In the absence of effective therapy and new strategies against viral spread the immunopharmacological down-modulation of cell-mediated immunity against HIV-triggered apoptotic self-destruction is probably the only meaningful approach for the prevention and treatment of AIDS.

ACKNOWLEDGEMENTS

It is our pleasure to thank Caroline F. Coleman for editorial and moral assistance. This work was supported in part by grant from the NIH RO1 AI31343 and T32 AI07382. The financial assistance of New York State's Unemployment Office is also appreciated.

REFERENCES

1. Rosenau W, Moon HD. Lysis of homologous cells by sensitized lymphocytes in tissue culture. J Natl Cancer Inst 27:471-83, 1961.
2. Martz E. Early steps in specific tumor lysis by sensitized mouse T-lymphocytes I. Resolution and characterization. J Immunol 115:261-7, 1975.
3. Riviere Y, Tanneau-Salvadori F, Regnault A, Lopez O, Sansonetti P, Guy B, Kieny MP, Fournel JJ, Montagnier L. Human immunodeficiency virus-specific cytotoxic responses of seropositive individuals: distinct types of effector cells mediate killing of targets expressing gag and env proteins. J Virol 63:2270-7, 1989.
4. Weinhold KJ, Lyerly HK, Stanley SD, Austin AA, Matthews TJ, Bolognesi DP. HIV-1 GP120-mediated immune suppression and lymphocyte destruction in the absence of viral infection. J Immunol 142:3091-7, 1989.
5. Pircher H, Brduscha K, Steinhoff U, Kasai M, Mizuochi T, Zinkernagel RM, Hengartner H, Kyewski B, Muller KP. Tolerance induction by clonal deletion of CD4+8+ thymocytes in vitro does not require dedicated antigen-presenting cells. Eur J Immunol 23:669-74, 1993.
6. Vollenweider I, Groscurth P. Ultrastructure of cell mediated cytotoxicity. Electr Micr Rev 4:249-67, 1991.
7. Smyth MJ, Ortaldo JR. Mechanisms of cytotoxicity used by human peripheral blood CD4+ and CD8+ T cell subsets. The role of granule exocytosis. J Immunol 151:740-7, 1993.
8. Apasov S, Redegeld F, Sitkovsky M. Cell-mediated cytotoxicity: contact and secreted factors. Current Opinion Immunol 5:404-10, 1993.
9. Liu CC, Joag SV, Kwon BS, Young JD. Induction of perforin and serine esterases in a murine cytotoxic T lymphocyte clone. J Immunol 144:1196-201, 1990.
10. Pasternak MS, Eisen HN. A novel series esterase expressed by cytotoxic T lymphocytes. Nature 314:743-5, 1985.
11. Shi L, Kam CM, Powers JC, Aebersold R, Greenberg AH. Purification of three cytotoxic lymphocyte granule serine proteases that induce apoptosis through distinct substrate and target cell interactions. J Exp Med 176:1521-9, 1992.
12. Pasternack MS, Bleier KJ, McInerney TN. Granzyme A binding to target cell proteins. Granzyme A binds to and cleaves nucleolin in vitro. J Biol Chem 266:14703-8, 1991.
13. Bourinbaiar AS, Phillips DM. Transmission of human immunodeficiency virus from monocytes to epithelia. J Acquir Immune Defic Syndr 4:56-61, 1991.
14. Phillips DM, Bourinbaiar AS. Mechanism of HIV spread from lymphocytes to epithelial cells. Virology 186:261-73, 1992.
15. Bourinbaiar AS, Nagorny R. Human immunodeficiency virus type 1 infection of choriocarcinoma-derived trophoblasts. Acta Virol 37:21-8, 1993.
16. Ueno R, Kuno S. Dextran sulphate, a potent anti-HIV agent in vitro having synergism with zidovudine. Lancet 1:1379, 1987.
17. Bourinbaiar AS, Nagorny R. Association of anti-HIV-1 effect of dextran sulfate with prevention of lymphocyte-to-trophoblast adhesion. Immunol Infect Dis 2:245-7, 1992.
18. Hildreth JE, Orentas RJ. Involvement of a leukocyte adhesion receptor (LFA-1) in HIV-induced syncytium formation. Science 244:1075-8, 1989.
19. Kalter DC, Gendelman HE, Meltzer MS. Inhibition of human immunodeficiency virus infection in monocytes by monoclonal antibodies against leukocyte adhesion molecules. Immunol Lett 30:219-27, 1991.
20. Fecondo JV, Pavuk NC, Silburn KA, Read DM, Mansell AS, Boyd AW, McPhee DA. Synthetic peptide analogs of intercellular adhesion molecule 1 (ICAM-1) inhibit HIV-1 replication in MT-2 cells. AIDS Res Human Retrovir 9:733-40, 1993.
21. Cohen J. Will media reports KO upcoming real-life trials. Science 264:1660, 1994.
22. Barr M. HIV therapeutic vaccines: The next stage. Treatment Issues, 7:1-8, 1993.
23. Prince AM, Horowitz B, Baker L, Shulman RW, Ralph H, Valinsky J, Cundell A, Brotman B, Boehle W, Rey F, et al. Failure of a human immunodeficiency virus (HIV) immune globulin to protect chimpanzees against experimental challenge with HIV. Proc Natl Acad Sci USA 85:6944-8, 1988
24. Hu SL, Fultz PN, McClure HM, Eichberg JW, Thomas EK, Zarling J, Singhal MC, Kosowski SG, Swenson RB, Anderson DC, et al. Effect of immunization with a vaccinia-HIV env recombinant on HIV infection of chimpanzees. Nature 328:721-3, 1987.
25. Nara PL, Smit L, Dunlop N, Hatch W, Merges M, Waters D, Kelliher J, Gallo RC, Fischinger PJ, Goudsmit J. Emergence of viruses resistant to neutralization by V3-specific antibodies in experimental human immunodeficiency virus type 1 IIIB infection of chimpanzees. J Virol 64:3779-91, 1990.

26. Martinez-A C, Marcos MA, de la Hera A, Marquez C, Alonso JM, Toribio ML, Coutinho A. Immunological consequences of HIV infection: advantage of being low responder casts doubts on vaccine development. Lancet 1:454-7, 1988.

27. Sabin AB. HIV vaccination dilemma. Nature 362:212, 1993.

28. Veljkovic V, Metlas R. Potentially negative effects of AIDS vaccines based on recombinant viruses carrying HIV-1 derived envelope gene. A warning on AIDS vaccine development. Vaccine 11:291-2, 1993.

29. Kliks SC, Shioda T, Haigwood NL, Levy JA. V3 variability can influence the ability of an antibody to neutralize or enhance infection by diverse strains of human immunodeficiency virus type 1. Proc Natl Acad Sci USA 90:11518-22, 1993.

30. Levy JA. Pathogenesis of human immunodeficiency virus infection. Microbiol Reviews 57:183-289, 1993.

31. Sastry KJ, Nehete PN, Venkatnarayanan S, Morkowski J, Platsoucas CD, Arlinghaus RB. Rapid in vivo induction of HIV-specific CD8+ cytotoxic T lymphocytes by a 15-amino acid unmodified free peptide from the immunodominant V3-loop of GP120. Virology 188:502-9, 1992.

32. Riddell SR, Gilbert MJ, Greenberg PD. CD8+ cytotoxic T cell therapy of cytomegalovirus and HIV infection. Current Opinion Immunol 5:484-91, 1993.

33. Bagasra O, Pomerantz RJ. The role of CD8-positive lymphocytes in the control of HIV-1 infection of peripheral blood mononuclear cells. Immunol Lett 5:83-92, 1993.

34. Koup RA, Sullivan JL, Levine PH, Brettler D, Mahr A, Mazzara G, McKenzie S, Panicali D. Detection of major histocompatibility complex class I-restricted, HIV-specific cytotoxic T lymphocytes in the blood of infected hemophiliacs. Blood 73:1909-14, 1989

35. Mackewicz CE, Ortega HW, Levy JA. CD8+ cell anti-HIV activity correlates with the clinical state of the infected individual. J Clin Invest 87:1462-6, 1991.

36. Langlade-Demoyen P, Ngo-Giang-Huong N, Ferchal F, Oksenhendler E. Human immunodeficiency virus (HIV) nef-specific cytotoxic T lymphocytes in noninfected heterosexual contact of HIV-infected patients. J Clin Invest 93:1293-7, 1994

37. Clerici M, Levin JM, Kessler HA, Harris A, Berzofsky JA, Landay AL, Shearer GM. HIV-specific T-helper activity in seronegative health care workers exposed to contaminated blood. JAMA 271:42-6, 1994.

38. Martz E. Can CTL control virus infections without cytolysis? The prelytic halt hypothesis. In: Sitkovsky MV, Henkart PA, eds. Cytotoxic cells. Recognition, Effector Function, Generation, and Methods. Birkhauser, Boston, 501-15, 1993.

39. Tsubota H, Lord CI, Watkins DI, Morimoto C, Letvin NL. A cytotoxic T lymphocyte inhibits acquired immunodeficiency syndrome virus replication in peripheral blood lymphocytes. J Exp Med 169:1421-34, 1989.

40. Brinchmann JE, Gaudernack G, Vartdal F. CD8+ T cells inhibit HIV replication in naturally infected CD4+ T cells. Evidence for a soluble inhibitor. J Immunol 144:2961-6, 1990.

41. Wiviott LD. Walker CM. Levy JA. CD8+ lymphocytes suppress HIV production by autologous CD4+ cells without eliminating the infected cells from culture. Cell Immunol 128:628-34, 1990.

42. Tenner-Racz K, Racz P, Thome C, Meyer CG, Anderson PJ, Schlossman SF, Letvin NL. Cytotoxic effector cell granules recognized by the monoclonal antibody TIA-1 are present in CD8+ lymphocytes in lymph nodes of human immunodeficiency virus-1-infected patients. Am J Pathol 142:1750-8, 1993. 43. Devergne O, Peuchmaur M, Crevon MC, Trapani JA, Maillot MC, Galanaud P, Emilie D. Activation of cytotoxic cells in hyperplastic lymph nodes from HIV-infected patients. AIDS 5:1071-9, 1991.

44. Laman JD, Claassen E, Van Rooijen N, Boersma WJ. Immune complexes on follicular dendritic cells as a target for cytolytic cells in AIDS. AIDS 3:543-4, 1989.

45. Bollinger RC, Quinn TC, Liu AY, Stanhope PE, Hammond SA, Viveen R, Clements ML, Siliciano RF. Cytokines from vaccine-induced HIV-1 specific cytotoxic T lymphocytes: effects on viral replication. AIDS Res Human Retrovir 9:1067-77, 1993.

46. Harrer T, Jassoy C, Harrer E, Johnson RP, Walker BD. Induction of HIV-1 replication in a chronically infected T-cell line by cytotoxic T lymphocytes. J Acquir Immune Defic Syndr 6:865-71, 1993.

47. Kobayashi N, Hamamoto Y, Yamamoto N. Production of tumor necrosis factors by human T cell lines infected with HTLV-1 may cause their high susceptibility to human immunodeficiency virus infection. Med Microbiol Immunol 179:115-22, 1990.

48. Toth FD, Mosborg-Petersen P, Kiss J, Aboagye-Mathiesen G, Zdravkovic M, Hager H, Ebbesen P. Differential replication of human immunodeficiency virus type 1 in CD8- and CD8+ subsets of natural killer cells: relationship to cytokine production pattern. J Virol 67:5879-88, 1993.

49. Andersen KB. Cleavage fragments of the retrovirus surface protein gp70 during virus entry. J Gen Virol 68:2193-202, 1987.

50. McCune JM, Rabin LB, Feinberg MB, Lieberman M, Kosek JC, Reyes GR, Weissman IL. Endopro-teolytic cleavage of gp160 is required for the activation of human immunodeficiency virus. Cell 53:55-67, 1988.

51. Vuillier F, Bianco NE, Montagnier L, Dighiero G. Selective depletion of low-density CD8+, CD16+ lymphocytes during HIV infection. AIDS Res Human Retrovir 4:121-9, 1988.

52. Mansour I, Doinel C, Rouger P. CD16+ NK cells decrease in all stages of HIV infection through a selective depletion of the CD16+CD8+CD3- subset. AIDS Res Human Retrovir 6:1451-7, 1990.

53. Carmichael A, Jin X, Sissons P, Borysiewicz L. Quantitative analysis of the human immunodeficiency virus type 1 (HIV-1)-specific cytotoxic T lymphocyte (CTL) response at different stages of HIV-1 infection: differential CTL responses to HIV-1 and Epstein-Barr virus in late disease. J Exp Med 77:249-56, 1993.

54. De Maria A, Pantaleo G, Schnittman SM, Greenhouse JJ, Baseler M, Orenstein JM, Fauci AS. Infection of CD8+ T lymphocytes with HIV. Requirement for interaction with infected CD4+ cells and induction of infectious virus from chronically infected CD8+ cells. J Immunol 146:2220-6, 1991.

55. Mercure L, Phaneuf D, Wainberg MA. Detection of unintegrated human immunodeficiency virus type 1 DNA in persistently infected CD8+ cells. J Gen Virol 74:2077-83, 1993.

56. Bell SJ, Cooper DA, Kemp BE, Doherty RR, Penny R. CD8+ T-cells from HIV-infected patients can either augment or abrogate HIV-specific lymphoproliferation. Clin Immunol Immunopathol 64:254-60, 1992.

57. Gruters RA, Terpstra FG, De Jong R, Van Noesel CJ, Van Lier RA, Miedema F. Selective loss of T cell functions in different stages of HIV infection. Early loss of anti-CD3-induced T cell proliferation followed by decreased anti-CD3-induced cytotoxic T lymphocyte generation in AIDS-related complex and AIDS. Eur J Immunol 20:1039-44, 1990.

58. Sirianni MC, Tagliaferri F, Aiuti F. Pathogenesis of the natural killer cell deficiency in AIDS. Immunol Today 11:81-2, 1990

59. Henderson LA, Qureshi NM, Rasheed S, Garry R. Human immunodeficiency virus-induced cytotoxicity for CD8 cells from some normal donors and virus-specific induction of a suppressor factor. Clin Immunol Immunopathol 48:174-86, 1988.

60. Muller C, Kukel S, Bauer R. Relationship of antibodies against CD4+ T cells in HIV-infected patients to markers of activation and progression: autoantibodies are closely associated with CD4 cell depletion. Immunology 79:248-54, 1993.

61. Callahan LN, Roderiquez G, Mallinson M, Norcross MA. Analysis of HIV-induced autoantibodies to cryptic epitopes on human CD4. J Immunol 149:2194-202, 1992.

62. Debure A, Chkoff N, Chatenoud L, Lacombe M, Campos H, Noel LH, Goldstein G, Bach JF, Kreis H. One-month prophylactic use of OKT3 in cadaver kidney transplant recipients. Transplantation 45:546-53, 1988.

63. Wee SL, Stroka DM, Preffer FI, Jolliffe LK, Colvin RB, Cosimi AB. The effects of OKT4A monoclonal antibody on cellular immunity of nonhuman primate renal allograft recipients. Transplantation 53:501-7, 1992.

64. Aksentijevich I, Sachs DH, Sykes M. Humoral tolerance in xenogeneic BMT recipients conditioned by a nonmyeloablative regimen. Transplantation. 53:1108-14, 1992.

65. Chatenoud L, Thervet E, Primo J, Bach JF. Anti-CD3 antibody induces long-term remission of overt autoimmunity in nonobese diabetic mice. Proc Natl Acad Sci USA 91:123-7, 1994.

66. Sharpe RJ, Schweizer RT. The LAV/HTLV-III virus may evade elimination by the immune system by inducing low zone tolerance to itself. Med Hypoth 20:421-7, 1986.

67. Ascher MS, Sheppard HW. AIDS as immune system activation. II. The panergic imnesia hypothesis. J Acquir Immune Defic Syndr 3:177-91, 1990.

68. Marker O, Thomsen AR. T-cell effector function and unresponsiveness in the murine lymphocytic choriomeningitis virus infection. I. On the mechanism of a selective suppression of the virus-specific delayed-type hypersensitivity response. Scand J Immunol 24:127-35, 1986

69. Moskophidis D, Lechner F, Pircher H, Zinkernagel RM. Virus persistence in acutely infected immuno-competent mice by exhaustion of antiviral cytotoxic effector T cells. Nature 362:758-61, 1993.

70. Bogner JR, Matuschke A, Heinrich B, Schreiber MA, Nerl C, Goebel FD. Expansion of activated T lymphocytes (CD3 + HLA/DR +) detectable in early stages of HIV-1 infection. Klin Wochenschrift 68:393-6, 1990.

71. Groux H, Torpier G, Monte D, Mouton Y, Capron A, Ameisen JC. Activation-induced death by apoptosis in CD4+ T cells from human immunodeficiency virus-infected asymptomatic individuals. J Exp Med 175:331-40, 1992.

72. Ferrari G, Ottinger J, Place C, Nigida SM Jr, Arthur LO, Weinhold KJ. The impact of HIV-1 infection on phenotypic and functional parameters of cellular immunity in chimpanzees. AIDS Res Human Retrovir 9:647-56, 1993.

73. Van Eendenburg JP, Yagello M, Girard M, Kieny MP, Lecocq JP, Muchmore E, Fultz PN, Riviere Y, Montagnier L, Gluckman JC. Cell-mediated immune proliferative responses to HIV-1 of chimpanzees vaccinated with different vaccinia recombinant viruses. AIDS Res Human Retrovir 5:41-50, 1989.

74. Zarling JM, Ledbetter JA, Sias J, Fultz P, Eichberg J, Gjerset G, Moran PA. HIV-infected humans, but not chimpanzees, have circulating cytotoxic T lymphocytes that lyse uninfected CD4+ cells. J Immunol 144:2992-8, 1990.

75. Schuitemaker H, Meyaard L, Kootstra NA, Dubbes R, Otto SA, Tersmette M, Heeney JL, Miedema F. Lack of T cell dysfunction and programmed cell death in human immunodeficiency virus type 1-infected chimpanzees correlates with absence of monocytotropic variants. J Infect Dis 168:1140-7,1993.

76. Saxinger C, Alter HJ, Eichberg JW, Fauci AS, Robey WG, Gallo RC. Stages in the progression of HIV infection in chimpanzees. AIDS Res Human Retrovir 3:375-85, 1987.

77. Gibbs CJ Jr, Peters R, Gravell M, Johnson BK, Jensen FC, Carlo DJ, Salk J. Observations after human immunodeficiency virus immunization and challenge of human immunodeficiency virus seropositive and seronegative chimpanzees. Proc Natl Acad Sci USA 88:3348-52, 1991.

78. Castro BA, Homsy J, Lennette E, Murthy KK, Eichberg JW, Levy JA. HIV expression in chimpanzees can be activated by CD8+ cell depletion or CMV infection. Clin Immunol Immunopathol 65:227-33, 1992.

79. Husch B, Eibl MM, Mannhalter JW. CD3, CD8 double-positive cells from HIV-1-infected chimpanzees show group-specific inhibition of HIV-1 replication. AIDS Res Human Retrovir 9:405-13, 1993.

80. Andrieu JM, Even P, Venet A, Tourani JM, Stern M, Lowenstein W, Androin C, Erne D, Masson D, Sors H, Israel-Biet D, Beldjord K. Effects of cyclosporin on T-cell subsets in human immunodeficiency virus disease. Clin. Immunol. Immunopathol. 47:181-98, 1988.

81. Klatzmann D, Laporte JP, Achour A, Brisson E, Gruest J, Montagnier L, Gluckman JC. Cyclosporine A treatment for human immunodeficiency virus-infected transplant recepients. Transplant Proc 19:1828, 1987.

82. Wainberg MA, Dascal A, Blain N, Fitz-Gibbon L, Boulerice F, Numazaki K, Tremblay M. The effect of cyclosporine A on infection of susceptible cells by human immunodeficiency virus type 1. Blood 72:1904-10, 1988.

83. Sawada M, Suzumura A, Marunouchi T, Down regulation of CD4 expression in cultured microglia by immunosuppressants and lipopolysaccharide. Biochem Biophys Res Comm 189:869-76, 1992.

84. Ameisen JC, Capron A. Cell dysfunction and depletion in AIDS: the programmed cell death hypothesis. Immunol Today 12:102-5, 1991.

85. Amendola A, Lombardi G, Oliverio S, Colizzi V, Piacentini M. HIV-1 gp120-dependent induction of apoptosis in antigen-specific human T cell clones is characterized by 'tissue' transglutaminase expression and prevented by cyclosporin A. FEBS Lett 339:258-64, 1994.

86. Karpas A, Lowdell M, Jacobson SK, Hill F. Inhibition of human immunodeficiency virus and growth of infected T cells by the immunosuppressive drugs cyclosporin A and FK 506. Proc Natl Acad Sci USA 89:8351-5, 1992.

87. Bell KD, Ramilo O, Vitetta ES. Combined use of an immunotoxin and cyclosporine to prevent both activated and quiescent peripheral blood T cells from producing type 1 human immunodeficiency virus. Proc Natl Acad Sci USA 90:1411-5, 1993.

88. Luban J, Bossolt KL, Franke EK, Kalpana GV, Goff SP. Human immunodeficiency virus type 1 Gag protein binds to cyclophilins A and B. Cell 73:1067-78, 1993.

89. Polacino PS, Liang HA, Firpo EJ, Clark EA. T-cell activation influences initial DNA synthesis of simian immunodeficiency virus in resting T lymphocytes from macaques. J Virol 67:7008-16, 1993.

90. Tindall B, Carr A, Goldstein D, Penny R, Cooper DA. Administration of zidovudine during primary HIV-1 infection may be associated with a less vigorous immune response. AIDS 7:127-8, 1993.

91. Stine KC, Tyler DS, Stanley SD, Bartlett JA, Bolognesi DP, Weinhold KJ. The effect of AZT on in vitro lymphokine-activated killer (LAK) activity in human immunodeficiency virus type-1 (HIV-1) infected individuals. Cell Immunol 136:165-72, 1991

92. Ascher MS, Sheppard HW. The panergic imnesia hypothesis. Part I: Update of current findings. In: Montagnier L, Gougeon M-L, eds. New concepts in AIDS pathogenesis. Marcel Dekker, New York, 291-9, 1993.

93. Dadaglio G, Michel F, Langlade-Demoyen P, Sansonetti P, Chevrier D, Vuillier F, Plata F, Hoffenbach A. Enhancement of HIV-specific cytotoxic T lymphocyte responses by zidovudine (AZT) treatment. Clin Exp Immunol 87:7-14, 1992.

94. Brack C, Mattaj IW, Gautschi J, Cammisuli S. Cyclosporin A is a differential inhibitor of eukaryotic RNA polymerases. Exp Cell Res 151:314-21, 1984.

95. Mahajan PB, Thompson, EA, Jr. Cyclosporin A inhibits rDNA transcription in lymphosarcoma P1798 cells. J Biol Chem 262:16150-6, 1987.

96. Copeland WC, Chen MS, Wang TS. Human DNA polymerase alpha and beta are able to incorporate anti-HIV deoxynucleotides into DNA. J Biol Chem 267:21495-4,1992.

97. Lacey SF, Reardon JR, Furfine JE, Kunkel ES, Bebenek K, Eckert KA, Kemp SD, Larder BA. Biochemical studies on the reverse transcriptase and RNase H activities from human immunodeficiency virus strains resistant to 3'-azido-3'- deoxythymidine. J Biol Chem 267:15789-94, 1992.

98. Yasutomi D, Odaka C, Saito S, Niizeki H, Kizaki H, Tadakuma T. Inhibition of programmed cell death by cyclosporin A; preferential blocking of cell death induced by signals via TCR/CD3 complex and its mode of action. Immunology 77:68-74, 1992.

99. Andrieu JM, Even P, Tourani JM, Beldjord K, Audroin C. Result of a 2-year exploratory study with cyclosporin A in human immunodeficiency virus infection. In: Andrieu JM, Bach JF, Even P, eds. Autoimmune aspects of HIV infection. London: Royal Society of Medicine Services Ltd. 191-4, 1988.

100. Cerny A, Merino R, Fossati L, de Cossodo S, Heusser C, Waldvogel FA, Morse III HC, Izui S. Effect of cyclosporin A and zidovudine on immune abnormalities observed in the murine acquired immunodeficiency syndrome. J Infect Dis 166:285-90, 1992.

101. Kotler DP, Weaver SC, Terzakis JA. Ultrastructural features of epithelial cell degeneration in rectal crypts of patients with AIDS. Am J Surg Pathol 10:531-8, 1986.

102. Gougeon ML, Laurent-Crawford AG, Hovanessian AG, Montagnier L. Direct and indirect mechanisms mediating apoptosis during HIV infection: contribution to in vivo CD4 T cell depletion. Sem Immunol 5:187-94, 1993.

103. Oyaizu N, McCloskey TW, Coronesi M, Chirmule N, Kalyanaraman VS, Pahwa S. Accelerated apoptosis in peripheral blood mononuclear cells (PBMCs) from human immunodeficiency virus type-1 infected patients and in CD4 cross-linked PBMCs from normal individuals. Blood 82:3392-400, 1993.

104. Gougeon ML, Garcia S, Heeney J, Tschopp R, Lecoeur H, Guetard D, Rame V, Dauguet C, Montagnier L. Programmed cell death in AIDS-related HIV and SIV infections. AIDS Res Human Retrovir 9:553-63, 1993

105. Gougeon ML, Colizzi V, Dalgleish A, Montagnier L. New concepts in AIDS pathogenesis. AIDS Res Human Retrovir 9:287-9, 1993.

106. Cohen DA, Fitzpatrick EA, Barve SS, Guthridge JM, Jacob RJ, Simmerman L, Kaplan AM. Activation-dependent apoptosis in CD4+ T cells during murine AIDS. Cell Immunol 151:392-403, 1993.

107. Meyaard L, Otto SA, Keet IP, Roos MT, Miedema F. Programmed death of T cells in human immunodeficiency virus infection. No correlation with progression to disease. J Clin Invest 93:982-8, 1994.

108. Meyaard L, Otto SA, Jonker RR, Mijnster MJ, Keet RP, Miedema F. Programmed death of T cells in HIV-1 infection. Science 257:217-9, 1992.

109. Mahalingam M, Peakman M, Davies ET, Pozniak A, McManus TJ, Vergani D. T cell activation and disease severity in HIV infection. Clin Exp Immunol 93:337-43, 1993.

110. Kimura M. Evolutionary rate at the molecular level. Nature 217:624-6, 1968.

111. Zychlinsky A, Zheng LM, Liu CC, Young JD. Cytolytic lymphocytes induce both apoptosis and necrosis in target cells. J Immunol 146:393-400, 1991.

112. Chen RH, Ivens KW, Alpert S, Billingham ME, Fathman CG, Flavin TF, Shizuru JA, Starnes VA, Weissman IL, Griffiths GM. The use of granzyme A as a marker of heart transplant rejection in cyclosporine or anti-CD4 monoclonal antibody-treated rats. Transplantation 55:146-53, 1993.

113. Forrest MJ, Jewell ME, Koo GC, Sigal NH. FK-506 and cyclosporin A: selective inhibition of calcium ionophore-induced polymorphonuclear leukocyte degranulation. Biochem Pharmacol 42:1221-8, 1991.

114. Hudig D, Powers JC. Use of protease inhibitors as probes for biological functions: Conditions, controls, and caveats. In: Sitkovsky MV, Henkart PA, eds. Cytotoxic cells. Recognition, Effector Function, Generation, and Methods. Birkhauser, Boston, 501-15, 1993.

115. Kido H, Fukutomi A, Katunuma N. Tryptase TL2 in the membrane of human T4+ lymphocytes is a novel binding protein of the V3 domain of HIV-1 envelope glycoprotein gp 120. FEBS Lett 286:233-6, 1991.

116. Hallenberger S, Bosch V, Angliker H, Shaw E, Klenk H-D, Garten W. Inhibition of cleavage activation of HIV-1 glycoprotein gp160. Nature 360:358-361, 1992.

117. Callebaut C, Krust B, Jacotot E, Hovanessian AG. T cell activation antigen, CD26, as a cofactor for entry of HIV in CD4+ cells. Science 262:2045-50, 1993.

118. Johnson ME, Lin Z, Padmanabhan K, Tulinsky A, Kahn M. Conformational rearrangements required of the V3 loop of HIV-1 gp120 for proteolytic cleavage and infection. FEBS Lett 337:4-8, 1994.

119. Bourinbaiar AS, Lee-Huang S, Krasinski K, Borkowsky W. Inhibitory effect of the oral immune response modifier, bestatin, on cell-mediated and cell-free HIV infection in vitro. Biomed Pharmacother 48:55-61, 1994.

120. Bourinbaiar AS, Nagorny R. Effect of serine protease inhibitor, N-α-tosyl-L-lysyl-chloromethylketone (TLCK), on cell-mediated and cell-free HIV-1 spread. Cell Immunol 155:230-6, 1994.

121. Werner A, Levy JA. Human immunodeficiency virus type 1 envelope gp120 is cleaved after incubation with recombinant soluble CD4. J Virol 67:2566-74, 1993.

122. Chang WT, Eisen H. Effects of N-α-tosyl-L-lysyl-chloromethyl- ketone on the activity of cytotoxic T lymphocytes. J Immunol 124:1028-32, 1980.

123. Pasternack MS, Sitkovsky MV, Eisen HN. The site of action of N-α-tosyl-L-lysyl-chloromethyl-ketone (TLCK) on cloned cytotoxic T lymphocytes. J Immunol 131:2477-83, 1983.

124. Redegeld FA, Chatterjee S, Berger NA, Sitkovsky MV. Poly-(ADP-ribose) polymerase partially contributes to target cell death triggered by cytolytic T lymphocytes. J Immunol 149:3509-16, 1992.

125. Kashman Y, Gustafson KR, Fuller RW, Cardellina JH 2d, McMahon JB, Currens MJ, Buckheit RW Jr, Hughes SH, Cragg GM, Boyd MR. The calanolides, a novel HIV-inhibitory class of coumarin derivatives from the tropical rainforest tree, Calophyllum lanigerum J Med Chem 35:2735-43, 1992.

126. Bourinbaiar AS, Tan X, Nagorny R. Effect of the oral anticoagulant, warfarin, on HIV-1 replication and spread. AIDS 7:129-30, 1993.

127. Bourinbaiar AS, Tan X, Nagorny R. Inhibitory effect of coumarins on HIV replication and cell-mediated or cell-free viral infection. Acta Virol 37:241-50, 1993.

128. Jozefonvicz J, Jozefowicz M. Interactions of biospecific functional polymers with blood proteins and cells. J Biomater Sci Polymer Ed 1:147-65, 1990.

129. Cushman M, Wang PL, Chang SH, Wild C, De Clercq E, Schols D, Goldman ME, Bowen JA. Preparation and anti-HIV activities of aurintricarboxylic acid fractions and analogues: direct correlation of antiviral potency with molecular weight. J Med Chem 34:329-37, 1991.

130. Helgason CD, Shi L, Greenberg AH, Shi Y, Bromley P, Cotter TG, Green DR, Bleackley RC. DNA fragmentation induced by cytotoxic T lymphocytes can result in target cell death. Exp Cell Res 206:302-10, 1993.

131. Bruley-Rosset M, Payelle B, Rappaport H. Acceleration of age-associated immune decline and mortality by early repeated administration of bestatin to C57BL/6 mice. J Biol Response Mod 5:176-90, 1986.

132. Gerschenson LE, Rotello RJ. Apoptosis and cell proliferation are terms of the growth equation. In: Tomei LD, Cope FO, eds. Apoptosis: The Molecular Basis of Cell Death. Cold Spring harbor Laboratory Press, Cold Spring Harbor, NY, 175-92, 1991.

133. Bourinbaiar AS, Nagorny R, Tan X. Pregnancy hormones, estrogen and progesterone, prevent HIV-1 synthesis in monocytes but not in lymphocytes. FEBS Lett 302:206-8, 1992.

134. Pierce JG. Eli Lilly lecture: The subunits of pituitary thyrotropin - their relationships to other glycoprotein hormones. Endocrinol. 89:1331, 1971.

135. Affronti LF, DeBlaker DF. Immunological detection of hCG-like substances in aerobic bacteria of both tumour and non-tumour origin. Microbios 48:173, 1986.

136. Maghnie M, Valtorta A, Moretta A, Priora C, Preti P. Effetto della terapia con gonadotropina corionica (hCG) sul sistema immunitario. Medicina 10:148-9, 1990.

137. Tapanainen JS, Tilly JL, Vihko KK, Hsueh AJ. Hormonal control of apoptotic cell death in the testis: gonadotropins and androgens as testicular cell survival factors. Mol Endocrinol 7:643-50, 1993

138. Harbour-McMenamin D, Smith EM, Blalock JE. Production of immunoreactive chorionic gonadotropin during mixed lymphocyte reactions: a possible selective mechanism for genetic diversity. Proc Natl Acad Sci USA 83:6834-38, 1986.

139. Milwidsky A, Finci-Yeheskel Z, Yagel S, Mayer M. Gonadotropin- mediated inhibition of proteolytic enzymes produced by human trophoblast in culture. J Clin Endocrinol Metabol 76:1101-5, 1993.

140. Bourinbaiar AS, Nagorny R. Effect of human chorionic gonadotropin (hCG) on reverse transcriptase activity in HIV-1 infected lymphocytes and monocytes. FEMS Microbiol Lett 96:27- 30, 1992.

141. Bourinbaiar AS, Nagorny R. Inhibitory effect of human chorionic gonadotropin (hCG) on HIV-1 transmission from lymphocytes to trophoblasts. FEBS Lett 309:82-4, 1992

142. Bourinbaiar AS, Lee-Huang S. Anti-HIV effect of beta subunit of human chorionic gonadotropin (βhCG) in vitro. Immunology Lett 44:13-18, 1995.

8

THE ROLE OF SURFACE CD4 IN HIV-INDUCED APOPTOSIS

Jacques Corbeil[*1] and Douglas D. Richman[1,2]

[1] University of California San Diego
Departments of Medicine and Pathology
La Jolla, California 92093-0679
[2] San Diego Veterans Affairs Medical Center
San Diego, California

INTRODUCTION

The decline in CD4+ T lymphocytes is one of the hallmarks of HIV infection (Levy, 1993; Rosenberg and Fauci,1991; Stein et al.,1992). A number of studies have found that the level of virus replication in asymptomatic infection is greater than previously thought and HIV may directly account for a significant proportion of the CD4+ T cell depletion seen in AIDS (Embretson et al., 1993; Pantaleo et al. 1993; Piatak et al.,1993; Scadden et al., 1992). HIV-induced apoptosis may be an important contributor to this depletion. Several mechanisms have been proposed to explain how HIV-1 infection may lead to apoptotic cell death (Ameisen and Capron,1991; Banda et al.,1992; Gougeon et al., 1993a; Groux et al., 1992; Laurent-Crawford et al., 1991; Meyaard et al., 1992; Terai et al.,1991); however, some uncertainty remains concerning the conditions that trigger this process and if the target cells needs to be HIV-infected (Ameisen, 1992; Cohen, 1993; Gougeon et al., 1993b; Gougeon and Montagnier, 1993; Weiss, 1993).

The limitation of certain experimental approaches and their interpretation has lead to some confusion with respect to the contribution of apoptosis in CD4+ T cells depletion seen in AIDS. The analysis of cells cultured from HIV-infected individuals may contribute to this confusion because other variables apart from HIV may impact on the extent of apoptosis. Ex vivo cultures of lymphocytes obtained from HIV-infected individuals are more susceptible to both spontaneous and activation-induced apoptosis than their normal counterparts (Ameisen. 1994). However, it should be noted that in any acute infection, for example infectious mononucleosis, cultured cells have a greater tendency to die spontaneously in culture (Uehara et al. 1992). This process is not specific to CD4+ T cells.

---

[*] Corresponding author: Dr. Jacques Corbeil, Departments of Medicine and Pathology, University of California San Diego, Clinical Science Building Room 325, 9500 Gilman Drive, La Jolla, California 92093-0679, U.S.A. Ph: (619) 552-7439; Fax: (619) 552-7445; E-Mail: jcorbeil@ucsd.edu.us.

Cell Activation and Apoptosis in HIV Infection
Edited by Jean-Marie Andrieu and Wei Lu, Plenum Press, New York, 1995

Cytotoxic CD8+ T cells activated by the disease state compose a sizeable fraction of cells which are eliminated by apoptosis. The fate of activated CD8+ T cells is to die by apoptosis in a relatively short time span, thereby preventing any deleterious effects to occur. This phenomenon is therefore not specific to AIDS pathogenesis (Carbonari et al. 1994). Furthermore, the activation signals used to induce apoptosis impact on the extent of apoptosis that can be detected. For example, PHA (10 μg/ml) readily stimulates the cells obtained from asymptomatic individuals (where most cells are not infected) to proliferate without causing apoptosis. On the other hand, with the same conditions, the use of PMA triggers apoptosis (Groux et al. 1991).

HIV-1 envelope protein gp120 alone does not cause apoptosis in an uninfected cell. To induce apoptosis of an uninfected cell requires gp120, cross-linking antibodies to gp120, and further crosslinking of gp120 and anti-gp120 antibody complexes with a secondary antibody (Banda et al.1992). This treatment still does not result in apoptosis without the addition of an anti-TCR antibody. These conditions would not occur in vivo.

Lastly, it should be noted that PBMC obtained from HIV-infected individuals in order to conduct ex vivo experiments represent populations of cells that have survived pathogenic processes, and have adapted to the presence of chronic antigenic stimulation, as well as other manifestations of the disease particularly cytokines dysregulation.

Our premise is that if signaling events alone explained CD4+ T cell depletion, HIV infection would not be a chronic process. Signaling events would be expected to rapidly deplete available CD4+ T cells, as susceptible cells, virions and antibodies to viral proteins are constantly circulating in abundant concentrations. Apoptosis is not a protracted phenomenon, when it is induced the cell is dead within 24 hours and phagocytosed by scavenger cells rapidly (Fadok et al. 1992). Furthermore, there is accumulating evidence that CD4 cell numbers correlate inversely with levels of plasma HIV RNA as suggested by ongoing antiretroviral therapy clinical trials (Lin et al. 1994).

HIV-infected CD4+ T cells probably represent the greater proportion of cells which undergo apoptosis in vivo. The balance between renewal and depletion tips toward the slow but progressive CD4 T cell reduction seen in AIDS. We propose that HIV infection induces a pre-apoptotic state in CD4+ T cells rendering them susceptible to apoptosis when reencountering either HIV or its cognate antigen (Corbeil et al. in press., Rey-Cuille et al. 1994, Schwartz et al., 1994). This requirement for HIV infection may explain the slow decline of CD4+ T cells in HIV-infected individuals.

In this review, we shall first describe some mechanisms shown to induce apoptosis by HIV and argue that the virus may utilize strategies to delay this process in order to optimize its propagation.

HOW HIV INFLUENCES T CELL RESPONSE TO STIMULATION?

Figure 1 illustrates some of the choices a CD4 T cell faces when encountering a stimulus. Choice A depicts the normal interaction between an antigen-presenting cell (APC) and a CD4+ T cell whereby presentation of an antigen in the context of class II MHC with the appropriate co-stimulatory signals (The interaction of B7-CD28 with the presence of IL-2) results in activation of the CD4+ T cell and its clonal expansion. Most effector cells are destined to die by apoptosis at a later time, and only a small fraction will become memory (CD45 RO+) T cells and persist. In the absence of the co-stimulatory signals (choice B), an anergic state is established such that the cell is no longer responsive to normal external stimuli. This state may persist and even be reversed but the duration has not been determined (range a few hours to months) and may eventually lead to apoptosis (apoptosis by neglect or default apoptosis) (Lenschow et al. 1993., Rocha et al. 1993.). Choice C illustrates a

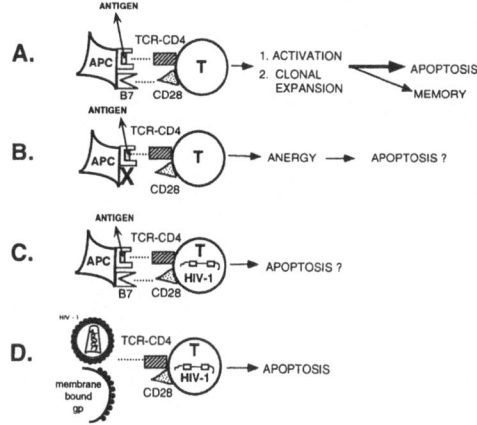

Figure 1. CD4+ T cell choices upon encountering HIV-1.

normal presentation to a HIV-infected T cell that in this particular case may result in apoptosis. This option has not been formally demonstrated yet. Some evidence has been gathered to validate the scenario presented in choice D. In this case, a HIV-infected T cell undergoes apoptosis when rechallenged through the CD4 receptor either by the virus alone or by another infected T cell with expressed gp120 on its cell surface.

HOW DOES HIV TRIGGER APOPTOSIS?

The CD4 signal transduction pathway is most probably involved in triggering HIV-induced apoptosis. The possibility for aberrant signal transduction due to multimerization of the CD4 receptor has been postulated (Schwartz et al. 1994; Laurent-Crawford et al. 1993a) which would either prevent further signaling or deliver an inadequate signal. The details of the intracellular signaling events initiated by such multimerization have not elucidated. HIV-induced apoptosis could be triggered by a CD4-mediated signal to a HIV-infected cell which is interpreted as inappropriate (Corbeil et al. in press). These two possibilities are not mutually exclusive. The propensity of a target cell to undergo apoptosis seemed to correlate with the amount of surface expression of the CD4 receptor. The ability to generate chronically HIV-infected cell lines may reflect this resistance to apoptosis (Nishino et al. 1994). For example, it is difficult to generate a CD4+ T cell line producing high levels of virus and which still express CD4 on the cell surface even with HIV-1 lacking the nef gene. Furthermore, HTLV-1 transformed CD4+ T cell lines such as MT-2 and C8166-45 are excellent cell lines to grow the virus to high titer for prolonged period of time possibly because these cell lines have no competent CD4 transduction pathways due to the lack of functional p56[lck] protein. Moreover, the association of p56[lck] with the cytoplasmic domain of CD4 downregulates the rate of replication of the virus ultimately reducing virion production (Tremblay et al.1994). These examples strongly suggest that high level of virus production and retention of CD4 expression are incompatible.

CONSEQUENCES OF SURFACE CD4 PERSISTENCE IN THE CONTEXT OF HIV INFECTION

There are many potentially deleterious consequences associated with retaining cell surface CD4 expression in the face of HIV-1 infection. First, accumulation of viral DNA through the process of superinfection has been demonstrated in acutely infected cultures of lymphoblastoid T cell lines in vitro and is associated with cytopathology (Pauza et al. 1990). Viral DNA may compete with genomic DNA for essential factors, and prevents the cell from replicating or dividing. Alternatively, the accumulation of specific viral proteins may block cell replication. The situation may not occur *in vivo* due to downregulation of CD4 and the requirement for high viral load. Moreover, evidence against this cytopathology being the causal factor of apoptosis has been documented in the case of HIV-1 (Laurent-Crawford et al. 1993b). Second, circulating gp120 may bind to the CD4 receptor and thus render such cells susceptible to cytotoxic T cell attack. It is still unclear if the gp120 has to be expressed on the cytoplasmic membrane to trigger such a response. Third, gp120 binding to CD4 can also deliver a negative signal to the cell, and if the amounts of gp120 are sufficiently elevated to occupy the receptor for extended period of time. This situation would result in a state of non-responsiveness possibly facilitated by the release of p56^{LCK} from the cytoplasmic tail of CD4. Cross-linking antibodies to gp120 also has been reported to induce a state of reversible anergy in T cells (Liegler et al. 1994). It has also been proposed that this situation may directly induce anergy and prevent cell stimulation. This would result in diminished virus production because the cell is no longer capable of cycling. Fourth, syncytium formation may also be a consequence of expression of both CD4 and gp120 in concentrations sufficient to induce fusion to other infected or uninfected cells. Although, syncytia have only been detected in the brain in cells of the monocyte/macrophage lineage, it is still not clear whether T cells could not exhibit such cytopathology in specific microenvironments, such as the lymph node where large amounts of virus and T cells are trafficking. Lastly, some evidence suggests that apoptosis would be enhanced if CD4 downmodulation were not to occur rapidly (Oyaizu et al. 1993). In conclusion, multiple lines of investigation indicate that high concentrations of surface CD4 on HIV-infected cells prevent persistent and chronic HIV infection, a state which would not be beneficial to the virus.

MECHANISMS BY WHICH HIV ACHIEVES CD4 RECEPTOR DOWNREGULATION

In the genome of HIV-1, three (*nef*, *vpu* and *env*) of its 10 genes modulate the expression of surface CD4. Expression of the *nef* gene, one of the first genes expressed after HIV-1 infection, rapidly results in the downmodulation of surface CD4 (Garcia et al. 1991., Aiken et al. 1994., Rhee et al. 1994). This downmodulation requires the presence of the myristoylated form of nef and the cytoplasmic tail of the CD4 receptor. The *env* gene product, gp160, and *vpu* act in concert later in the viral cycle to further reduce CD4 surface expression. Gp160 in concert with the *vpu* protein act as a trap and retain the CD4 protein in the endoplasmic reticulum, thus facilitating its digestion. CD4 downregulation is very efficient, promptly repressing surface expression by 90-95% (Figure 2). This built-in redundancy is highly suggestive of the importance of the CD4 downregulation to successful viral replication and propagation of HIV.

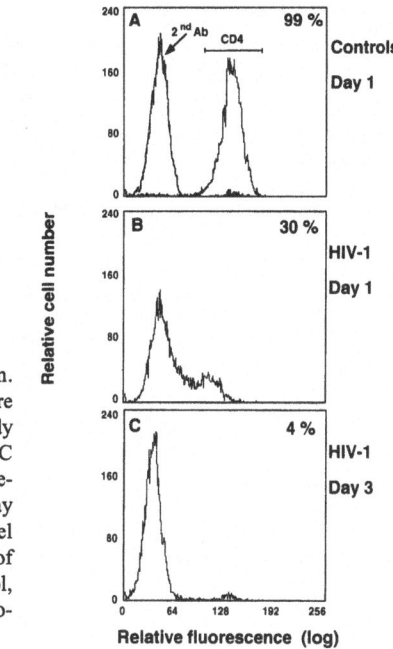

CD4 expression

Relative fluorescence (log)

Figure 2. CD4 downregulation upon HIV-1$_{LAI}$ infection. Aliquots were taken at day 1 and 3. The controls (panel A) were uninfected SupT1 cells stained either with the anti-CD4 antibody OKT4 and FITC labelled goat anti mouse or with the FITC labelled goat anti-mouse antibody only (2nd Ab). Panel A represents the amount of cell surface expression of CD4 after 1 day post-infection where 30% of the cells still expressed CD4. Panel C represent SupT1 cells, 3 day after infection, where only 4% of the cells retained CD4 expression on their surface. The control, uninfected SupT1 cells, at day 3 were similar to day 1 (reproduced with permission).

VIRAL INHIBITION OF APOPTOSIS AS A SURVIVAL STRATEGY FOR PERSISTENCE

One protective host response to the presence of a virus may be for the infected cell to commit suicide, thereby aborting continuing virus replication. An increasing number of viruses have been shown to induce apoptosis in target cells. These viruses include alphaviruses, FIV, HIV-1, HIV-2, HTLV, influenza virus, parvovirus B19 and probably many others. This may not represent a problem for highly infectious viruses which can quickly move to another individual and find new target cells. However, viruses with less efficient means of transmission must develop ways to persist for longer periods of time in their host in order to propagate. Rather than a process used by the virus to produce pathology, apoptosis of infected cells may then represent a strategy utilized by the cell to limit viral replication. This latter possibility seems more logical.

Many viruses have developed means to repress apoptosis upon infection of their target cells (Table 1). These mechanisms include downregulation of surface receptors (CD4), upregulation of cellular genes involved in progression into the cell cycle and upregulation of the cellular anti-apoptotic gene bcl-2. Bcl-2 is involved in maintaining cell survival and is capable of preventing apoptosis induced by a large number of stimuli which usually induce death by apoptosis. The proto-oncogene p53 is involved in cell cycling by regulating the entry into mitosis. This proto-oncogene is particularly important when DNA damage is present in the cell by maintaining the cell in G1 to allow sufficient time to proceed with repairs. Its inactivation may result in the cell's progress through the cycle before undergoing corrective DNA modification (Martin et al. 1994).

On the other hand some viruses induce apoptosis of their target cells if mechanisms in place to prevent apoptosis are insufficient or absent (gene mutation, slower response,

Table 1. Viral products which modulate apoptosis

Gene	Virus	Function	References
vpu,nef, gp160	HIV-1	down-modulates CD4	Aiken et al. 1994 Rhee et al. 1994
tat	HIV-1	Upregulates bcl-2 upregulation of cellular genes?	Zauli et al. 1993
BCRF-1 (v IL-10)	EBV	Upregulates bcl-2	Steward et al. 1992 Henderson et al. 1993 Tarodi et al. 1994
LMP-1	EBV	Upregulates bcl-2	Henderson et al. 1991 Gregory et al. 1991 Nakagomi et al. 1994
E1B	Adenovirus	Prevent E1A and TNF induced apoptosis	White et al. 1991 White et al. 1992 Debbas et al. 1993
crm A	Cow pox virus	inhibits ICE-induced apoptosis	Ray et al. 1992 Gagliardini et al. 1994
p35	Baculovirus	inhibits apoptosis	Clem et al. 1991 Crook et al. 1993 Kamita et al. 1993 Sugimoto et al. 1994
v-abl	Abelson virus	inhibits activation-induced apoptosis	Evans et al. 1993
Large T antigen	SV40	inhibition of p53	McCarthy et al. 1994

stimuli too intense). For example, alphavirus becomes neurovirulent upon a single aminoacid change in the E2 glycoprotein (Ubol et al. 1994).

CONCLUSION

Apoptosis may be a protective host cell response to abort continuing viral replication. Viruses, including HIV, have evolved various mechanisms to suppress apoptosis of their target cells. Apoptosis in the context of HIV infection may be considered beneficial to the host and strategies directed at preventing infection and reducing viral burden may be more effective at preventing the CD4 T cell depletion seen in AIDS than trying to circumvent apoptosis in HIV-infected patients as has been suggested (Estaquier et al. 1994).

ACKNOWLEDGEMENTS

The authors thank Drs. Seamus J. Martin and David J. Looney for comments and discussion. J.C. is supported by a Fellowship of the Commonwealth of Australia AIDS Research Committee. D.D.R. is supported by grants AI-27670, AI-30457 and AI-29164 from the National Institutes of Health, and the Research Center for AIDS and HIV Infection of the San Diego Veterans Affairs Medical Center.

REFERENCES

Aiken, C., Konner, J., Landau, N.R., Lenburg, M.E., and Trono, D. 1994. Nef induces CD4 endocytosis: requirement for a critical dileucine motif in the membrane-proximal CD4 cytoplasmic domain. Cell. 76:853-64.

Ameisen, J. C., and Capron, A. 1991. Cell dysfunction and depletion in AIDS: the programmed cell death hypothesis. Immunol. Today. 12:102-105.

Ameisen, J. C. 1992. Programmed cell death and AIDS: from hypothesis to experiment. Immunol. Today. 13:388-391.

Ameisen, J. C. 1994. Programmed cell death (apoptosis) and cell survival regulation:relevance to AIDS and cancer. AIDS. 8:1197-1213

Banda, N.K., Bernier, J., Kurahara, D.K., Kurrle, R., Haigwood, N.,Sekaly, R.P., and Finkel, T.H. 1992. Crosslinking CD4 by human immunodeficiency virus gp120 primes T cells for activation-induced apoptosis. J. Exp. Med. 176:1099-1106.

Carbonari, M., Cibati, M., Cherchi, M., Sbarigia, D., Pesce, A.M., Dell'Anna, L., Modica, A., and Fiorilli, M. 1994. Detection and characterization of apoptotic peripheral blood lymphocytes in human immunodeficiency virus infection and cancer chemotherapy by a novel flow immunocytometric method. Blood. 83:1268-77.

Clem, R. J., and Miller, L. K. 1993. Apoptosis reduces both the in vitro replication and the in vivo infectivity of a baculovirus. J. Virol. 67: 3730-8.

Cohen, J. 1993. What causes the immune system collapse seen in AIDS? Science. 260:1256.

Corbeil, J., and Richman, D.D. 1994. Productive infection and subsequent CD4-gp120 interaction at cellular membrane required for HIV-induced apoptosis of CD4+ T cell. J. Gen. Virology. In press.

Crook, N. E., Clem, R. J., and Miller, L. K. 1993. An apoptosis-inhibiting baculovirus gene with a zinc finger-like motif. J Virol. 67: 2168-74.

Debbas, M,. and White, E. 1993. Wild-type p53 mediates apoptosis by E1A, which is inhibited by E1B. Genes and Development. 7:546-54.

Embretson, J., Zupancic, M., Ribas, J.L., Burke, A., Racz, P., Tenner-Racz, K., and Haase, A.T. 1993. Massive covert infection of helper T lymphocytes and macrophages by HIV during the incubation period of AIDS. Nature. 362:359-362.

Estaquier, J., Idziorek T., De Bels F., Barré-Sinoussi F., Hurtrel, B., Aubertin, A-M., Venet, A., Mehtali, M., Muchmore, E., Michel, P., Mouton, Y., Girard, M., and Ameisen, J.C. 1994. Programmed cell death and AIDS: Significance of T-cell apoptosis in pathogenic and non-pathogenic primate lentiviral infections. Proc. Natl. Acad. sci. (USA) , 91:9431-9435.

Evans, C. A., Owen-Lynch, P. J., Whetton, A. D., and Dive, C. 1993. Activation of the Abelson tyrosine kinase activity is associated with suppression of apoptosis in hemopoietic cells. Cancer Res. 53:1735-8.

Fadok, V.A., Voelker, D.R., Campbell, P.A., Cohen, J.J., Bratton, D.L., and Henson, P.M. 1992. Exposure of phosphatidylserine on the surface of apoptotic lymphocytes triggers specific recognition and removal by macrophages. J. Immunol.148:2207-16.

Gagliardini, V., Fernandez, P. A., Lee, R. K., Drexler, H. C., Rotello, R. J., Fishman, M. C., and Yuan, J. 1994. Prevention of vertebrate neuronal death by the crmA gene. Science. 263: 826-8.

Garcia, J.V., and Miller, A.D. 1991. Serine phosphorylation-independent downregulation of cell-surface CD4 by nef. Nature. 350:508-11.

Gougeon, M.L., Garcia, S., Heeney, J., Tschopp, R., Lecoeur, H., Guétard, D., Rame, V., Dauguet, C., and Montagnier, L. 1993a. Programmed cell death in AIDS-related HIV and SIV infections. Aids Res. Hum. Retroviruses. 9:553-563.

Gougeon, M.L., Laurent-Crawford, A.G., Hovanessian, A.G., and Montagnier, L. 1993b. Direct and indirect mechanisms mediating apoptosis during HIV infection.contribution to in vivo CD4 T cell depletion. Sem. Immunol. 5:187-194.

Gougeon, M. L., and Montagnier, L. 1993. Apoptosis in AIDS. Science. 260:1269-1270.

Gregory, C.D., Dive, C., Henderson. S., Smith, C.A., Williams, G.T., Gordon, J., and Rickinson, A.B. 1991. Activation of Epstein-Barr virus latent genes protects human B cells from death by apoptosis. Nature, 349:612-4.

Groux, H., Monte, D., Bourrez, J.M., Capron, A., and Ameisen J.C. 1991. Activation of CD4+ T-lymphocytes in asymptomatic HIV infected patients induce the program action of lymphocyte death by apoptosis. Comptes Rendus Acad. Sci.(Paris) 312:599-606.

Groux, H., Torpier, G., Monte, D., Mouton, Y., Capron, A., and Ameisen, J.C. 1992. Activation-induced death by apoptosis in CD4+ T cells from human immunodeficiency virus-infected asymptomatic individuals. J. Exp. Med. 175:331-340.

Henderson, S., Huen, D., Rowe, M., Dawson, C., Johnson, G., and Rickinson, A. 1993. Epstein-Barr virus-coded BHRF1 protein, a viral homologue of Bcl-2, protects human B cells from programmed cell death. Proc. Natl. Acad. Sci. U S A. 90: 8479-83.

Henderson, S., Rowe, M., Gregory, C., Croom-Carter, D., Wang, F., Longnecker, R., Kieff, E., and Rickinson, A. 1991. Induction of bcl-2 expression by Epstein-Barr virus latent membrane protein 1 protects infected B cells from programmed cell death. Cell. 65:1107-15.

Kamita, S. G., Majima, K., and Maeda, S. 1993. Identification and characterization of the p35 gene of Bombyx mori nuclear polyhedrosis virus that prevents virus-induced apoptosis. J. Virol. 67: 455-63.

Laurent-Crawford, A.G., Krust, B., Muller, S., Rivière, Y., Rey-Cuille, M.A., Bechet, J.M., Montagnier, L., and Hovanessian, A.G. 1991. The cytopathic effect of HIV is associated with apoptosis. Virol.185:829-839.

Laurent-Crawford, A.G., Krust, B., Rivière, Y., Desgranges, C., Muller, S., Kieny, M.P., Dauguet, C., and Hovanessian, A.G. 1993a. Membrane expression of HIV envelope glycoproteins triggers apoptosis in CD4 cells. Aids Res. Hum. Retroviruses. 9:761-773.

Laurent-Crawford, A.G., and Hovanessian, A.G. 1993b. The cytopathic effect of human immunodeficiency virus is independent of high levels of unintegrated viral DNA accumulated in response to superinfection of cells. J. Gen.Virol.74:2619-28.

Lenschow, D.J., and Bluestone, J.A. 1993. T cell co-stimulation and in vivo tolerance. Cur. Op. Immunol. 5:747-52.

Levy, J.A. 1993. Pathogenesis of human immunodeficiency virus infection. Microbiol. Rev. 57:183-289.

Liegler, T.J., and Stites, D.P. 1994. HIV-1 gp120 and anti-gp120 induce reversible unresponsiveness in peripheral CD4 T lymphocytes. J. Acquir. Imm. Def. Syn. 7:340-8.

Lin, H.J., Myers, L.E., Yen-Lieberman, B., Hollinger, F.B., Henrard, D., Hooper, C.J., Kokka, R,. Kwok, S., Rasheed, S., Vahey, M., et al. 1994. Multicenter evaluation of quantification methods for plasma human immunodeficiency virus type 1 RNA. J. Infect. Dis.170:553-62.

Martin, S.J., Green, D.R., and Cotter, T.G. 1994. Dicing with death: dissecting the components of the apoptosis machinery. TIBS. 19:26-30.

McCarthy, S. A., Symonds, H. S., and Van Dyke, T. 1994. Regulation of apoptosis in transgenic mice by simian virus 40 T antigen-mediated inactivation of p53. Proc Natl Acad Sci U S A. 91: 3979-83.

Meyaard, L., Otto, S.A., Jonker, R.R., Mijnster, M.J., Keet, R.P.,Miedema, F. 1992. Programmed death of T cells in HIV-1 infection. Science. 257:217-219.

Nakagomi, H., Dolcetti, R., Bejarano, M.T., Pisa, P., Kiessling, R., and Masucci, M.G. 1994. The Epstein-Barr virus latent membrane protein-1 (LMP1) induces interleukin-10 production in Burkitt lymphoma lines. Int. J. Cancer. 57:240-4.

Nishino, Y., Nakaya, T., Fujinaga, K., Kishi, M., Azuma, I., and Ikuta, K. 1994. Persistent infection of MT-4 cells by human immunodeficiency virus type 1 becomes increasingly likely with in vitro serial passage of wild-type but not nef mutant virus. J. Gen. Virol. 75:2241-51.

Oyaizu, N., McCloskey, T. W., Coronesi, M., Chirmule, N., Kalyanaraman, V. S., and Pahwa, S. 1993. Accelerated apoptosis in peripheral blood mononuclear cells (PBMCs) from human immunodeficiency virus type-1 infected patients and in CD4 cross-linked PBMCs from normal individuals. Blood. 82: 3392-400.

Pantaleo, G., Graziosi, C., Demarest, J.F., Butini, L., Montroni, M., Fox, C.H., Orenstein, J. M., Kotler, D.P., and Fauci, A.S. 1993. HIV infection is active and progressive in lymphoid tissue during the clinically latent stage of disease. Nature. 362:355-358.

Pauza, C.D., Galindo, J.E., and Richman, D.D. 1990. Reinfection results in accumulation of unintegrated viral DNA in cytopathic and persistent human immunodeficiency virus type 1 infection of CEM cells. J. Exp. Med. 172:1035-42.

Piatak, M. Jr., Saag, M.S., Yang, L.C., Clark, S.J., Kappes, J.C., Luk, K.C., Hahn, B.H., Shaw, G.M., and Lifson, J.D. 1993. High levels of HIV-1 in plasma during all stages of infection determined by competitive PCR. Science. 259:1749-1754.

Ray, C.A., Black, R.A., Kronheim, S.R., Greenstreet, T.A., Sleath, P.R., Salvesen, G.S., and Pickup, D.J.1992. Viral inhibition of inflammation: cowpox virus encodes an inhibitor of the interleukin-1 beta converting enzyme. Cell. 69:597-604.

Rey-Cuille, M.A., Galabru, J., Laurent-Crawford, A., Krust, B., Montagnier, L., and Hovanessian, A.G. 1994. HIV-2 EHO isolate has a divergent envelope gene and induces single cell killing by apoptosis. Virol. 202:471-6.

Rhee, S.S., and Marsh, J.W. 1994. Human immunodeficiency virus type 1 nef-induced down-modulation of CD4 is due to rapid internalization and degradation of surface CD4. J. Virol. 68:5156-5163.

Rocha, B., Tanchot, C., and Von Boehmer, H. 1993. Clonal anergy blocks in vivo growth of mature T cells and can be reversed in the absence of antigen. J. Exp. Med. 177:1517-21.

Rosenberg, Z.F., and Fauci, A.S. 1991. Immunopathogenesis of HIV infection. FASEB J. 5:2382-2390.

Scadden, D.T., Wang, Z., and Groopman, J.E. 1992. Quantitation of plasma human immunodeficiency virus type 1 RNA by competitive polymerase chain reaction. J. Infect. Dis. 165:1119-1123.

Schwartz, O., Alizon, M., Heard, J.M., and Danos, O. 1994. Impairment of T cell receptor-dependent stimulation in CD4+ lymphocytes after contact with membrane-bound HIV-1 envelope glycoprotein. Virol. 198:360-365.

Stein, D.S., Korvick, J.A., and Vermund, S.H. 1992. CD4+ lymphocyte cell enumeration for prediction of clinical course of human immunodeficiency virus disease. J. Infect. Dis. 165:352-363.

Stewart, J.P., and Rooney, C.M. 1992. The interleukin-10 homolog encoded by Epstein-Barr virus enhances the reactivation of virus-specific cytotoxic T cell and HLA-unrestricted killer cell responses. Virol. 191:773-82.

Sugimoto, A., Friesen, P. D., and Rothman, J. H. 1994. Baculovirus p35 prevents developmentally programmed cell death and rescues a ced-9 mutant in the nematode Caenorhabditis elegans. EMBO J. 13: 2023-8.

Tarodi, B., Subramanian, T., and Chinnadurai, G. 1994. Epstein-Barr virus BHRF1 protein protects against cell death induced by DNA-damaging agents and heterologous viral infection. Virol. 201: 404-7.

Terai, C., Kornbluth, R.S., Pauza, C.D., Richman, D.D., and Carson, D.A. 1991. Apoptosis as a mechanism of cell death in cultured T lymphoblasts acutely infected with HIV-1. J. Clin. Invest. 87:1710-1715.

Tremblay, M., Meloche, S., Gratton, S., Wainberg, M.A., and Sekaly, R.P. 1994. Association of p56lck with the cytoplasmic domain of CD4 modulates HIV-1 expression. Embo J.13:774-83.

Ubol, S., Tucker, P.C., Griffin, D.E., and Hardwick, J.M.1994. Neurovirulent strains of Alphavirus induce apoptosis in bcl-2-expressing cells: role of a single amino acid change in the E2 glycoprotein. Proc. Natl. Acad. Sci.U.S.A, 91:5202-6.

Uehara, T., Miyawaki, T., Ohta, K., Tamaru, Y., Yokoi, T., Nakamura, S., and Taniguchi, N.1992. Apoptotic cell death of primed CD45RO+ T lymphocytes in Epstein-Barr virus-induced infectious mononucleosis. Blood, 80:452-8.

Weiss, R.A. 1993. How does HIV cause AIDS? Science. 260:1273-1279.

White, E., Sabbatini, P., Debbas, M., Wold, W.S., Kusher, D.I., and Gooding, L.R. 1992. The 19-kilodalton adenovirus E1B transforming protein inhibits programmed cell death and prevents cytolysis by tumor necrosis factor alpha. Mol. Cell. Biol. 12:2570-80.

White, E., Cipriani, R., Sabbatini, P., AND Denton, A. 1991. Adenovirus E1B 19-kilodalton protein overcomes the cytotoxicity of E1A proteins. J. Virol. 65:2968-78.

Zauli, G., Gibellini, D., Milani, D., Mazzoni, M., Borgatti, P., La Placa M., Capitani, S. 1993. Human immunodeficiency virus type 1 Tat protein protects lymphoid, epithelial, and neuronal cell lines from death by apoptosis. Cancer Res. 53: 4481-5.

9

MECHANISM OF APOPTOSIS IN PERIPHERAL BLOOD MONONUCLEAR CELLS OF HIV-INFECTED PATIENTS

Naoki Oyaizu,* Thomas W. Mc Closkey, Soe Than, Rong Hu, and
Savita Pahwa

The Department of Pediatrics
North Shore University Hospital-Cornell University Medical College
Manhasset, New York, New York 11030

ABSTRACT

Lymphocytes from patients with HIV-infection have been shown to undergo accelerated spontaneous apoptosis. Binding of CD4 molecules by HIV envelope protein gp120 and anti-gp120 antibodies can lead to crosslinking of CD4 molecules (CD4XL) *in vitro* and conceivably *in vivo*. We have recently shown that CD4XL *in vitro*, when performed in unfractioned peripheral blood mononuclear cells (PBMC) on normal HIV seronegative donors, is by itself sufficient to induce T cell apoptosis (Blood 82:3392, 1993). To further examine the mechanisms involved in apoptosis, we have examined the expression of Fas antigen (Fas) using 3 color flow cytometry. Fas is a cell surface molecule known to mediate apoptosis-triggering signals. We induced CD4XL in PBMC obtained from normal donors, either by anti-CD4 mAb Leu3a or by HIV-1 envelope protein gp160. PBMC subpopulations were examined for Fas Ag expression and for apoptosis induction by flow cytometry. CD4XL was found to result in increased Fas expression as well as Fas mRNA in lymphocytes and the up-regulated Fas Ag was closely correlated with apoptotic cell death. CD4XL in PBMC also resulted in induction of the cytokines INF-τ and TNF-α in the absence of IL-2 and IL-4 secretion. Both these cytokines contributed to Fas Ag up-regulation and antibodies to TNF-α and INF-τ abrogated CD4XL-induced Fas up-regulation and T-cell apoptosis. These findings suggest that CD4XL occuring *in vivo* might play an important role in inducing an abberant cytokine profile (which has been observed in HIV infected individuals) and also in triggering of T-cell apoptosis.

---

* Address correspondence and reprint request to Dr. N. Oyaizu/ Dr. S. Pahwa, Room 303, Biomedical Research Building, NSUH-CUMC, 350 Community Drive, Manhasset, New York, NY 11030. Tel: (516) 562-1071; Fax: (516) 562-2866.

INTRODUCTION

More than ten years into the epidemic, the mechanism whereby Human Immunodeficiency Virus type 1 (HIV-1) infection leads to the profound loss of CD4+ T cells remains enigmatic. We and others have demonstrated that T cells of HIV-infected individuals show enhanced susceptibility to cell death by apoptosis (1-4). In the absence of activating agents, accelerated cell death through apoptosis occurs in cultured lymphocytes of HIV-infected patients. Further we have recently shown that crosslinking of CD4 molecules induces T cell apoptosis in peripheral blood mononuclear cells (PBMC) of HIV-seronegative healthy donors (3). However, the underlying mechanisms for the accelerated T cell apoptosis in HIV infection are currently speculative and need to be elucidated. This study was focused to investigate the mechanism of CD4XL-induced T-cell apoptosis. We chose to examine the role of Fas Ag and participation of cytokines in this process.

Fas antigen (Ag), recently designated as CD95, is transmembrane glycoprotein identical to the APO-1 Ag and belongs to the nerve growth factor (NGF)/tumor necrosis factor (TNF) receptor family of surface molecules (5-7). Addition of anti-Fas antibody results in cytolytic activity of certain cells expressing this antigen (5). Several recent studies have suggested that Fas/APO-1 Ag, which is preferentially expressed on CD45RO+ T cells (8), may mediate apoptosis. Human lymphocytes activated with IL-2 undergo apoptosis after anti-Fas mAb treatment (9). In addition, anti-Fas mAb treatment has been shown to induce selective killing of cells chronically infected with HIV (10). Our studies show that in vitro CD4XL, when performed in normal PBMC results in increased lymphocyte apoptosis and increased expression of Fas Ag . Moreover, the up-regulated Fas Ag correlates closely with apoptotic cell death. Many studies have shown that patients with HIV infection have cytokine dysregulation. We examined the cytokines IL-2, IL-4, INF-τ and TNF-α in supernatants of CD4XL PBMC. CD4XL was found to result in induction of INF-τ and TNF-α in the absence of IL-2 and IL-4 secretion, and both of the induced cytokines contribute to Fas Ag up-regulation/lymphocyte apoptosis, which were blocked by neutralizing antibodies to these cytokines. These findings provide new insights for elucidating the mechanism of accelerated T cell apoptosis and explain the aberrant cytokine profile observed in HIV-infected individuals. At the same time, our observations implicate crosslinking of CD4 in vivo as a major contributor to this mechanism of accelerated cell death in HIV infection.

MATERIALS AND METHODS

Cells and Culture Conditions

Peripheral blood mononuclear cells (PBMC) were were isolated from heparinized venous blood by Ficoll-Hypaque density gradient centrifugation. In the cell selection experiments, purified T cells were prepared by rosette formation with sheep red blood cells followed by Petri dish adherent cell depletion as described (15). These cells were >97% CD2-positive and contained <1% CD14-positive monocytes as determined by flow cytometry. RPMI 1640 (Gibco Laboratories, Grand Island, NY) supplemented with 10% heat-inactivated FCS (Gibco), 2mM L-glutamine (Whittaker Bioproducts, Inc., Walkersville, MD), 100 U/ml penicillin G and 100 ug/ml streptomycin was used for all cultures.

Antibodies and Reagents

Reagents and sources were as follows: monoclonal antibody (mAb) to human Fas (IgM, clone CH-11, UBI, Lake Placid, NY); mAb to CD4 (Leu3a; IgG1, Becton Dickinson, Mountain View, CA); mAb to CD1a (IgG1, AMAC Inc, Westbrook, ME); mAb to CD3 (IgG2a, mAb 454, Ref. 11 a gift from Dr. N. Chiorazzi, North Shore Univ. Hospital, Manhasset, NY), goat anti-mouse immunoglobulin, (GAM; Tago, Inc., Burlingame CA); purified mouse IgM (Pharminogen, San Diego, CA); genistein (ICN Biochemicals, Cleveland, OH); and cyclosporin A (CsA, Sandoz, East Hanover, NJ). Preparation of native envelope protein gp160 was described in detail previously (12). Rabbit anti-gp120 (HIV-1_{IIIB}) polyclonal antibodies were obtained from American Bio-Technologies, Cambridge, MA.

Recombinant Cytokines and Anti-cytokine Antibodies

Recombinant human INF-τ (rINF-τ), monoclonal anti-human INF-τ antibody (α-INF-τ mAb) and polyclonal rabbit anti-human TNF-α antibody (α-TNFα Ab) were obtained from Genzyme (Cambridge, MA); recombinant human TNF-α from Dr. K. J. Tracey (Picower Institute, Manhasset, NY); recombinant human IL-2 (rIL-2) from Boehringer Mannheim (Indianapolis, IN).

Induction of CD4 Crosslinking

Procedure for induction of CD4XL was as described (3). In brief, cells were treated with Leu3a or an isotype matched control antibody for 1 h at 4°C. Cells were then cultured in 24-well Nunc plates coated with goat anti-mouse immunoglobulin (GAM). Treatment of cells with gp160 following culture on immobilized anti-gp120 antibodies was performed in a procedure identical to Leu3a/GAM treatment. In some experiments, cells were treated with genistein or CsA prior to anti-CD4 mAb treatment (30 min pre-incubation and continued presence throughout the culture period at concentrations of 30 ug/ml of genistein and 300 ng/ml of CsA, respectively).

Immunofluorescence Staining and Flow Cytometry

For study of Fas Ag expression, cells were stained with anti-Fas mAb followed by FITC-conjugated secondary antibody (FITC-goat anti-mouse IgM; Jackson). For three colour immunofluorescence analyses, anti-Fas stained cells were subsequently stained with Per-CP-conjugated anti-CD3 mAb (Becton Dickinson, Mountain View, CA) followed by phycoerythrin (PE)-conjugated anti-CD8 mAb (Coulter, Hialeah, FL). All incubations of cells with antibodies were for 10 min at room temperature followed by washing with HBSS and fixing in 1% paraformaldehyde. The stained cells were analyzed on a flow cytometer (Epics Elite, Coulter Electronics). Flow cytometric analysis was accomplished in the following manner: A lymphocyte gate was drawn on a histogram of forward vs. right angle light scatter. Fluorescence emissions were collected at 525-nm for FITC (green), 575-nm for PE (orange), and 675-nm for Per-CP (red), respectively. On this histogram, appropriate gates were drawn to capture certain populations (CD3+8-, CD3+8+) as required. Single parameter green histograms representing Fas Ag expression in each gated population were evaluated by comparing them with the background histograms containing control mAb using Coulter's cytologic nalysis program (Overton's Cumulative Subtraction Algorithm: OVERSUB) which was implemented to assess percent of cells positive for Fas Ag expression over background obtained from irrelevant antibody/FITC-GAM-stained samples.

Measurement of Apoptosis by Flow Cytometry

The percentage of cells undergoing apoptosis was quantitated by a modification of the flow cytometric method as described (13). Briefly, 2×10^6 cells were fixed in 70% ethanol. The cells were then stained with propidium iodide (PI, 100 ug/ml HBSS, Molecular Probes, Eugene, OR). The PI fluorescence of individual cells was measured using a flow cytometer. A distinct cell cycle region of apoptosis (Ao) could be identified below the Go/G1 diploid peak. Percentage of cells in the Ao region were estimated. The same sample was also evaluated morphologically (4) for percentage of apoptotic cells, utilizing cytocentrifuge-preparations and a fluorescent microscope. Cell death was also evaluated by trypan blue exclusion.

Determination of Cytokine Concentrations

Cytokine concentrations were quantitated by using commercial ELISA kits (for IL-2 from R&D Systems, Minneapolis MN; for INF-τ, IL-4 and TNF-α from Genzyme) according to the manufacturer's instructions.

Statistical Analysis

Statistical significance was assessed by Student's t-test.

RESULTS

CD4 Crosslinking-Upregulates Apoptosis and Fas Ag Expression

As shown in Table 1, *in vitro* induction of CD4XL in PBMC from normal donors, either by anti-CD4 mAb Leu3a/GAM or by HIV gp120/α-gp120 antibodies, resulted in significant induction of lymphocyte apoptosis (3). Induction of CD4XL also results in increased Fas Ag expression in lymphocytes (Table 1, Ref14). Basal levels of Fas Ag expression was unchanged in medium-treated controls during the 3-day culture period whereas CD4XL resulted in increased number/intensity of Fas Ag positive cells beginning

Table 1. Effects of CD4XL on Lymphocyte Apoptosis Induction and Fas Ag Expression in Unfractioned PBMC and in Purified T Cells

Pretreatment		Cell Population			
		PBMC		purified T cells	
step 1	step 2	% Ao Cells	%Fas±T Cells	% Ao Cells	%Fas±T Cells
—	—	16.2 ± 7.8	58 ± 4	19.0 ± 4.7	67 ± 3
—	GAM	21.9 ± 6.7	64 ± 2		
α CD1	GAM	23.3 ± 4.6	60 ± 6		
Leu3a	GAM	51.5 ± 11.0*	94 ± 1*	23.8 ± 1.7	97 ± 3*
gp120	α -gp120 Ab	33.1 ± 10.5**			

CD4XL was induced in unfractioned PBMC and in purified T cells from mormal donors. Following culture for 3 days, cells were harvested and analysed for apoptosis and for Fas Ag expression by flow cytometry. % Ao cells denote the percentage of cells found in Ao peak (mean + AD) determined in PI-stained cells. Percentage of Fas Ag expressing cell in CD3+ subpopulation (%Fas+ T cells) are also indicated. Statistically significant increase in the degree of apoptosis as compared to no-pretreatment controls (-/-) at (* p< 0.01, ** p<0.05) was determined by Student's t test.

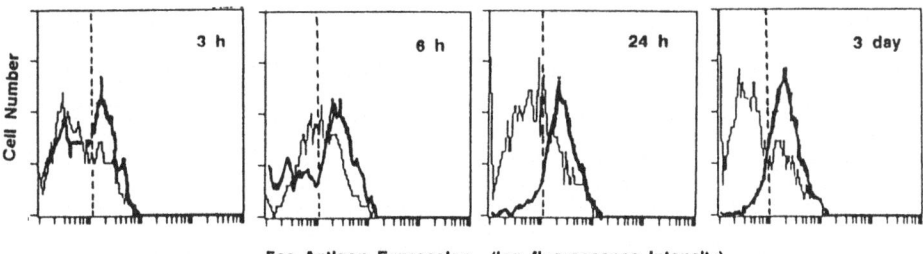

Fas Antigen Expression   (log fluorescence intensity)

Figure 1. Time course study of CD4xl-induced Fas Ag expression. PBMC were treated with medium (thin line) or with Leu3a/GAM to induce CD4XL (thick line) as described in the Methods. PBMC were then cultured for the indicated periods and analyzed for Fas Ag expression by flow cytometry. Dashed line indicates control samples treated with irrelevant antibody. The increase of Fas positive cells in CD4 crosslinked samples as compared with time matched medium controls was 24% at 3h, 34% at 6h, 42% at 24 h, and 46% at 3 d, respectively as evaluated by the OVERSUB program.

as early as 3 h after treatment, reaching a sub-plateau level by 24 h and becoming maximal on day 3 (Fig. 1). By employing three-color immunofluorescence analysis, CD4XL was found to induce augmented Fas Ag expression not only in CD3+8- (presumed CD4+ T cells) but also in CD8+ T cells (Fig. 2). Further, we confirmed by RT-PCR that CD4XL resulted in Fas mRNA up-regulation (Ref. 14). Treatment of PBMC with HIV-1 envelope protein

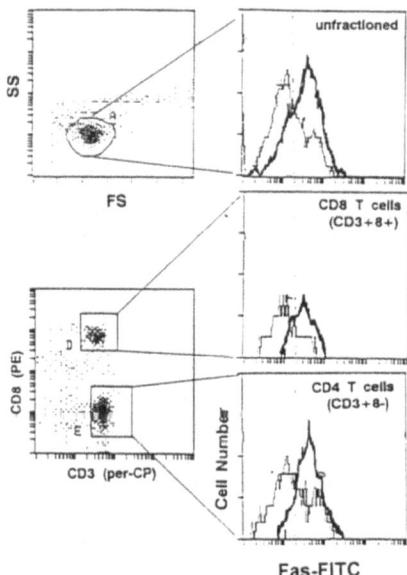

Fas-FITC

Figure 2. CD4 crosslinking results in augmented Fas Ag expression in CD4 T cells, CD8 T cells. PBMC which had been treated with medium (thin line) or with Leu3a/GAM (thick line) were cultured for 3 days. Cells were harvested and subjected to three-colour immunofluorescence. Top picture shows a lymphocyte gate for Fas Ag expression in unfractioned lymphocytes. Appropriate gates were drawn to capture certain populations (CD3+8-, CD3+8+) as shown and single parameter green histograms representing Fas Ag expression in each gated population was evaluated. The vertical line indicates the position of control samples treated with irrelevant antibody. Reprinted by permission from Blood, Vol 84, No 8, 1994 pp2622-2631, Fig 1.

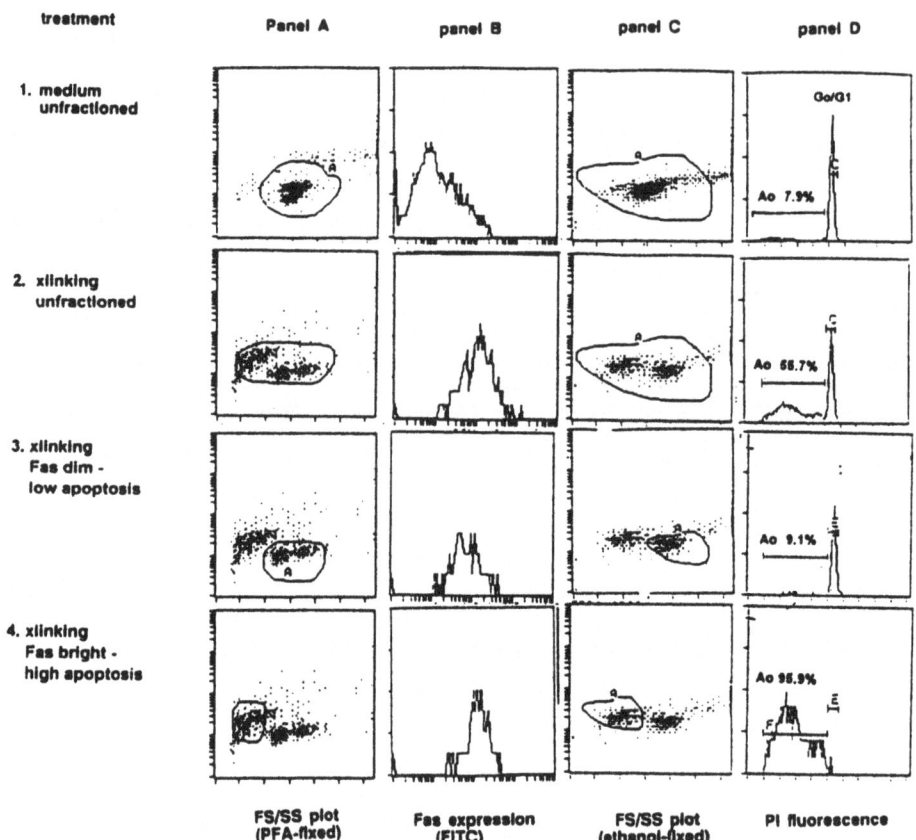

Figure 3. Fas Ag expression correlates with apoptotic cell death. PBMC were treated with medium (row 1) or with Leu3a/GAM (rows 2-4) for 3 days. Cells were harvested, fixed in paraformaldehyde (PFA) and stained for Fas Ag expression. The same samples were also fixed in ethanol and stained with propidium iodide (PI). Panels A and C indicate plots of FSC/SSC in PFA-fixed samples (panel: A) and ethanol-fixed samples (panel C), respectively. Fas Ag expression (panel B) and DNA content with PI staining (panel D) were analyzed in the gated regions indicated in panels A and C by flow cytometry, respectively. Percentages of cells found in sub-Go/G1 diploid Ao peak are indicated. Reprinted by permission from Blood, Vol 84, No 8, 1994 pp2622-2631, Fig 7.

gp160 and anti-gp120 antibodies also resulted in augmentation of Fas Ag expression (Ref. 14).

Fas Ag Expression Correlates with Apoptotic Cell Death

As shown in Fig. 3 (Ref 14), medium-treated resting lymphocytes are composed of a relatively homogenous cell population in the plot of forward scatter (FS: indicating cell volume) versus side scatter (SS: indicating cell density) in both paraformaldehyde (PFA)-(panel A-1; for Fas staining) and ethanol-(panel C-1; for the PI staining) fixed samples. An additional population that accumulated in the CD4XL PBMC was comprised of cells with decreased volume and increased density (DV/ID, panels A-4, C-4). Loss of the cellular volume and increase of density is one of the characteristic features accompanying apoptosis (15). In fact, this latter population represents cells undergoing apoptosis as confirmed by the

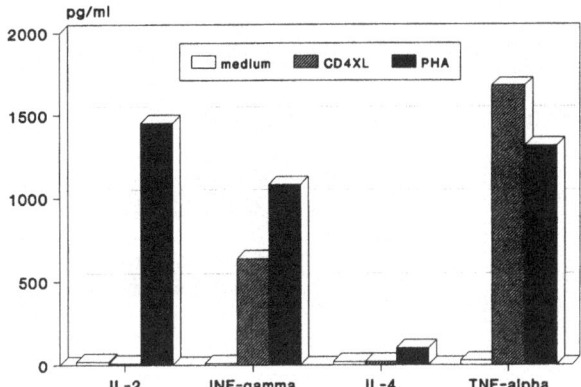

Figure 4. Cytokine levels of 72 h cell culture supernatants (except PHA-stimulated supernatants for IL-2 which have been collected at 48 h) were measured by ELISA. Levels below which signals were undetectable: IL-2; 10 pg/ml; INF-τ 100 pg/ml; IL-4 45 pg/ml; and TNF-α 10 pg/ml. Data represents mean ± SD of four different experiments.

emergence of cells in the sub-Go/G1 peak (Ao, panel D-4). In contrast, the normal volume and normal density cell population (NV/ND, panels A-3, C-3) contained few apoptotic cells (panel D-3). Interestingly, the DV/ID cell population preferentially expressed augmented Fas Ag (Fas bright: panel B-4), whereas the NV/ND cell population was composed of Fas dim positive cells (Fas dim: panel B-3). These observations indicate that the increased Fas Ag expression correlates with apoptotic cell death.

CD4 Crosslinking Induces INF-τ and Tnf-α Secretion

Crosslinking of CD4 molecules was found to result in increased Fas Ag expression not only on CD4+ T cells but also on CD4-negative cell populations such as CD8+ T cells. These findings suggest that some soluble factor(s) might be involved in CD4XL-mediated Fas Ag up-regulation. To test the possibility that CD4XL augments Fas Ag expression via a mechanism of cytokine secretion, we evaluated the cytokines IL-2, IL-4, INF-τ and TNF-α in the supernatants of CD4 crosslinked PBMC samples. As shown in Fig 4, CD4 crosslinking was found to induce significant INF-τ and TNF-α secretion in the absence of IL-2 and IL-4 secretion. In addition, we examined the effects of cyclosporin A (CsA) and genistein, a known inhibitor of PTK, on CD4XL-induced Fas up-regulation.on CD4XL-mediated Fas Ag up-regulation. Both CsA and genistein were found to block CD4XL-induced Fas up-regulation (Ref 14). These results implicate CsA-sensitive soluble factor(s) as mediators of Fas Ag up-regulation and the involvement of TPK in the CD4XL-mediated Fas Ag up-regulation.

Role of TNF-α and INF-τ in CD4XL-Induced Fas Up-regulation and Apoptosis Induction

Figure 5A shows the Fas Ag expression on peripheral blood lymphocytes in response to exogenously added recombinant INF-τ and TNF-α. Both of the cytokines were found to augment Fas Ag expression in a dose dependent manner. In contrast, treatment of resting PBMC with these cytokines either singly or in combination did not induce significant apoptosis (Ref. 14). The CD4XL-induced Fas Ag up-regulation was inhibited dose dependently in the presence of either anti-INF-τ mAb or anti-TNF-α Ab (Fig. 5B). These results indicate that CD4 XL-mediated Fas Ag expression can be ascribed, at least in part, to its ability to induce INF-τ and TNF-α secretion. Finally, we examined the effects of neutralizing

Naoki Oyaizu et al.

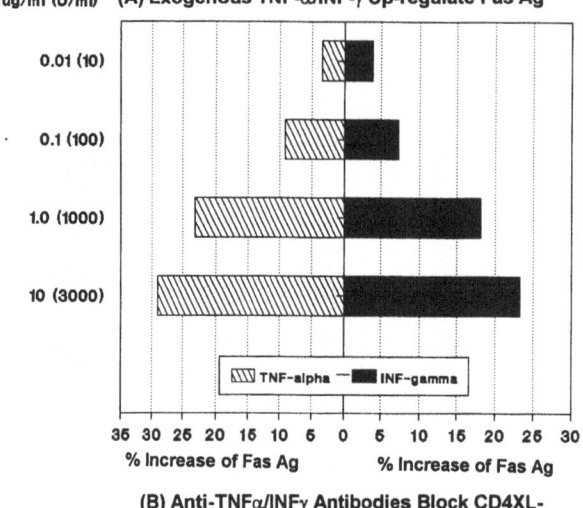

ug/ml (U/ml)   **(A) Exogenous TNF-α/INF-γ Up-regulate Fas Ag**

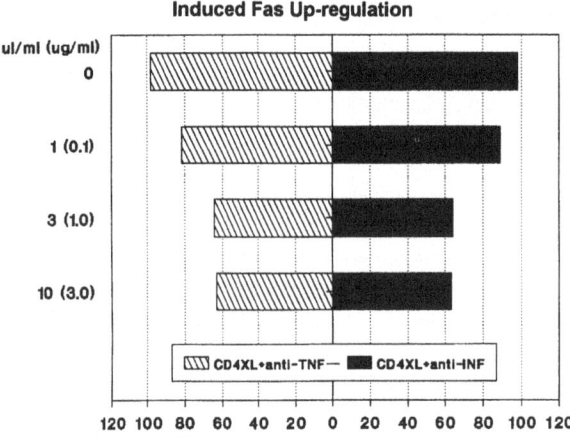

Figure 5. (A) PBMCs were cultured without or with various concentrations of recombinant TNF-α (ug/ml: hatched bar) or INF-τ (U/ml: closed bar) for 3 days and analyzed for Fas Ag expression. Percent increase of Fas Ag expression over the no-cytokine addition medium controls was calculated using the OVERSUB program to normalize the variation of base Fas Ag expression between individuals. (B) CD4XL was performed in PBMCs from 3 different individuals with Leu3a/GAM in the absence or presence of various concentrations of anti-TNF-α (ul/ml: hatched bar) or anti-INF-τ (ug/ml: closed bar) antibodies and cells were cultured for 3 days. Data represents mean ± SD of three experiments.

antibodies to TNF-α and INF-τ on lymphocyte apoptosis that is observed in PBMC following CD4XL (Ref 3, Fig 2). Addition of anti-INF-τ and anti-TNF-α antibodies were both found to block CD4XL-induced lymphocyte apoptosis (Fig 6); anti-TNF-α antibody blocked this more effectively in comparison to anti-INF-τ antibody.

DISCUSSION

In this study, we have focused on Fas Ag expression and cytokine induction in response to CD4XL since CD4XL was found to induce lymphocyte apoptosis in PBMC. We show here that induction of CD4XL *in vitro* performed in normal PBMC by anti-CD4 mAb Leu3a or by HIV-1 envelope protein gp160, results in enhanced apoptosis and up-regulation of Fas Ag expression in T cells. This CD4XL-mediated Fas Ag up-regulation did not require the presence of accessory cells (Table 1, Ref. 14) while apoptosis induction was dependent on their presence. Both apoptosis and Fas Ag up-regulation by CD4XL were sensitive to CsA and to the TPK inhibitor genistein (Ref 14). Further, we observed that CD4XL induces

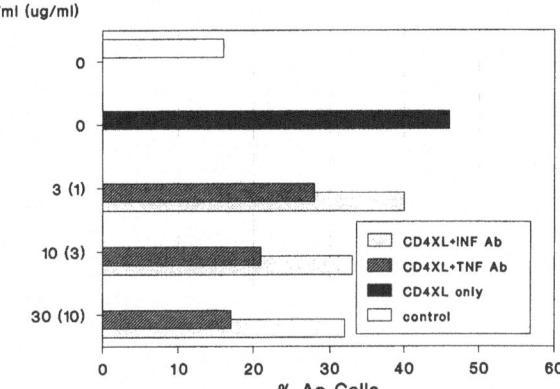

Figure 6. PBMCs with (closed bar) or without CD4XL (control: open bar) were cultured for 3 days and analyzed for apoptosis. Various concentration of anti-TNF-α [TNFAb (ul/ml): hatched bar] or anti-INF-τ [INFAb (ug/ml): dotted bar] antibodies were added to the CD4 crosslinked PBMCs. After PI staining, "% Ao cells" were assessed by flow cytometry as described.

INF-τ and TNF-α secretion in the absence of IL-2 and IL-4 secretion. Both INF-τ and TNF-α were found to augment Fas Ag expression and antibodies to these cytokines both blocked CD4XL-mediated Fas Ag up-regulation and T-cell apoptosis. We also show that the Fas Ag "bright" population correlates closely with the population undergoing apoptosis.

The CD4+ T cell depletion cannot be attributed solely to the cytocidal and/or syncytia-forming ability of HIV, as it is out of proportion to the numbers of cells that are productively infected. An alternative mechanism that has been proposed is that HIV could induce CD4+ T cell destruction indirectly through a mechanism resulted in apoptosis (16). Indeed, T cells from HIV-infected patients have been shown to undergo accerelated apoptosis (1-4). Proposed explanations for the observed T cell apoptosis in HIV infection are currently speculative and include the following: (i) interaction of gp120 with CD4 triggers CD4+ T cells to undergo apoptosis subsequent to TCR-elicited signals (16), (ii) HIV-1 encodes one or more superantigen sequences, thereby inducing particular TCR Vß-expressing cell expansion followed by cell death (17), (iii) HIV upregulates cytokines with known apoptosis-inducing ability such as TNF-α and TGF-ß (2, 18-19). All these possibilities, either alone or in combination, can be involved in inducing apoptosis, and our present data clearly indicate that CD4XL-induced abberant cytokine secretion plays a critical in this process.

A major observation of in our studies of CD4XL is that it results in apoptosis and Fas Ag up-regulation in peripheral blood lymphocytes. Several lines of evidence suggest that Fas Ag plays a pivotal role in the induction of peripheral T cell apoptosis. Mice homozygous for the lpr mutation (lpr/lpr) develop a remarkable T-cell accumulation and exhibit an autoimmune syndrome (20). The lpr mutation has been shown to affect the structural gene for the mouse Fas Ag (21). Although defective Fas Ag expression in lpr mice was initially proposed to be responsible for escaping negative selection in the thymus, there is increasing evidence to suggest that clonal deletion in the thymus of lpr mice is largely normal and that Fas Ag might play a pivotal role in maintaining peripheral tolerance by inducing mature T cell apoptosis (22-25). Experiments with Fas-defective T cells from lpr mice have shown that although cytokine induction is normal, there is no TCR-driven apoptosis in these T cells (24, 25). Further the recent characterization of Fas-ligand (Fas-L) mRNA as being expressed in freshly isolated splenocytes, but not in thymocytes (26), and the recent demonstration of the mutation of Fas-L in gld mice (27, 28), which also resulted in massive lymphadenopathy, support this notion.

The second major observation in the studies of CD4XL is that of aberrant cytokine induction by CD4XL, consisting of INF-τ and TNF-α without IL-2 or IL-4. This discordant cytokine secretion pattern has been previously described in murine Th1 clones stimulated by immobilized anti-TCR/CD3 mAbs in the absence of accessory cells (29), and in human PHA lymphoblasts (composed of 98% CD2+ cells) stimulated by immobilized anti-CD3 mAb (30). Both of the systems have been shown to induce T cell apoptosis and the observed apoptosis was blocked either by the addition of anti-INF-τ mAb or by exogenous IL-2. An intriguing finding was the ability of CD4XL to induce TNF-α secretion in addition to INF-τ. Each of the cytokines, INF-τ and TNF-α, was able to augment Fas Ag expression independently and both cytokines acted additively together. Previously, INF-τ has been shown to up-regulate murine Fas mRNA expression (31). A recent study demonstrated that activation of Fas Ag and TNF receptor resulted in synergistic signaling for apoptosis (32). In fact, we have demonstrated that anti-INFτ and anti-TNFα antibodies are both able to block CD4XL-induced lymphocyte apoptosis (Ref 14).

The cellular interactions resulted for induction of apoptosis are unclear. Studies by Newell (33) and by Banda (34) have shown that CD4XL in purified CD4+ T cells is insufficient for apoptosis induction, but "primes" the cells for apoptosis. A second stimulus via the TCR is required for T-cell apoptosis induction. Our studies have shown that requirement for an apoptosis inducing second stimulus for T cells can be by-passed if CD4XL is performed in PBMC rather than purified T cells (3). In contrast, up-regulation of Fas Ag expression was independent of the requirment for accessory cells. Furthermore, the cytokines TNF-α and/or INF-τ were by themselves not sufficient to induce apoptosis in non-transformed peripheral T cells although they could up-regulate Fas Ag. These results indicate that the important role of accessory cells or of TCR stimulation in inducing T-cell apoptosis. Based on these findings and our results, we believe that CD4XL in PBMC is able to induce not only TNF-α and INF-τ secretion but also induces other factor(s) required for T cell apoptosis. The latter factor(s) could not be induced by the simple addition of TNFα/INFτ. The most likely candidate of this factor(s) is Fas-L, a novel member of TNF family. Fas-L is an activation-inducible molecule and Fas-L mRNA has been shown to be abundantly induced in splenocytes upon stimulation with phorbol ester and calcium ionophore (26). Taken together, CD4XL may by itself be sufficient to induce Fas-L in macrophage, but not in T cells, and Fas-L induction in purified T cells may require additional TCR stimulation.

It should be noted that the abberant cytokine profile induced by CD4XL agrees perfectly with that actually observed in HIV infection. Serum levels of INF-τ, TNF-α, and IL-6 have been reported to be increased in many patients (35-37). We have previously reported that gp120/160 is able to induce IL-6 (38) and TNF-α (unpublished observation) secretion in cloned T cells through interaction with CD4 molecules. High expression of INF-τ mRNA and very low levels of IL-2 mRNA have been found in T lymphocytes infiltrating lymph nodes of HIV-infected individuals (39). In addition, Fan et al. recently reported elevated levels of INF-τ and TNF-α mRNA with lowered IL-2 mRNA expression in PBMC from HIV-infected patients (40). In the setting of HIV infection, the likelihood of CD4XL occurring *in vivo* is extreamely high. The presence of circulatory (41) as well as cell associated-gp120/160 (42) predominantly in the form of immune complexes, the frequent detection of anti-CD4 T cell antibodies (43), and the heavy load of HIV/anti-HIV complexes which are trapped in the follicular dendritic cell network in the lymph nodes (44-46), could all contribute towards CD4XL and thereby induce aberrant cytokine secretion and Fas Ag up-regulation. In fact, we have observed significantly increased Fas Ag expression in T cells from HIV-infected patients (McCloskey T et al. submitted) Interestingly, HIV gp120 has been found to bear sequence homology to CD4 molecule (SLWDQ sequence) (47) and to Fas Ag (VEINCTR sequence) (48). It may therefore be hypothesized that immune responses to HIV envelope proteins by themselves might also contribute to T cell depletion. For example, anti-gp120(SLWDQ) antibodies (Ab) may cross-react with CD4 molecules and thereby

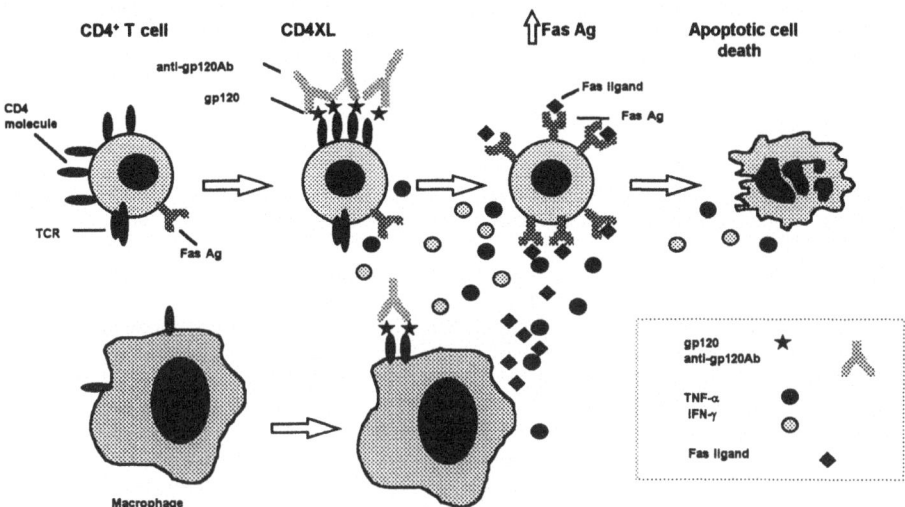

Figure 7. A hypothetical model for CD4XL-induced lymphocyte apoptosis.

induce CD4XL which results in Fas Ag up-regulation; at the same time other anti-gp120(VE-INCTR) Ab may act as Fas-L, thus creating a vicious cycle in inducing T cell apoptosis.

In conclusion, the present study strongly suggests that CD4XL might contribute to HIV pathogenesis by inducing aberrant cytokine secretion, Fas Ag up-regulation and apoptosis induction. Based on our observation, we propose the following hypothetical model to explain an pathophisiologic mechanism of observed accelerated apoptosis in HIV-infection (Fig. 7). Namely, CD4+ T cells (regardless of whether they are infected with HIV or not) are subject to CD4XL through interaction with gp120/anti-gp120 and/or by anti-gp120(SLWDQ)/CD4 cross-reacting antibodies, which leads to INF-τ and TNF-α secretion and consequent Fas Ag up-regulation on T cells in an autocrine or pracrine manner. At the same time, these CD4XL reagents act on CD4+ monocyte/macrophage which lead to Fas-L induction/secretion. Macrophage-derived Fas-L and/or anti-gp120 (VEINCTR)/Fas cross-reacting Ab act on T-cells which express augumented Fas Ag to trigger apoptosis. Now this model is ready to test both in *in vivo* and in *in vitro* experimental system. This model is not restricted to CD4+ T cells. Unexpectedly, CD4XL was found to induce augmented Fas Ag expression not only in CD4+ T cells but also in CD8+ T cells as well. The increased Fas Ag expression in CD8+ T cells may also account for the reported accelerated CD8+ T cell apoptosis in HIV infection (1, 4). Finally, considering the ongoing vaccine trials utilizing HIV envelope proteins, stringent monitoring is stressed, and the hazardous potential of envelope proteins needs to be seriously taken into consideration. Our findings suggest that therapies aimed at controlling abberant cytokine, especially drugs which selectively block TNF-α secretion, should prove beneficial in blocking disease progression in patients with HIV-infection.

ACKNOWLEDGMENTS

The authors wish to thank Dr. Vaniambadi S. Kalyanaraman for the kind gift of gp120/160, Dr. Nicholas Chiorazzi for the mAb 454; Dr. Kevin J. Tracey and Ms. Ona Bloom for providing recombinant TNF-α, Ms. Maria Coronesi for technical assistance and Dr. Xue

Ping for art works. This work was supported by National Institutes of Health grants AI28281, HD26606 and DA05061.

REFERENCES

1. Groux H, Torpier G, Monte D, Mouton Y, Carpon A, Ameisen JC: Activation-induced death by apoptosis in CD4+ T cells from human immunodeficiency virus-infected asymptomatic individuals. 1992 J Exp Med 175:331-340.

2. Meyaard L, Otto SA, Jonker RR, Mijnster MJ, Keet RPM, Miedema F: Programmed death of T cells in HIV-1 infection. 1992 Science 257:217-219

3. Oyaizu N, McCloskey TW, Coronesi M, Chirmule N, Kalyanaraman VS, Pahwa S. Accelerated apoptosis in peripheral blood mononuclear cells (PBMC) from human immunodeficiency virus type-1 infected patients and in CD4 cross-linked PBMCs from normal individuals. 1993 Blood 82:3392-3400

4. Lewis DE, NgTang DS, Adu-Oppong A, Schober W, Rogers JR: Anergy and apoptosis in CD8+ T cells from HIV-infected persons. J. Immunol. 1994, 153:412-420.

5. Yonehara S, Ishii A, Yonehara M: A cell-killing monoclonal antibody (anti-Fas) to a cell surface antigen co-downregulated with the receptor of tumor necrosis factor. 1989 J Exp Med 169:1747-1756.

6. Trauth BC, Klas C, Peters AMJ, Matzku S, Moller P, Falk W, Debatin K-M, Krammer PH: Monoclonal antibody-mediated tumor regression by induction of apoptosis. 1989 Science 245:301-305.

7. Ito N, Yonehara S, Ishii A, Yonehara M, Mizushima S, Sameshima M, Hase A, Seto Y, Nagata S: The polypeptide encoded by the cDNA for human cell surface antigen fas can mediate apoptosis. 1991 Cell 66:233-243

8. Miyawaki T, Uehara T, Nibu R, Tsuji T, Yachie A, Yonehara S, Taniguchi, N: Differential expression of apoptosis-related Fas antigen on lymphocyte subpopulation in human peripheral blood. 1992 J Immunol 149:3753-3758

9. Owen-Schaub LB, Yonehara S, Crump III WL, Grimm EA: DNA fragmentation and cell death is selectively triggered in activated human lymphocytes by Fas antigen engagement. Cellular Immunol 1992 140:197-205

10. Kobayashi N, Hamamoto Y, Yamamoto N, Ishii A, Yonehara M, Yonehara S: Anti-Fas monoclonal antibody is cytocidal to human immunodeficiency virus-infected cells without augmenting viral replication. 1990 Proc Natl Acad Sci USA 87:9620-9624.

11. Stohl W, Posnett DN, Chiorazzi N: Induction of T cell-dependent B cell differentiation by anti-CD3 monoclonal antbodies. 1987 J Immunol 138:1667-1673.

12. Kalyanaraman VS, Rodrigues V, Veronese F, Rahman R, Lusso P, DeVico AL, Copeland T, Oroszlan S, Gallo RC, Sarngadharan MG: Characterization of the secreted, native gp120 and gp160 of the human immunodeficiency virus type 1. 1990 AIDS Res Retroviruses 6:371-380

13. Nicoletti I, Migliorati G, Pagliacci MC, Riccardi C: A rapid simple method for measuring thymocyte apoptosis by propidium iodide staining and flow cytometry. J Immunol. Method. 1991 139:271-279.

14. Oyaizu N, McCloskey TW, Coronesi M, Chirmule N, Karyanaraman VS, Pahwa S. Accelerated apoptosis in peripheral blood mononuclear cells (PBMCs) from human immunodeficiency virus type-1 infected patients and in CD4 cross-linked PBMCs from normal individuals. Blood. 1993 82:3392-3400.

15. Dive C, Gregory CD, Phipps DJ, Evans DL, Milner AE, Wylee AH: Analysis and discrimination of necrosis and apoptosis (programmed cell death) by multiparameter flow cytometry. 1992 Bioch et Bioph Acta 1133:275

16. Ameisen JC, Capon A. Cell dysfunction and depletion in AIDS: the programmed cell death hypothesis. 1991 Immunol. Today 12:102-105.

17. Laurence J, Hodtsev AS, Posnett DN: Superantigen implicated in dependence of HIV-1 replication in T cells on TCR Vß expression. 1992 Nature 358:255

18. Rosenberg, ZF, Fauci AS: Immunopathogeneic mechanisms of HIV infection: cytokine induction of HIV expression. 1990 Immunol. Today 11:176

19. Kenow JW, Wachsman W, McCutchan JA, Cronin M, Carson DA, Lotz M: Transforming growth factor ß and noncytopathic mechanisms of immunodeficiency in human immunodeficiency virus infection. 1990 Proc. Natl. Acad. Sci. U.S.A. 87:8321

20. Andrews BS, Eisenberg RA, Theofilopoulos AN, Izui S, Wilson CB, McConahey PJ, Murphy ED, Roths JB, Dixon FJ: Spontaneous murine lupus-like syndromes. Clinical and immunopathological manifestations in several strains. 1978 J Exp Med 148:1198

21. Watanabe-Fukunaga R, Brannan CI, Copeland NG, Jenkins NA, Nagata S: Lymphoproliferation disorder in mice explained by defects in Fas antigen that mediates apoptosis. 1992 Nature 356:314-317.

22. Singer PA, Balderas RS, McEvilly RJ, Bobardt M, Theofilopoulos AN: Tolerance-related Vß clonal deletions in normal CD4-8-, TCR-α/ß+ and abnormal lpr and gld cell population. 1989 J Exp Med 170:1869-1877.

23. Herron LR, Eisenberg RA, Roper E, Kakkanaiah VN, Cohen PL, Kotzin BL: Selection of the T cell receptor repertoire in lpr mice. 1993 J Immunol 15:3450-3459.

24. Russel JH, Rush B, Weaver C, Wang R: Mature T cells of autoimmune lpr/lpr mice have a defect in antigen-stimulated suicide. 1993 Proc Natl Acad Sci USA 90:4409-4413.

25. Bossu P, Singer GG, Andres P, Ettinger R, Marshak-Rothstein A Abbas AK: Mature CD4+ T lymphocytes from MRL/lpr mice are resistant to receptor-mediated tolerance and apoptosis. 1993 J Immunol 151:7233

26. Suda T, Takahashi T, Golstein P, Nagata S: Molecular cloning and expression of the Fas ligand, a novel member of the tumor necrosis factor family. 1993 Cell. 75:1169-1178

27. Takahashi T, Tanaka M, Brannan CI, Jenkins NA, Copeland NG, Suda T, Nagata S. Generalized lymphoproliferative disease in mice. caused by a point mutation in the Fas ligand. 1994 Cell. 76:969-976.

28. Lynch DH, Watson ML, Alderson MR, Baum PR, Miller RE, Tough T, Gibson M, Davis-Smith T, Smith CA, Hunter K, Bhat D, Din W, Goodwin RG, Seldin MF: The mouse Fas-ligand gene is mutated in gld mice and is part of TNF family gene cluster. 1994 Immunity, 1:131-136.

29. Liu Y, Janeway Jr. CA: Interferon τ plays a critical role in induced cell death of effector T cell: A possible third mechanism of self-tolerance. 1990 J Exp Med 172:1735

30. Groux H, Monte D, Plouvier B, Ameisen A-C: CD3-mediated apoptosis of human medullary thymocytes and activated peripheral T cells: respective roles of interleukin-1, interleukin-2, interferon-τ and accessory cells. 1993 Eur J Immunol. 23:1623-1629

31. Watanabe-Fukunaga R, Brannan CI, Itoh N, Yonehara S, Copeland NG, Jenkins NA, Nagata S: The cDNA structure, expression, and chromosomal assignment of the mouse Fas antigen. 1992 J Immunol 148:1274

32. Wong GHW, Goeddel DV: Fas antigen and p55 TNF receptor signal apoptosis through distinct pathways. 1994 J.Immunol. 152:1751

33. Newell MK, Haughn LJ, Maroun CR, Julius MH: Death of mature T cells by separate ligation of CD4 and the T-cell receptor for antigen. 1990 Nature 347:286-289

34. Banda NK, Bernier J, Kurahara DK, Kurrle R, Haigwood N, Sekaly R-P, Finkel TH: Crosslinking CD4 by human immunodeficiency virus gp120 primes T cells for activation-induced apoptosis. 1994 J Exp Med 176:10991106.

35. Fuchs D, Hausen A, Reibnegger G, Werner ER, Werner-Felmayer G, Dierich, MP, Wachter H: Interferon-τ concentration are increased in sera from individuals infected with human immunodeficiency virus type 1. 1989 J Acquired Immune Defic Syndr. 2:158

36. Lahdevirta J, Maury CPJ, Teppo A-M, Repo H: Elevated levels of circulating cachectin/tumor necrosis factor in patients with acquired immunodeficiency syndrome. 1988 American J Med 85:289

37. Breen EC, Rezai AR, Nakajima K, Beall GN, Mitsuyasu RT, Hirano T, Kishimoto T, Martinez-Maza O: Infection with HIV is associated with elevated IL-6 levels and production. 1990 J Immunol 144:480

38. Oyaizu N, Chirmule N, Ohnishi Y, Kalyanaraman VS, Pahwa S. Human immunodeficiency virus type 1 envelope glycoprotein gp120 and gp160 induce interleukin-6 production in CD4+ T-cell clones. 1991 J Virol 65:6277-6282.

39. Emille D, Permutter M, Maillot MC, Crevon MC, Brousse N, Delfraissy JF, Dormont J, Galanaud P: Production of interleukins in human immunodeficiency virus-1-replicating lymph nodes. 1990 J Clin Invest 86:148-159

40. Fan J, Bass HZ, Fahey JL: Elevated INF-τ and decreased IL-2 gene expression are associated with HIV infection. 1993 J Immunol 151:5031-5040.

41. Oh S-K, Cruikshank WW, Raina J, Blanchard GC, Adler WH, Walker J, Kornfeld H: Identification of HIV-1 envelope glycoprotein in the serum of AIDS and ARC patients. 1992 J Acquired Immune Defic Syndr 5:251

42. Amadori A, Silvestro GD, Zamarchi R, Veronese ML, Mazza MR, Schiavo G, Panozzo M, Rossi AD, Ometto L, Mous J, Barelli A, Borri A, Salmaso L, Chieco-Bianchi L: CD4 epitope masking by gp120/anti-gp120 antibody complexes. A potential mechanism for CD4+ cell function down-regulation in AIDS patients. 1992 J Immunol 148:2709-2716

43. Weimer R, Daniel V, Zimmermann R, Schimpf K, Opelz G: Autoantibodies against CD4 cells are associated with CD4 helper defects in human immunodeficiency virus-infected patients. 1991 Blood 77:133-140

44. Spiegel J, Herbst H, Niedobitek G, Foss HD, Stein H: Follicular dendritic cells are a major reservoir for human immunodeficiency virus type 1 in lymphoid tissues facilitating infection of CD4+ T-helper cells. 1992 Am J Pathol 140:15

45. Pantaleo G, Graziosi C, Demarest JF, Butini L, Montroni M, Fox CH, Orenstein JM, Kotler DP, Fauci AS: HIV infection is active and progressive in lymphoid tissue during the clinically latent stage of disease. 1993 Nature 362:355-358

46. Embretson J, Zupancic M, Ribas JL, Burke A, Racz P, Tenner-Racz K, Haase AT: Massive covert infection of helper T lymphocytes and macrophages by HIV during the incubation period of AIDS. 1993 Nature 362:359-362

47. Zagury JF, Bernard J, Achour A, Astigen A, Lachgar A, Fall L, Carelli C, Ising W, Mbika JP, Picard O, Carlotti M, Callebaut I, Mornon JP, Burny A, Feldman M, Bizzini B, Zagury D: Identification of CD4 and major histocompatibilty complex functional peptide sites and their homology with oligopeptides from human imunodeficiency virus type 1 glycoprotein gp120: Role in AIDS pathogenesis. 1993 Proc Natl Acad Sci USA 90:7573-7577

48. Szawlowski PWS, Hanke T, Randall RE: Sequence homology between HIV-1 gp120 and the apoptosis mediating protein Fas. 1993 AIDS 7:1018. (letter)

10

PROGRAMMED DEATH OF T CELLS IN THE COURSE OF HIV INFECTION

Linde Meyaard and Frank Miedema

Department of Clinical Viro-Immunology
Central Laboratory of the Netherlands Red Cross
   Blood Transfusion Service and
Laboratory for Experimental and Clinical Immunology
University of Amsterdam
Plesmanlaan 125, 1066 CX
Amsterdam, The Netherlands

INTRODUCTION

Infection with the human immunodeficiency virus (HIV) is characterized by an asymptomatic phase of variable length and a decline in CD4+ T-cell numbers, eventually leading to the acquired immune deficiency syndrome (AIDS). Importantly, even before CD4+ T-cell numbers start to decline, functional abnormalities of T cells can be demonstrated in asymptomatically infected individuals. Both CD4+ and CD8+ T-cell function such as IL-2 production and proliferation in response to recall antigens and CD3 antibodies is affected (Shearer et al.1984; Miedema et al.1988; Schellekens et al.1990). One of the enigmas of AIDS pathogenesis is the mechanism by which HIV is capable of perturbing immune functions in a stage of infection where the number of infected cells is low (Schnittman et al.1989). In the past few years, several possible mechanisms have been investigated, including specific loss of memory cells, induction of anergy by antigen presenting cell dysfunction or dysregulation of the Th1/Th2 cytokine balance (reviewed in (Miedema et al.1994)). Following the hypothesis by Ameisen et al (Ameisen et al.1991), who proposed apoptosis as a mechanism for CD4+ T-cell depletion and loss of cellular immune function, several groups, including our group, have investigated PCD of (CD4+) T cells as a possible cause of T-cell dysfunction and CD4+ T-cell depletion in HIV-infected individuals.

PCD IN THE COURSE OF INFECTION

PBMC from HIV-infected persons, cultured overnight display the typical morphology characteristic for PCD when analyzed by electron microscopy (Meyaard et al.1992). Cells have extensive peripheral chromatin condensation, dilation of the endoplasmatic reticulum and preservation of mitochondrial structures, all features of PCD (Wyllie et

Cell Activation and Apoptosis in HIV Infection
Edited by Jean-Marie Andrieu and Wei Lu, Plenum Press, New York, 1995

al.1980). Low molecular weight DNA fractions isolated from lysed cells and subjected to gel electrophoresis, exhibit the DNA cleavage pattern specific for apoptosis. The fragmentation can be prevented by Zn^{2+}, which inhibits endonuclease activity (Duke et al.1983). PCD can be enhanced by activation in vitro with TCR/CD3 (Meyaard et al.1992). PCD occurs in both CD4+ and CD8+ T cells and phenotypical analysis suggests that CD8+ cells are dying at higher percentages (Meyaard et al.1992; Meyaard et al.1994).

In primary HIV infection the increased percentage of T cells dying due to apoptosis after overnight culture is high (up to 60 %) and parallels increased numbers of CD8+ cells. Because they form the largest fraction of T-cells, numerically the majority of cells dying during primary infection are activated, CD8+CD45RO+ cells. However, all CD8+ T-cell subsets contain cells dying due to PCD and there is no evidence for preferential death in one specific subset of cells (Meyaard et al.1994). In the asymptomatic phase of HIV infection there is a variable but, compared to HIV-negative controls, consistently increased percentage of cells dying due to PCD (Meyaard et al.1992; Meyaard et al.1994). In our hands, PCD does not correlate with CD4+ T-cell numbers in asymptomatic individuals, nor with T-cell function as measured by proliferation to CD3 mAb, arguing against dramatic changes in the extent of PCD with progression to disease. Longitudinal analysis of four individuals through infection, from seroconversion to AIDS, also demonstrated a variation but not a consistent increase or decrease in the number of cells in apoptosis over time. There is no correlation of the numbers of cells dying due to PCD after in vitro culture with virus load or presence of SI and NSI HIV-variants (Meyaard et al.1994).

PCD RESULTS FROM GENERALIZED VIRUS-INDUCED IMMUNE ACTIVATION?

Many studies now have demonstrated death of T cells from HIV-infected individuals die due to apoptosis upon in vitro culture (Groux et al.1992; Meyaard et al.1992; Gougeon et al.1993a; Oyaizu et al.1993; Pandolfi et al.1993; Meyaard et al.1994; Lewis et al.1994). PCD can be enhanced not only by activation in vitro with TCR/CD3 mab, but also with lectins, superantigens or ionomycin (Meyaard et al.1992; Groux et al.1992; Gougeon et al.1993a; Oyaizu et al.1993). In line with our initial observations, PCD was reported to occur in both CD4+ and CD8+ T cells (Gougeon et al.1993a; Lewis et al.1994) and all CD8+ T-cell subsets contain cells dying due to PCD and there is no evidence reported yet to indicate preferential death in one specific subset of cells (Meyaard et al.1994; Lewis et al.1994).

In HIV-infected chimpanzees, that do not develop clinical symptoms, the proportion of T cells dying due to PCD does not exceed that in non-infected animals (Gougeon et al.1993a; Schuitemaker et al.1993). This could imply either a direct role for PCD in HIV pathogenesis in humans, or that PCD is a reflection of immuno pathogenic events. Several hypothesis on the cause of increased PCD of T cells in human HIV infection, and the contribution to AIDS pathogenesis have been proposed, including direct virus infection of cells, CD4-ligation by gp120 and excessive immune activation.

Infection of T cells and T-cell lines with HIV in vitro results in cell death associated with apoptosis (Terai et al.1991; Laurent-Crawford et al.1991; Martin et al.1994). Direct virus-induced cell death can, however be excluded as the main cause of PCD of peripheral T cells in asymptomatic HIV infection. Not only is the frequency of infected cells during asymptomatic infection too low to explain the extent of cell death observed, there seems to be no clear cut relation between virus load during both acute and asymptomatic infection and increases in PCD (Meyaard et al.1994). However, in later stages of infection, with a high viral burden in T cells in lymph nodes, direct infection of cells leading to apoptosis might contribute in some extent to CD4+ T-cell depletion. Moreover, HIV infection of thymocytes might lead to increased apoptotic death in the thymus, thereby affecting regeneration of the peripheral T-cell compartment (Bonyhadi et al.1993).

The initial hypothesis with regard to PCD in HIV infection was that interaction of soluble HIV envelope protein gp120 with CD4 could prime T cells for PCD (Ameisen et al.1991). Mature murine lymphocytes die from PCD after stimulation via TCR/CD3 when CD4 was previously ligated by CD4 antibodies (Newell et al.1990). Furthermore, addition of gp120 in vitro has been shown to impair T cell function (Oyaizu et al.1990; Manca et al.1990; Cefai et al.1990). Indeed in human cells, cross-linking of CD4 mAb or bound gp120 on human CD4+ T cells followed by signalling through the TCR results in apoptosis in vitro (Banda et al.1992; Oyaizu et al.1993). These data point to a role for gp120 in inducing T-cell deficiency and apoptosis. gp120-CD4 ligation might be a mechanism for apoptosis of CD4+ T-cells in vivo. The contribution to the PCD observed, however, is hard to asses.

A CD4-dependent mechanism for PCD is not likely to be the only explanation. First, both CD4+ and CD8+ cells, with a preference for CD8+ cells, are dying due to apoptosis (Meyaard et al.1992; Gougeon et al.1993a) and secondly, during primary HIV-infection, the number of cells dying exceeds by far the percentage of CD4+ cells present at that time (Meyaard et al.1994). CD8+ T cells from HIV-infected individuals have increased expression of activation markers as CD38, HLA-DR and CD57 suggestive for continuous immune activation (Stites et al.1989; Salazar-Gonzalez et al.1985). CD8+ cells expressing activation markers have severely decreased proliferative responses and clonogenic potential (Pantaleo et al.1990) and are reported to die in culture (Prince et al.1991). Because the percentage of cells dying due to PCD in primary HIV infection parallels the CD8+ T-cell expansion, it is tempting to speculate that PCD in HIV infection reflects turn over of activated immune cells, although PCD is not confined to a specific subset expressing activation markers (Meyaard et al.1994; Lewis et al.1994).

PCD as a result of massive immune activation following acute virus infection is not specific for HIV infection since it was also demonstrated for CMV infection in man (Van den Berg et al.1994) and acute LCMV infection in mice (Razvi et al.1993), correlating with hypo-responsiveness as a result of hyperactivation of T cells in vivo. Similar findings have been reported for Epstein-Barr virus infection in humans (Moss et al.1985; Uehara et al.1992), where both CD4+ and CD8+ cells die upon culture. Dying cells were confined to the CD45RO+ population and cell death could be prevented by culture in the presence of cytokines like IL-2 (Bishop et al.1985; Uehara et al.1992). Also in that condition, PCD was suggested to affect the population of activated T cells which expands during the acute phase of the infection.

We propose that PCD in acute HIV infection is a reflection of immune activation leading to high turn-over of cells as is observed in acute virus infections in general. High numbers of apoptotic cells in the early stage of infection are followed by moderately increased numbers of cells dying during the asymptomatic phase, as is also observed in the asymptomatic phase of feline immunodeficiency virus infection in cats (Bishop et al.1993). In asymptomatic HIV infection, PCD reflects a continuous activation leading to priming for death and deletion of responding T cells.

As in other viral infections, PCD in acute HIV infection might be a reflection of immune activation by a so far unknown mechanism leading to decreased expression of survival genes and increased expression of apoptosis genes and turn-over of immune cells. The increased numbers of cells dying during the asymptomatic phase might be the result of continuous activation and priming for death to maintain T-cell homeostasis.

Although PCD in early asymptomatic infection is probably reflecting the activated immune system rather than being a critical pathogenic mechanism, virus-induced apoptosis might contribute to CD4+ cell depletion. First by infection of thymocytes, thus affecting the renewal of the T-cell compartment and secondly, when the viral burden increases, by HIV-induced apoptosis of peripheral CD4+ T cells.

It has been proposed that therapeutic intervention with agents that block T-cell apoptosis might be beneficial for HIV-infected patients (Gougeon et al.1993b). However, PCD is more the outcome rather than the basis of AIDS pathogenesis, while effective immune therapy should aim for early events leading to immune dysfunction. Moreover, cell death is a physiological phenomenon which normally occurs in the immune system and other systems to maintain homeostasis. Intervention in this process might be more harmful than beneficial for the patient. Immune therapy therefore, should aim at preserved Th cell responses leading to controlled virus replication by preservation of HIV-specific cytotoxic T-cell responses (Klein et al.1994).

ACKNOWLEDGEMENTS

Our work is supported by grant 90-015 from the Dutch Ministry of Public Health and is conducted as a part of the Amsterdam Cohort Studies on AIDS.

REFERENCES

Ameisen, J.C. and Capron, A. 1991. Cell dysfunction and depletion in AIDS: the programmed cell death hypothesis. *Immunol.Today* 12:102-105.

Banda, N.K., Bernier, J., Kurahara, D.K., Kurrle, R., Haigwood, N., Sekaly, R-P. and Helman Finkel, T. 1992. Crosslinking CD4 by Human Immunodeficiency Virus gp120 primes T cells for activation-induced apoptosis. *J.Exp.Med.* 176:1099-1106.

Bishop, C.J., Moss, D.J., Ryan, J.M. and Burrows, S.R. 1985. T lymphocytes in infectious mononucleosis. II. Response in vitro to interleukin-2 and establishment of T cell lines. *Clin.Exp.Immunol.* 60:70-77.

Bishop, S.A., Gruffydd-Jones, T.J., Harbour, D.A. and Stokes, C.R. 1993. Programmed cell death (apoptosis) as a mechanism of cell death in peripheral blood mononuclear cells from cats infected with feline immunodeficiency virus (FIV). *Clin.Exp.Immunol.* 93:65-71.

Bonyhadi, M.L., Rabin, L., Salimi, S., Brown, D.A., Kosek, J., McCune, J.M. and Kaneshima, H. 1993. HIV induces thymus depletion in vivo. *Nature* 363:728-732.

Cefai, D., Debre, P., Kaczorek, M., Idziorek, T., Autran, B. and Bismuth, G. 1990. Human immunodeficiency virus-1 glycoproteins gp120 and gp160 specifically inhibit the CD3/T cell-antigen receptor phosphoinositide transduction pathway. *J.Clin.Invest.* 86:2117-2124.

Duke, R.C., Chervenak, R. and Cohen, J.J. 1983. Endogenous endonuclease-induced DNA-fragmentation: An early event in cell-mediated cytolysis. *Proc.Natl.Acad.Sci.USA* 80:6361-6365.

Gougeon, M., Garcia, S., Heeney, J., Tschopp, R., Lecoeur, H., Guetard, D., Rame, V., Dauguet, R. and Montagnier, L. 1993a. Programmed cell death in AIDS-related HIV and SIV infections. *AIDS Res.Hum.Retroviruses* 9:553-563.

Gougeon, M. and Montagnier, L. 1993b. Apoptosis in AIDS. *Science* 260:1269-1270.

Groux, H., Torpier, G., Monté, D., Mouton, Y., Capron, A. and Ameisen, J.C. 1992. Activation-induced death by apoptosis in CD4+ T cells from Human Immunodeficiency Virus-infected asymptomatic individuals. *J.Exp.Med.* 175:331-340.

Klein, M.R., van Baalen, C.A., Kerkhof-Garde, S.R., Bende, R.J., Schuitemaker, H., Keet, I.P.M., Eeftinck Schattenkerk, J.K.M., Osterhaus, A.D.M.E. and Miedema, F. 1994. HIV-1 specific CTL responses correlate with clinical course of HIV-1 infection: Persistent anti-Gag CTL activity during prolonged survival. *submitted for publication*

Laurent-Crawford, A.G., Krust, B., Muller, S., Rivière, Y., Rey-Cuillé, M.A., Béchet, J.-M., Montagnier, L. and Hovanessian, A.G. 1991. The cytopathic effect of HIV is associated with apoptosis. *Virology* 185:829-839.

Lewis, D.E., Ng Tang, D.S., Adu-Oppong, A., Schober, W. and Rodgers, J.R. 1994. Anergy and apoptosis in CD8+ T cells from HIV-infected individuals. *J.Immunol.* In press

Manca, F., Habeshaw, J.A. and Dalgleish, A.G. 1990. HIV envelope glycoprotein, antigen specific T-cell responses, and soluble CD4. *Lancet* 335:811-815.

Martin, S.J., Matear, P.M. and Vyakarnam, A. 1994. HIV-1 infection of human CD4+ T cells in vitro. Differential induction of apoptosis in these cells. *J.Immunol.* 152:330-342.

Meyaard, L., Otto, S.A., Jonker, R.R., Mijnster, M.J., Keet, R.P.M. and Miedema, F. 1992. Programmed death of T cells in HIV-1 infection. *Science* 257:217-219.

Meyaard, L., Otto, S.A., Keet, I.P.M., Roos, M.Th.L. and Miedema, F. 1994. Programmed death of T cells in HIV-1 infection: no correlation with progression to disease. *J.Clin.Invest.* 93:982-988.

Miedema, F., Petit, A.J.C., Terpstra, F.G., Schattenkerk, J.K.M.E., De Wolf, F., Al, B.J.M., Roos, M.Th.L., Lange, J.M.A., Danner, S.A., Goudsmit, J. and Schellekens, P.Th.A. 1988. Immunological abnormalities in human immunodeficiency virus (HIV)-infected asymptomatic homosexual men. HIV affects the immune system before CD4+ T helper cell depletion occurs. *J.Clin.Invest.* 82:1908-1914.

Miedema, F., Meyaard, L., Koot, M., Klein, M.R., Roos, M.Th.L., Groenink, M., Fouchier, R.A.M., Van 't Wout, A.B., Tersmette, M., Schellekens, P.Th.A. and Schuitemaker, H. 1994. Changing virus-host interactions in the course of HIV-1 infection. *Imm.Rev.* In press

Moss, D.J., Bishop, C.J., Burrows, S.R. and Ryan, J.M. 1985. T lymphocytes in infectious mononucleosis.I.T cell death in vitro. *Clin.Exp.Immunol.* 60:61-69.

Newell, M.K., Haughn, L.J., Maroun, C.R. and Julius, M.H. 1990. Death of mature T cells by separate ligation of CD4 and the T-cell receptor for antigen. *Nature* 347:286-288.

Oyaizu, N., Chirmule, N., Kalyanaraman, V.S., Hall, W.W., Good, R.A. and Pahwa, S. 1990. Human immunodeficiency virus type 1 envelope glycoprotein gp120 produces immune defects in CD4+ T lymphocytes by inhibiting interleukin 2 mRNA. *Proc.Natl.Acad.Sci.USA* 87:2379-2383.

Oyaizu, N., McCloskey, T.W., Coronesi, M., Chirmule, N., Kalyanaraman, V.S. and Pahwa, S. 1993. Accelerated apoptosis in peripheral blood mononuclear cells (PBMCs) from human immunodeficiency virus type-1 infected patients and in CD4 cross-linked PBMCs from normal individuals. *Blood* 82:3392-3400.

Pandolfi, F., Oliva, A., Sacco, G., Polidori, V., Liberatore, D., Mezzaroma, I., Kurnick, J.T. and Aiuti, F. 1993. Fibroblast-derived factors preserve viability in vitro of mononuclear cells isolated from subjects with HIV-1 infection. *AIDS* 7:323-329.

Pantaleo, G., Koenig, S., Baseler, M., Clifford Lane, H. and Fauci, A.S. 1990. Defective clonogenic potential of CD8+ T lymphocytes in patients with AIDS. Expansion in vivo of a nonclonogenic CD3+CD8+DR+CD25-T cell population. *J.Immunol.* 144:1696-1704.

Prince, H.E. and Jensen, E.R. 1991. HIV-related alterations in CD8 cell subsets defined by in vitro survival characteristics. *Cell.Immunol.* 134:276-286.

Razvi, E.S. and Welsh, R.M. 1993. Programmed cell death of T lymphocytes during acute viral infection: a mechanism for virus-induced immune deficiency. *J.Virol.* 67:5754-5765.

Salazar-Gonzalez, J.F., Moody, D.J., Giorgi, J.V., Martinez-Maza, O., Mitsuyasu, R.T. and Fahey, J.L. 1985. Reduced ecto-5'-nucleotidase activity and enhanced OKT 10 and HLA-DR expression on CD8 lymphocytes in the aquired immune deficiency syndrome: evidence of CD8 cell immaturity. *J.Immunol.* 135:1778-1785.

Schellekens, P.Th.A., Roos, M.Th.L., De Wolf, F., Lange, J.M.A. and Miedema, F. 1990. Low T-cell responsiveness to activation via CD3/TCR is a prognostic marker for AIDS in HIV-1 infected men. *J.Clin.Immunol.* 10:121-127.

Schnittman, S.M., Psallidopoulos, M.C., Lane, H.C., Thompson, L., Baseler, M., Massari, F., Fox, C.H., Salzman, N.P. and Fauci, A.S. 1989. The reservoir for HIV-1 in human peripheral blood is a T cell that maintains expression of CD4. *Science* 245:305-308.

Schuitemaker, H., Meyaard, L., Kootstra, N.A., Otto, S.A., Dubbes, R., Tersmette, M., Heeney, J.L. and Miedema, F. 1993. Lack of T-cell dysfunction and programmed cell death in human immunodeficiency type-1 infected chimpanzees correlates with absence of monocytotropic variants. *J.Infect.Dis.* 168:1140-1147.

Shearer, G.M., Payne, S.M., Joseph, L.J. and Biddison, W.E. 1984. Functional T lymphocyte immune deficiency in a population of homosexual men who do not exhibit symptoms of acquired immune deficiency syndrome. *J.Clin.Invest.* 74:496-506.

Stites, D.P., Moss, A.R., Bacchetti, P., Osmond, D., McHugh, T.M., Wang, Y.J., Hebert, S. and Colfer, B. 1989. Lymphocyte subset analysis to predict progression to AIDS in a cohort of homosexual men in San Francisco. *Clin.Immunol.Immunopathol.* 52:96-103.

Terai, C., Kornbluth, R.S., Pauza, C.D., Richman, D.D. and Carson, D.A. 1991. Apoptosis as a mechanism of cell death in cultured T lymphoblasts acutely infected with HIV-1. *J.Clin.Invest.* 87:1710-1715.

Uehara, T., Miyawaki, T., Ohta, K., Tamaru, Y., Yokoi, T., Nakamura, S. and Taniguchi, N. 1992. Apoptotic cell death of primed CD45RO+ T lymphocytes in Epstein-Barr virus induced infectious mononucleosis. *Blood* 80:452-458.

Van den Berg, A.P., Meyaard, L., De Leij, L.H.F.M., Otto, S.A., Mesander, G., Van Son, W.J., Klompmaker, I.J., Miedema, F. and The, T.H. 1994. Decreased T-cell proliferative capacity and increased rate of programmed cell death of lymphocytes in human cytomegalovirus infection. *submitted for publication*

Wyllie, A.H., Kerr, J.F.K. and Currie, A.R. 1980. Cell death: The significance of apoptosis. *Int.Rev.Cytol.* 68:251-306.

11

T CELL APOPTOSIS AS A CONSEQUENCE OF CHRONIC ACTIVATION OF THE IMMUNE SYSTEM IN HIV INFECTION

Marie-Lise Gougeon

Unité d'Oncologie Virale
Département SIDA et Rétrovirus
Institut Pasteur
28 rue du Dr. Roux
75724 Paris Cedex 15
France

I. INTRODUCTION

The hallmark of AIDS is the progressive disappearance of CD4+ helper T lymphocytes which, in addition to be the targets of the virus play a major role in the immune system. Although it is likely that the active replication of the virus in lymphoid organs is at least associated with CD4+ T cell depletion, it has become clear that indirect mechanisms have to be considered to explain the extent of immunosuppression. HIV disease is now considered as a multifactorial process and the immunopathogenic mechanisms involved appear to be very complex. In the present review, some of the indirect mechanisms potentially involved in AIDS pathogenesis will be discussed, focusing on the causes and consequences of a persistant and inappropriate activation of the immune system leading to paralysis (anergy) or self destruction (apoptosis) of non-infected patients' T cells (1-4).

II. HIV-INDUCED IMMUNE DEFICIENCY

A number of factors seem to be involved in HIV-induced immune deficiency. Direct cytopathic effect (CPE) of HIV on CD4+ T cells might contribute to the immune CD4 T cell depletion. Indeed simultaneous analysis of viral burden in the blood and lymphoid organs indicated that HIV is sequestrated in lymph nodes both as an extracellular virus trapped in the follicular dendritic cell network of the germinal centers and as intracellular virus usually in a latent form (5,6). Furthermore during the apparently latent period between infection with HIV and the overt symptoms of AIDS, HIV is actively replicating in lymphoid organs (6) despite a low viral burden and low replication in PBL, indicating that a state of true microbiological latency does not exist.

Cell Activation and Apoptosis in HIV Infection
Edited by Jean-Marie Andrieu and Wei Lu, Plenum Press, New York, 1995

The cytopathic effect of HIV in CD4+ T cells is associated with apoptosis (7,8) and it was shown that apoptosis is tightly associated with the formation of syncytia and is triggered by the binding of CD4 to the viral envelope glycoprotein (gp120) (9). Another potential mechanism for CD4+ cell loss is the covering of cells carrying the CD4 molecule with gp120. These uninfected cells are then recognized as virus-infected cells by NK (Natural Killer) effector cells or CTL (Cytotoxic T Lymphocytes) and subsequently destroyed, even though they are not infected by the virus (10,11). Therefore cytotoxic CD8+ cells might kill normal CD4+ cells as well as those infected with HIV (12,13). Anti-lymphocyte antibodies may also play a role in immune deficiency. Autoantibodies to the CD4 protein have been detected in HIV-infected individuals and might be involved in CD4+ lymphocyte death (14).

Besides the direct effects of HIV on CD4+ cells, viral proteins released by infected cells could interfere with the normal events in signal transduction. Indeed very early in the course of the disease, before CD4 cell depletion, functional defects of helper T cells are observed in patients' lymphocytes, characterized by the impairment of in vitro T-cell receptor (TcR)-dependent activation (15,16). Extracellular signals mediated by gp120 via CD4 molecule may affect signal transduction. For example gp120 signalling has been shown to be involved in the induction of anergy (17) or in the programming for cell death of non-infected CD4+ T cells (18).

Paradoxically, concomitantly to the inhibition of lymphocyte activation (anergy) of helper CD4+ T cells in patients, a chronic activation of the immune system is observed: expression of T cell activation antigens on CD4+ and CD8+ T cells, spontaneous B cell hyperactivation, lymph node hyperplasia early in the course of infection, increased cytokine expression etc... The persistence of virus and viral replication throughout the course of HIV disease may play a primary role in the maintenance of this chronic activation and it has been proposed that superantigens (either of bacterial origin or encoded by HIV) may contribute to this activation. The potential influence of superantigens in AIDS pathogenesis is also discussed in the present article.

III. CHRONIC ACTIVATION AND APOPTOSIS

Apoptosis (Programmed Cell Death) is an active suicide mechanism that constitutes the principal form of cell death for lymphocytes. In general the cell undergoing apoptosis sustains profound structural changes and one of these is a nuclear collapse associated with condensation of chromatin which tends to marginate in crescents around the nuclear envelope. The nuclear collapse indicates extensive damage to chromatin which is degraded into single and multiple oligonucleosomes. This fragmentation of DNA is enzymatic and generally occurs after activation of a calcium-dependent endogenous endonuclease (19).

There are several examples of PCD in T lymphocytes. This process is involved in the negative intrathymic selection of the T cell repertoire, which leads to the clonal deletion of autoreactive T cells and to the establishment of self tolerance (20). Mature T cells generally respond to TCR-dependent stimulation by proliferation and differentiation. However under certain circumstances apoptosis is thought to mediate the death of antigen-activated mature T cells (21-23).

Spontaneous apoptosis can be observed in mature peripheral T cells in the context of acute viral infection such as EBV-induced infectious mononucleosis or VZV infection (24-25). In these viral infections, both CD4 and CD8 T cells undergo apoptosis upon a few-hour culture. Similarly these two T cell subsets were shown to die spontaneously of apoptosis when isolated from asymptomatic HIV-infected individuals (26-29). FACScan phenotyping of CD4+ and CD8+ T cells dying of apoptosis after 24 hours of culture indicated that a significative fraction of them expressed the activation markers CD45R0 or HLA-DR.

Spontaneous apoptosis of CD45R0- and HLA-DR- expressing CD4 and CD8 T cells was also described in EBV or VZV-infected patients where these circulating T cell subsets were found specifically expanded during the acute phase of infection (24-25). Since apoptosis of these cells in viral infections can be prevented by cytokines, IL-2 in EBV-infected patients (25) or IL-1α + IL-2 in HIV-infected patients (28) it suggests that after T cell activation in vivo, the expanded population is destined to perish unless some factors, such as cytokines, promote their survival.

Spontaneous apoptosis of CD4 and CD8 T cells is observed at all stages of HIV-infection but it is more pronounced at the AIDS stage. We found a significative inverse correlation between the extent of apoptosis and the ex-vivo absolute number of CD4 but it is noteworthy that an extensive phenotyping of cells undergoing apoptosis in patients at different stages of the disease indicated a statistically significant increase of apoptosis in CD4 T cells along with the evolution of the disease. Although CD8 T cells comprise the major population undergoing apoptosis at the AIDS stage (since very few CD4 T cells are left at this stage), they do not show a greater fragility as opposed to CD4 T cells (30). The causes of the increased CD4 fragility at the late stages of HIV-infection have to be determined.

The T cell lymphocytosis associated with acute viral infections is transient as the absolute number of circulating T lymphocytes and the relative proportion of CD4+ and CD8+ cels return to normal upon resolution of the disease. It probably occurs via a rapid clearance by apoptosis of the majority of activated T cell blasts in vivo which allows a balance between cell death and survival. In the case of a chronic infection such as the retroviral HIV-infection, persistence of immune activation generating suicide sensitive CD45RO+ T cells, expressing low bcl-2 (30), would induce regular deletion of memory CD4+ and CD8+ T cells, contributing to the immune deficiency. The disappearance of such cells is particularly dramatic if the immune system from HIV-infected individuals is not capable of spontaneous regeneration. Indeed there is evidence that in HIV-infected individuals the thymus is severely damaged. Thus even if the bone-marrow precursor cells are still present in HIV-infected individuals it is questionable whether the reconstitution of normal immune function would occur in the absence of an intact thymic microenvironment. A number of questions related to the possible impairment in T cell renewal are still unanswered such as : Do CD8+ T cells die in vitro as a consequence of their hyperactivation but would survive in the patients? Do CD8+ T cells die in vivo but are replaced? Does the selective loss of CD4+ T cells during HIV-infection is also the consequence of impairment of renewal of this population?

In addition to inducing a dramatic functional and physical loss of virus-specific immunocompetent cells, persistence of immune activation may also have viral consequences such as a more efficient virus spread in activated cells and expression of virus in cells latently infected with HIV (31, 32). It was proposed that HIV may induce itself a strong immune activation by encoding for a superantigen, by analogy with the murine retroviruses MMTV (33). Although there is no direct evidence today that HIV encodes for a protein harboring a superantigenic activity, several recent reports suggested that superantigens may be involved in the pathogenesis of AIDS .

IV. SUPERANTIGENS IN HIV-INFECTION

T cells recognize, in addition to the conventional antigens, another category of ligands, the superantigens, on the basis of the expressed Vβ on their T cell receptor. Exogenous bacterial superantigens comprise a set of protein toxins produced by *Staphylococcus*, *Streptococcus* or *Mycoplasma* that are recognized, in the context of MHC class II molecules, by T cells expressing particular TCR Vβ gene families, causing strong T cell activation associated with toxic shock and autoimmune diseases (34,35). Moreover super-antigens of retroviral origin encoded by MMTV and MuLV were shown, for the former to be responsible for activation and subsequent deletion of CD4+ T cell subsets expressing corresponding Vβ elements (33, 36) and for the latter to be involved in the murine acquired immunodeficiency syndrome (MAIDS) (37).

Since HIV-1 is a retrovirus it was suggested that it might encode for a superantigen expressed by activated infected cells causing, in conjunction with class II genes, cell anergy and deletion of noninfected Vβ specific CD4+ T cells (38). Several recent reports have discussed attempts to indirectly revealing the presence of an HIV-associated superantigen by looking for consistent amplifications and/or deletions in the ex-vivo peripheral TCR Vβ repertoire of HIV-infected individuals: a more restricted Vβ repertoire was found in HIV-infected patients with advanced disease (39) and a significant increase of peripheral CD4+ T cells of the Vβ5.3 subfamily was reported in asymptomatic subjects (40). Perturbations in the Vβ repertoire were also found in several pairs of monozygotic twins discordant for HIV with identical MHC (41). This last study allows meaningful comparisons of the Vβ repertoires since one of the major factors that influence the nature of the peripheral TCR Vβ repertoire is the MHC class II haplotype of the individual (42).

Instead of analysing the ex-vivo repertoire in peripheral T lymphocytes from HIV-infected individuals, we choosed a more functional approach: since in vivo murine studies have shown that anergy of a given Vβ subset gives evidence of a previous activation of this subset by a superantigen we have searched for a selective Vβ anergy in patients' T cells. We analyzed the Vβ usage of peripheral T cells from asymptomatic HIV-infected subjects in response to the bacterial superantigen Streptococcal erythrogenic toxin A (ETA), known to stimulate the Vβ8 and Vβ12 subsets. We demonstrated the existence, in a large fraction (around 60%) of HIV-infected individuals, of a Vβ specific anergy affecting both CD4+ and CD8+ T cells expressing the Vβ8 TCR element (43,44). Several observations are in favour of a direct involvement of HIV in this Vβ specific anergy (44): 1-anergy can be observed very early in the course of HIV-infection, a few weeks post-infection (CDC stage I); 2-comparison of clinical status of responder vs anergic patients showed no correlation with previous viral or bacterial infections suggesting that the Vβ anergy is not induced by opportunistic pathogens; 3- a strong proliferation was induced by in vitro stimulation of normal peripheral lymphocytes with inactivated HIV and concomitantly the selective expansion of Vβ8+ T cells was reproducibly detected. Characterization of the Vβ8 specific activity associated to HIV is currently under investigation.

Except for the acute pathogenic variant of simian immunodeficiency virus (SIV) PBj14 (45) no report has shown until now the ability of HIV to activate normal peripheral T cells. Since a selective expansion of superantigenic reactive T cells is known to precede anergy, one can speculate that in vivo infection of CD4+ cells will induce viral protein expression that, in association with MHC class II molecules, will activate in a superantigenic way followed by anergy subsets bearing the cognate Vβ determinants. It is interesting to note that the putative viral superantigen involved in the Vβ8 anergy has no selective tropism for CD4+ T cells since both CD4+ and CD8+ T cells are found anergic in patients and both are responsive to the in vitro Vβ8 specific activation by HIV. A recent report described the dependence of HIV-1 replication on a superantigen and it concerned particularly the V§12+ CD4+ cell subset which replicated more efficiently HIV in vitro and which was found enriched for gp120 expressing cells in vivo (46). Our study is probably concerned with another superantigen. Interestingly enough, as found by others, we could not confirm the massive deletions of a large proportion of Vβ families described (39) including the V§8 subset. Therefore, in HIV-infection it is likely that superantigens, if indeed they are present and have an impact on pathogenesis, act as potent activators of T cells contributing to virus dissemination and progressive immune failure (via anergy and apoptosis), rather than as factors directly responsible for deletion of selective subsets of T cells.

V. CONCLUSIONS

The immunopathogenic mechanisms underlying HIV-infection are more complex that was thought several years ago; viral burden is substantial particularly in lymphoid organs, inappropriate immune activation contributes to the pathogenic process, profound immune suppression finally occurs associated with the destruction of the immune environment, preventing the spontaneous regeneration of the immune system. Therefore any strategy must consider the complexity of these pathogenic mechanisms and should not be unidirected (1).

REFERENCES

1. Fauci AS (1993) Multifactorial nature of HIV disease: implications for therapy. Science 262:1011-1018
2. Gougeon ML and Montagnier L (1993) Apoptosis in AIDS. Science 260:1269-1270
3. Levy JA (1993) Pathogenesis of human immunodeficiency virus infection. Microb. Rev. 57: 183-289
4. Gougeon ML (1995) Does apoptosis contribute to CD4 T cell depletion in human immunodeficiency virus infection? Cell Death and Differentiation 2:1-8
5. Embretson J, Zupancic M, Ribas J.L., et al. (1993) Massive covert infection of helper T lymphocytes and macrophages by HIV during the incubation period of AIDS. Nature, 362:359-362
6. Pantaleo G, Graziosi C. Demarest J.F. et al. (1993) HIV infection is active and progressive in lymphoid tissue during the clinically latent stage of disease. Nature, 362:355-358
7. Terai C, Kornbluth, RS, Pauza CD, Richman DD, Carson DA (1991) Apoptosis as a mechanism of cell death in cultured T lymphoblasts acutely infected with HIV-1. J.Clin.Invest. 87: 1710-1715
8. Laurent-Crawford AG, Krust B, Muller S, Rivire Y, Rey-Cuill MA, Bchet JM, Montagnier L, Hovanessian A (1991). The cytopathic effect of HIV is associated with apoptosis. Virology 185: 829-839
9. Laurent-Crawford AG, Krust B, Rivire Y, Muller S, Kieny MP, Dauguet C, Hovanessian AG (1992) Membrane expression of HIV envelope glycoproteins triggers apoptosis in CD4 cells. AIDS Res Hum Retrov
10. Lanzavecchia A, Roosnek E, Gregory T et al. (1988). T cells can present antigen such as HIV gp120 targeted to their own surface molecules. Nature, 334, 530-532
11. Weinhold KJ, Lyerly HK, Stanley SD, et al. (1989) HIV-1-gp120 mediated immune response and lymphocyte destruction in the absence of viral infection. J. Immunol. 142, 3091-3097
12. Pantaleo G, De Maria A, Koenig S et al. (1990) CD8+ T lymphocytes of patients with AIDS maintain normal broad cytoloytic function despite the loss of HIV-specific cytotoxicity. Proc. Nat. Acad Sci USA 87: 4818-4822
13. Riviere Y, Tanneau-Salvadori F, Regnault A et al. (1989) HIV-specific cytotoxic responses of seropositive individuals : distinct types of effector cells mediate killing of targets expressing gag and env proteins. J. Virol. 63: 2270-2277
14. Chams V, Jouault T, Fenouillet E, Gluckman JC, Klatzmann D (1988) Detection of anti-CD4 autoantibodies in the sera of HIV-infected patients using recombinant soluble CD4 molecules. AIDS, 2, 353-361
15. Shearer GM and M Clerici (1991) Early T-helper cell defect in HIV infection. AIDS 5: 245-253
16. Miedema F, Petit AJC, Terpstra FG et al (1988). Immunological abnormalities in human immunodeficiency virus (HIV) infected asymptomatic homosexual men. HIV affects the immune system before CD4+ T helper cell depletion. J. Clin. Invest 82: 1908-1915
17. Di Rienzo AM, Furlini G, Olivier R, Ferris S, Heeney J, Montagnier L. (1993) Different proliferative response of human and chumpanzee lymphocytes after contact with HIV-1. Eur J Immunol. 24:34-40
18. Banda NM, Bernier J, Kurahara DK et al. (1992) Cross-linking by HIV gp120 primes T cells for activation-induced apoptosis J Exp Med 176: 1099-1106
19. Arends MJ , Morris RG,Wyllie A.H. (1990). Apoptosis. The role of the endonuclease AM. J. Pathol. 136: 593-608

20. Jenkinson EJ, Kingston CA, Smith CA, Williams GT, Owen JJT (1989). Antigen-induced apoptosis in developing T cells: a mechanism for negative selection of the TCR repertoire. Eur. J. Immunol. 19:2175-2180

21. Kawabe Y, Ochi A (1991) Programmed cell death and extrathymic reduction of Vβ8+CD4+ T cells in mice tolerant to Staphylocccus aureus enterotoxin B. Nature 349:245-248

22. Webb S, Morris C, Sprent J (1990) Extrathymic tolerance of mature T cells: clonal elimination as a consequence of autoimmunity. Cell 63:1249-1256

23. Newell MK, Haughn LJ, Maroun CR, Julius M (1990). Death of mature T cells by separate ligation of CD4 and the T cell receptor for antigen. Nature 347:286-288

24. Uehara T, Miyawaki T, Ohta K et al. (1992). Apoptotic cell death of primed CD45R0+ T lymphocytes in Epstein-Barr virus-induced infectious mononucleosis. Blood 80:452-458

25. Akbar AN, Borthwick N, Salmon M et al. (1993) The significance of low bcl-2 expression by CD45R0 T cells in normal individuals and patients with acute viral infections. The role of apoptosis in T cell memory. J Exp Med 178 427-438

26. Gougeon ML, Olivier R, Garcia S, Guétard D, Dragic T, Dauguet C, Montagnier L. (1991) Evidence for an engagement process towards apoptosis in lymphocytes of HIV infected patients. C. R. Acad. Sci. Paris 312: 529-537

27. Gougeon ML, Garcia S, Gutard D, Olivier R , Dauguet C, Montagnier L. (1992) Apoptosis as a mechanism of cell death in peripheral lymphocytes from HIV1-infected individuals in Immunology of HIV infection (Janossy G, Autran B, Miedema F, eds) pp. 115-126, A.G. Karger , Basel

28. Gougeon ML, Garcia S, Heeney, J., Tschopp, R. Lecoeur, H, Guetard, D, Rame, V, Dauguet, C. Montagnier L. (1993). Programmed cell death of T lymphocytes in AIDS related HIV and SIV infections. AIDS Res. Hum. Retrov. 9:553-563

29. Meyaard L, Otto, S.A. Jonker R.R. Mijnster M.J., Keet, R. Miedema, F. (1992). Programmed death of T cells in HIV-1 infection. Science, 257:217-219

30. Gougeon ML, Lecoeur H, Boudet F, Dulioust A, Enouf MG, Crouvoisier M, Montagnier L. (1995) Apoptosis as a consequence of the general state of immune activation in HIV-infection. Influence on bcl-2 expression. In "Retroviruses of Human AIDS and Related Animal Diseases" (M. Girard and L. Valette Eds), Fondation M. Merieux,8 me colloque des Cents Gardes, In press

31. Rosenberg ZF, Fauci AS (1990) Immunopathogenic mechanisms of HIV infection: cytokine induction of HIV expression. Immunol. Today 11: 176-180

32. Poli G and Fauci AS (1992) The effects of cytokines and pharmacologic agents on chronic HIV infection. AIDS Res Hum Retrov 8:191-197

33. Choi Y, Kappler JW, Marrack P (1991) A superantigen encoding in the open reading frame of the 3' long terminal repeat of mouse mammary tumour virus. Nature 350:203-207

34. Kappler J B, Kotzin, L. Herron, E. Gelfand, R. Bigler, A. Boylston, S. Carrel, D. Posnett, Y. Choi, and P. Marrack. (1989) V beta-specific stimulation of human T cells by staphylococcal toxins. Science. 244: 811.

35. Marrack, P., and J. Kappler.(1990). The staphylococcal enterotoxins and their relatives. Science. 248: 1066.

36. Korman, A.J., P. Bourgarel, T. Meo, and G.E. Rieckhof. (1992). The mouse mammary tumor virus long terminal repeat encodes a type II transmembrane glycoprotein. *EMBO. J.* 11: 1901.

37. Hugin A, M. Vacchio, and H. Morse. 1991. A virus-encoded "superantigen" in a retrovirus-induced immunodeficiency syndrome of mice. Science. 252: 424.

38. Janeway C (1991) Immune recognition. Mls: makes a little sense. Nature. 349: 459-460

39. Imberti, L., A. Sottini, A. Bettinardi, M. Puoti, and D. Primi. 1991. Selective depletion in HIV infection of T cells that bear specific T cell receptor V beta sequences. Science. 254: 860.

40. Dalgleish, A., S. Wilson, M. Gompels, C. Ludlam, B. Gazzard, A. Coates, and J. Habeshaw (1992) T-cell receptor variable gene products and early HIV-1 infection. Lancet. 339: 824.

41. Soudeyns, H., N. Rebai, G.P. Pantaleo, C. Ciurli, T. Boghossian, R.P. Skali, and A.S. Fauci. (1993). The T cell receptor V§ repertoire in HIV-1 infection and disease. Seminars in Immunology. 5: 175.

42. Gulwani-Akolkar B, DN Posnett, CH Janson, J Grunwald, H Wigzell, P Akolkar, PK Gregersen, and J Silver. (1991) T cell receptor V-segment frequencies in peripheral blood T cells correlate with human leucocyte antigen type. J. Exp. Med. 174: 1139.

43. Dadaglio G, Garcia S, Montagnier L, Gougeon ML (1994) Selective anergy of V§8+ T cells in human immunodeficiency virus-infected individuals. J Exp Med 179:413-424

44. Dadaglio G, Poccia F, Garcia S, Mller-Alouf H, Roue R, Montagnier L, Gougeon ML. (1993). V§ specific T cell clonal anergy in HIV-infected individuals with possible involvement of an HIV component. In

Retroviruses of human AIDS and related Animal Diseases (M. Girard and L. Valette Eds), p. 17-22, Fondation M.Mrieux

45. Fultz PN (1991) Replication of an acutely lethal simian immunodeficiency virus activates and induces proliferation of lymphocytes. J. Virol. 65: 4902-4910

46. Laurence, J., A.S. Hodtsev, and D.N. Posnett (1992) Superantigen implicated in dependence of HIV-1 replication in T cells on TCR V beta expression. Nature. 358: 255.

12

APOPTOSIS DURING HIV INFECTION

A Cytopathic Effect of HIV or an Important Host-Defense Mechanism against Viruses in General?

Seamus J. Martin* and Douglas R. Green

Division of Cellular Immunology
La Jolla Institute for Allergy and Immunology
11149 N. Torrey Pines Road
La Jolla, California 92037

INTRODUCTION

After several years of searching for an acceptable explanation for the early immune dysfunction seen in HIV-positive individuals with normal CD4 counts, recent reports indicate that these defects may be due to the inappropriate triggering of activation-induced cell death or apoptosis in T cells from such individuals when stimulated with specific antigen or certain mitogens (Groux *et al.*, 1992; Meyaard *et al.*, 1992; Gougeon and Montagnier, 1992; Oyaizu *et al.*, 1993). Thus, the progressive depletion of the CD4+ T cell population during HIV infection may be rationally explained as a sequential loss of antigen responsiveness as the patient encounters individual antigens and each clone of specific T cells are deleted. In this model of HIV pathogenesis, the virus is thought to somehow prime T cells for apoptosis, either as a result of gaining entry to the cell, by binding of a viral component or antibodies elicited by such components to the cell, or by causing dysregulation of the cytokine network. This model has provoked much interest, not least because apoptosis is widely perceived as a 'special' form of cell death since there appears to be a cellular apparatus which, once activated, is concerned with killing the cell from within (Duvall and Wyllie, 1985; Martin *et al.*, 1994a). The fact that such an apparatus exists has raised the possibility that it may be open to manipulation, making it possible to delay or even prevent cell death in some cases. However, whether inhibition of T cell apoptosis during HIV infection (if this is indeed possible) would necessarily be of benefit to a HIV-infected individual depends entirely on whether one percieves the apoptosis recorded in this context to be a beneficial or deleterious consequence of viral infection. In this article, we discuss the various possible routes to apoptosis during HIV infection and suggest that many of the cell deaths seen during infection with HIV, as well as with many other viruses, are entirely beneficial to the host since they limit replication and spread of the virus. Indeed, active suppression of host cell

---

* Address to Dr Seamus J. Martin at the above address or by Fax at 619 558 3525.

Cell Activation and Apoptosis in HIV Infection
Edited by Jean-Marie Andrieu and Wei Lu, Plenum Press, New York, 1995

Table 1. Viral genes that modulate apoptosis of their host cell

Virus	Gene/protein	Effect on apoptosis	Reference
Abelson murine leukemia virus	Abl	Represses	Evans et al., 1993
			McGahon et al., 1994
Adenovirus	E1A	Induces	White et al., 1991
Adenovirus	E1B	Represses	White et al., 1991
African swine fever virus	LMW5-HL	Undefined, homology to Bcl-2 and BHRF-1	Neilan et al., 1993
Autographa californica baculovirus	p35	Represses	Clem et al., 1991
Cowpox Virus	crmA	Represses, inhibits Interleukin-1β converting enzyme (ICE) activity	Gagliardini et al., 1994
Cydia pomonella granulosis virus	iap	Represses	Crook et al., 1993
Epstein-Barr Virus	LMP1	Represses, upregulates Bcl-2	Henderson et al., 1991
Epstein-Barr Virus	BHRF1	Represses, directly	Henderson et al., 1993
HIV-1	Tat	Represses, upregulates Bcl-2	Zauli et al., 1993
HTLV-1	Tax	Induces	Yamada et al.,

apoptosis (by viral genes), particularly during the early stages of HIV infection, may be an important mechanism of viral persistance.

IS APOPTOSIS DURING HIV INFECTION HOST CELL-DRIVEN OR VIRUS-DRIVEN?

Because we can detect apoptosis when we culture cells from HIV-positive individuals (Groux et al., 1992; Meyaard et al., 1992; Gougeon and Montagnier, 1992; Oyaizu et al., 1993) or upon infection of CD4+ T cells in vitro (Terai et al., 1991; Laurent-Crawford et al., 1991; Martin et al., 1994b), does it logically follow that this is inappropriate for the host cell and somehow good for the virus? Most reports on HIV-associated apoptosis to date would appear to have adopted this line of reasoning. However, apoptosis as a direct consequence of HIV infection may actually be a host strategy for containing the spread of the virus, since an infected cell undergoing apoptosis could be looked upon as killing itself in an attempt to limit replication of the virus within and therefore spare its neighbours. Since some of the genes implicated in the control of apoptosis appear to have been well conserved through evolution, at least from nematodes to man (see Vaux et al., 1994 for review), the ability to trigger apoptosis upon viral infection may actually be a primitive host-defense mechanism. The fact that man has evolved more sophisticated means of defending himself from infectious agents would not necessarily mean that cell suicide would cease to be a valuable means of defense against viruses. In fact, many of the weapons in our immune arsenal appear to be used for exactly the same purpose; i.e. to track down and destroy infected cells or invaders. Thus, for example, cytotoxic T lymphocytes (CTLs) attack and kill their target cells, as do natural killer (NK) cells, activation of complement by antibody also results in lysis of the target, and recent studies imply that Fas-ligand bearing CTL cells may have a role in eliminating unwanted or allogenic Fas-antigen positive cells by inducing apoptosis in these cells (Kagi et al., 1994).

Alternatively, one could take the view that apoptosis as a result of viral infection is a pathogenic effect of the virus upon the cell rather than the cell's response to the viral infection. However, since it has recently been discovered that many viruses possess genes that are capable of modulating apoptosis of their host cells (Table 1), this would suggest that the ability to control the cell death apparatus in the host is important to the virus and would imply that the ability of the host cell to undergo apoptosis upon infection is an important host-defense mechanism.

As one can see, in many of these cases, the viral gene acts as a repressor of cell death, thus it prevents the cell from dying under conditions in which it would normally do so. Epstein Barr virus actually appears to have two strategies for doing this: first, EBV carries a gene, BCRF-1, that encodes the BHRF-1 protein, a homologue of the *bcl-2* gene (Henderson *et al.*, 1993) which is well known to be a potent inhibitor of apoptosis (Korsmeyer, 1992), the second strategy used by EBV, is to induce the upregulation of endogenous *bcl-2* in the host cell, which it does using the late membrane protein-1 (LMP1) gene (Henderson *et al.*, 1991; Gregory *et al.*, 1991). Several other viruses, including insect baculoviruses, have also been found to possess genes that can repress apoptosis of their host cells (Clem *et al.*, 1991; White *et al.*, 1991; Crook *et al.*, 1993; Neilan *et al.*, 1993; Evans *et al.*, 1993; Gagliardini et al., 1994; McGahon *et al.*, 1994). But in situations where a virus possess a death repressor gene, does this result in any selective advantage for the virus? Data from the insect baculovirus system would seem to indicate that this is the case (Clem and Miller, 1993).

In this example, insect baculoviruses (Autographa california) carrying defective forms of a death repressor gene (p35) produced significantly lower amounts of viral progeny than baculoviruses which contained a functional p35 gene. These authors conclude that the host apoptotic response provides protection against viral infection. Similar data with p35 mutants was also reported by other workers (Lerch and Friesen, 1993).

Thus there is good reason to believe that many of the apoptotic cell deaths which occur as a consequence of HIV infection may well be a normal part of the host immune response against the virus. Taking this idea a step further, one prediction would be that HIV variants that manage to establish a productive infection must have some way of overcoming this host-defense mechanism. Is there actually any evidence for this? A recent report would seem to indicate that there is (Zauli *et al.*, 1993). These workers have found that HIV-1 *tat* can act as a repressor of apoptosis when transfected into a variety of human cell lines, apparently by upregulating the expression of *bcl-2*. However, it is not yet clear whether Bcl-2 can repress HIV-induced apoptosis, although this is currently being investigated (Martin, S.J. and Corbeil, J. unpublished data). Assuming for the moment that *bcl-2* can indeed block HIV-induced cell death, this observation could be interpeted to imply that HIV variants that express high levels of Tat protein would persist more successfullly than variants expressing low levels of this protein. With this line of reasoning, apoptosis is probably a good thing in early HIV infection.

It is therefore fairly plausible that by inhibiting (by pharmacological means) the triggering of apoptosis in HIV-primed T cells, one may actually facilitate virus proliferation, resulting in infection of even more T cells and death of these cells by other means (discussed later). Such an approach may lead to an acceleration of T cell depletion and therefore more rapid progression to AIDS. In addition, although there is undoubtedly a large amount of apoptosis ongoing during HIV infection, there are several alternative routes to T cell depletion during HIV infection which cannot be overlooked (Fig. 1A-F), as well as other observations which have been made with regard to apoptosis of cells from HIV-positive patients which complicate interpetation of the data. Careful consideration of these issues is therefore required before we approach strategies aimed at suppressing or modulating apoptosis with a view to stemming the tide of T cell loss *in vivo*.

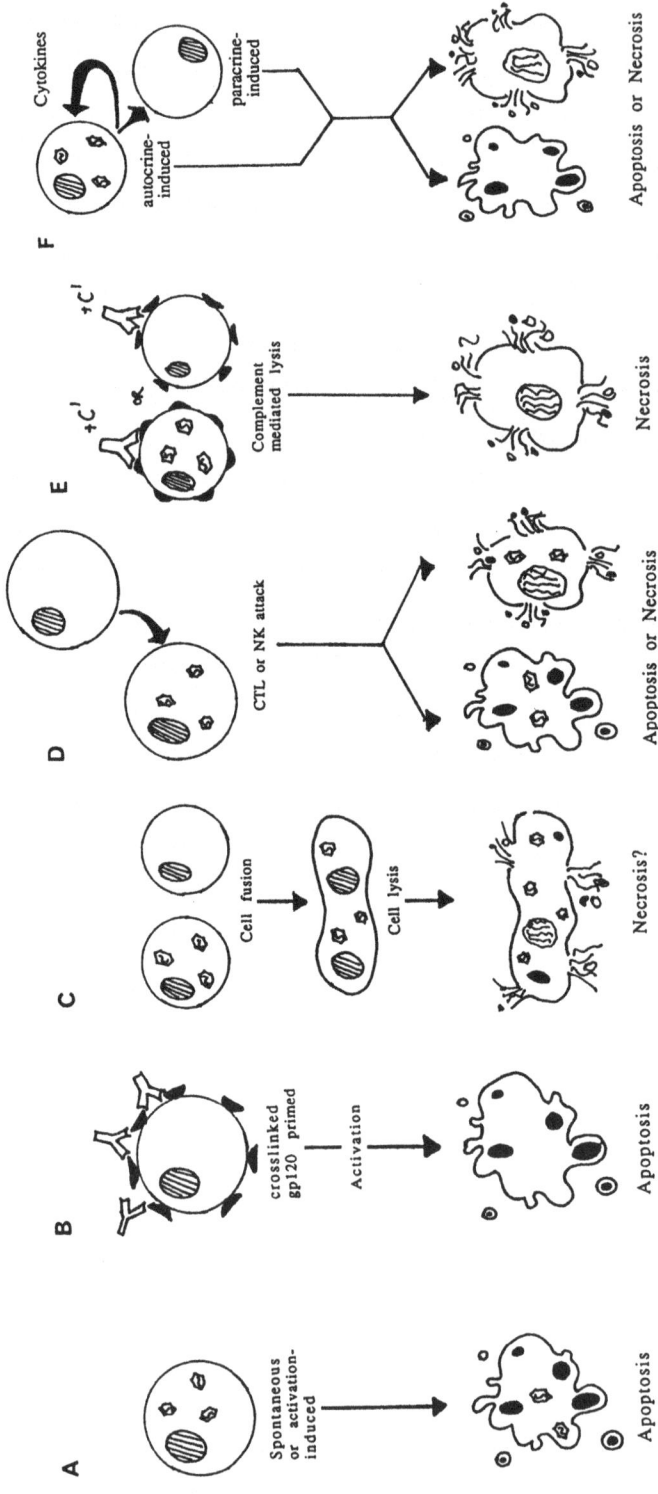

Figure 1. Routes to T cell death during HIV infection. (A) Spontaneous or activation-induced apoptosis as a direct result HIV infection, (B) Activation-induced apoptosis of uninfected cell as a result of crosslinking of CD4 by soluble gp120 (shed by infected cells) and anti-gp120 mAb, (C) Syncytium formation followed by cell lysis (D) CTL or NK attack of infected cell, (E) Antibody and complement attack of infected cell or a cell which has bound a viral component (such as free gp120), (F) HIV-induced overproduction of cytokines may trigger death of infected cells or bystander cells.

ROUTES TO APOPTOSIS DURING HIV INFECTION

It is still unclear how important priming of T cells for apoptosis may be as a mechanism of T cell depletion during HIV infection. Although several recent studies have demonstrated significant levels of activation-induced apoptosis after *in vitro* stimulation of peripheral blood mononuclear cells from HIV patients with various mitogens (Groux *et al.*, 1992; Meyaard *et al.*, 1992; Gougeon and Montagnier, 1992; Oyaizu *et al.*, 1993), or spontaneous apoptosis of these cells during *in vitro* culture (Gougeon and Montagnier, 1992) **(Fig. 1A)**, it is obviously difficult to relate these findings directly to what is happening *in vivo*. Since the normal final consequence of a stimulatory signal which results in proliferation and differentiation of T cells appears to be apoptosis (Martin, 1993b; Martin *et al.*, 1994b; Salmon *et al.*, 1994) (except in those cells destined to become memory cells), it is not unusual that T cells from HIV-infected individuals die by apoptosis *per se*. What is unusual is that these cells appear to die in the absence of proliferation, as evidenced by their decreased responsiveness to specific antigen and certain mitogens in ^{3}H-thymidine uptake assays (Groux *et al.*, 1992), and memory cell formation appears to be impaired. However, proliferative responses can be restored with the use of mAbs to the B7 receptor, CD28 (Miedema *et al.*, 1991, Groux *et al.*, 1992) which would seem to indicate a defect in antigen presentation rather than in the T cell itself. This would not account for the increased fragility of T cells from HIV-infected patients when simply cultured *in vitro* however (Gougeon and Montagnier, 1992), nor does it explain the increased apoptosis of purified populations of these cells when stimulated with agents such as ionomycin (Gougeon and Montagnier, 1992) or anti-CD3 mAbs (Meyaard *et al.*, 1992) which are not necessarily dependent on costimulatory signals from antigen presenting cells. It is possible that these cells have been primed for apoptosis *in vivo*, e.g. as a consequence of persistent activation by cytokines, which have been shown to be overproduced during HIV-infection (Vyakarnam *et al.*, 1991). Chronic immune activation could also account for apoptosis of many more cells than those which are directly infected.

Does HIV Directly or Indirectly Prime T Cells for Apoptosis?

A surprising finding in some of the recent studies was that CD8$^+$ T cells were found to undergo apoptosis to an even greater extent than CD4$^+$ T cells when activated *in vitro* (Meyaard et al., 1992; Gougeon and Montagnier, 1992; Gougeon *et al.*, 1993; Carbonari *et al.*, 1994) which obviously does not correlate with what happens in the HIV patient during the course of the infection. Once again, this could be a reflection of the widespread immune activation ongoing in HIV infection, resulting in rapid expansion and turnover of cells, particularly virus-specific CD8+ CTLs.

Because early studies failed to detect many HIV-infected cells in the peripheral blood of HIV-positive individuals, a situation we now know to be not quite true (Pantaleo *et al.*, 1993), many workers have sought to explain HIV immunopathology by looking for indirect ways in which the virus may prime celld for death. The most popular candidate for indirect priming is gp120, the viral envelope glycoprotein, since it is so easily shed from the virus and binds specifically to the CD4 molecule (Moore *et al.*, 1990). As an extension of the observation that crosslinking of CD4 followed by stimulation through the T cell receptor leads to apoptosis of murine T cells (Newell *et al.*, 1990), it was suggested that gp120 may prime human T cells for a similar fate (Ameisen and Capron, 1991). Evidence in support of this hypothesis remains weak, however, some investigators do observe some potential of gp120-crosslinked or antibody-crosslinked CD4 to prime human T cells for apoptosis upon activation (Banda *et al.*, 1992; Oyaizu *et al.*, 1993)

(**Fig. 1B**), while others do not (Martin *et al.*, 1994b; Liegler and Stites, 1994). Another problem with regard to gp120-mediated cell death is the scarcity of free gp120 in peripheral blood available to prime T cells for apoptosis, compared with the amounts used in the *in vitro* studies mentioned above. Since the observations concerning proliferative defects and apoptosis of cells from HIV-infected individuals were made on peripheral blood cells, it seems an unlikely explanation of these phenomena. It is possible that trafficking cells which have picked up gp120 in a highly infected lymph node may be deleted by this mechanism, but this still leaves us with no explanation for the observed apoptosis of the CD8+ T cell population, if indeed this occurs *in vivo*. As stated in the previous section, *in vivo* priming of both CD4+ and CD8+ T cells due to persistent activation by cytokines may also be a plausible explanation for apoptosis upon further stimulation. However, if this is the case then it suggests that either the CD8$^+$ T cell population is more resistant to this effect *in vivo* or that the renewal potential of the CD4+ T cell population is impaired as compared with the CD8+ T cell population.

Do HIV-Induced Syncytia Die by Apoptosis or Necrosis?

HIV variants have been grouped into two broad categories, syncytium-inducing (SI) or non syncytium-inducing (NSI), depending on the nature of their cytotoxic properties *in vitro* (Miedema *et al.*, 1990). During syncytium formation, an HIV infected cell bearing membrane associated gp120 binds to the CD4 molecule of an uninfected T cell and fuses with this cell. The process can be repeated many times, resulting in a giant multinucleate cell or syncytium (**Fig. 1C**), and provides an attractive explanation of how a few infected cells can promote the destruction of many uninfected T cells. Syncytia are a very common cytopathic effect of many HIV isolates *in vitro* (Lifson *et al.*, 1986a,b), but as with all *in vitro* observations an important issue is whether syncytium formation occurrs at an appreciable rate *in vivo*. Theoretically, at sites of T cell accumulation such as the lymph nodes, a single infected cell should be capable of triggering syncytium formation. However, while syncytia have been recorded in the spleen and brains of AIDS patients on autopsy, these have found to be composed largely of macrophages. Nonetheless, studies have shown that SI variants of HIV appear to be the ones associated with disease progression to AIDS (Miedema *et al.*, 1990). Therefore, circumstantially at least, the presence of HIV varients with the ability to promote syncytium formation seems to be correlated with CD4 cell depletion and progression to AIDS.

From a conceptual standpoint, we believe that syncytium-inducing variants of HIV probably kill their hosts by inducing necrosis. This view is taken after a consideration of the process of apoptotic cell death. Apoptosis is generally considered to be a mechanism for eliminating aged or excess cells from a multicellular organism in a controlled fashion without unnecessarily activating defense mechanisms by provoking inflammation (Kerr *et al.*, 1972). Therefore, when cells die via apoptosis they undergo a process of internal self-destruction which prevents leakage of cellular constituents, and rapidly leads to their recognition and engulfment by neighbouring cells or tissue macrophages (Wyllie *et al.*, 1980; Savill *et al.*, 1993). To aid their removal, apoptotic cells frequently shrink and fragment into many membrane-bound vesicles, termed apoptotic bodies. Necrosis on the other hand is a much more disordered process. Cells undergoing necrosis generally undergo high amplitude cell swelling which leads to cell lysis and spillage of a host of damaging cellular constituents which can kill neighbouring cells and provoke inflammation (Wyllie *et al.*, 1980).

With regard to the issue of how syncytia die once formed, we believe this to be necrosis for the following reason. Syncytia, due to their grossly abnormal size, cannot be phagocytosed unless they fragment into smaller membrane-bound vesicles, termed apoptotic bodies. Even if these cells fragment their DNA in the appropriate fashion (Laurent-Crawford *et al.*, 1991) and are recognized as being 'apoptotic' by neighbouring phagocytes, due to their grossly increased size it is highly unlikely that they could be engulfed. It is our experience from *in vitro* observations that syncytia do not collapse into apoptotic bodies, unlike other cells dying by apoptosis (S.J. Martin, unpublished observations). Syncytia therefore almost certainly undergo cell lysis, i.e. necrosis, thereby spilling out infectious virus and exacerbating the infection. Therefore, would-be attempts to minimise T cell killing during HIV-infection by blocking apoptosis are unlikely to succeed with syncytium-inducing strains of HIV, that is, if syncytia are indeed formed at an appreciable rate *in vivo*. These strains would have to be dealt with by blocking their ability to promote cell fusion (Martin, 1993a).

CTL-Induced Killing

Another important pathway to T cell depletion during HIV-infection may be class I-restricted cytotoxic T cell killing of virus-infected cells (Nixon *et al.*, 1988) (**Fig. 1D**). Whether CTLs are of benefit during HIV-infection or whether they actually exacerbate the situation has still not been established. For the moment, we should probably give CTLs the benefit of the doubt, since these are important effector cells in controlling other viral infections such as EBV. There is much evidence that CTLs generally kill their targets via an apoptotic mechanism, although there is also some evidence which suggests that CTLs may kill in some cases by inducing necrosis in their targets (Zychlinsky *et al.*, 1991). For cells that are considered to be specialised in the control of virus infection, it makes more sense that CTLs induce apoptosis rather than necrosis in their targets since lysis of a target cell which may be loaded with infective virus is surely less attractive for the host than a mechanism which kills the infected cell and ensures its recognition and phagocytosis without releasing cellular contents. Interfering with the apoptotic process in CTL targets would not be likely to be of benefit to the host unless the virus itself had no direct cytopathic effects, as in lymphocytic choriomeningitis virus (LCMV) infection in mice for example (Zinkernagel, 1988).

OTHER ROUTES TO CELL DEATH DURING HIV INFECTION

There are also other ways in which HIV may cause the depletion of T cells, several of which result in necrosis rather than apoptosis. Obvious ways such as antibody and complement-mediated cell lysis are undoubtedly necrotic in mechanism (**Fig. 1E**). Antibody-dependant cellular cytoxicity may take the form of necrosis or apoptosis, depending on the effector cell in question.

As previously mentioned, dysregulation of the cytokine network by HIV may also have important consequences for the viability of both infected cells as well as uninfected bystander cells. Excessive production of several cytokines including; TNF-α, TNF-β, and IFN-γ, has been demonstrated in HIV-infected patients in response to *in vitro* activation with mitogenic stimuli (Vyakarnam *et al.*, 1991). Secretion of high levels of these cytokines may not only have deleterious effects on infected cells themselves but could also lead to inappropriate activation of bystander cells which may result in death of these cells or may prime cells to die upon further activation. TNF has been shown to kill sensitive cells by triggering either apoptosis or necrosis, depending on the cell type in question (Laster *et al.*, 1988). Thus overproduction of cytokines by HIV-infected cells could result in either apoptosis or necrosis of susceptible cells (**Fig. 1F**).

CONCLUSION

While the fact that cells from HIV-infected patients appear more predisposed to undergoing apoptosis *in vitro* and that HIV can directly induce death of CD4+ T cells infected *in vivo* is clearly an important advance in our understanding of the possible mechanisms of pathogenicity of the virus, the implications of these results need to be considered carefully before we draw conclusions as to the impact of apoptosis in the T cell depletion seen during infection. In particular, we need to establish whether the apoptotic response is a benefical one, as it appears to be after CTL attack of infected target cells, or whether it is an inappropriate and damaging response to stimulation as a consequence of the immune dysregulation triggered by HIV. The role of SI variants of HIV in T cell depletion is still unclear and may be particularly important given the correlation between these variants and disease progression. Whether SI and NSI HIV variants kill by different modes remains unanswered. In addition, the role of cytokines in the cytopathic properties of HIV and their role in contributing to the chronic immune activation of cells from HIV-positive individuals requires further investigation.

ACKNOWLEDGEMENTS

SJM is in receipt of a Wellcome Trust International Travelling Prize Fellowship. Research in DRG's laboratory is supported by grant AI31591 from the NIH and CB-82 from the American Cancer Society. We thank Professors J.H.L Playfair and I.M. Roitt, and Drs. D. Briggs, J. McCullough, A. Vyakarnam and G.A.W. Rook for their comments on an earlier version of this manuscript and Dr. J. Corbeil for comments and discussion.

REFERENCES

Ameisen, J.C. and Capron, A. (1991) Cell dysfunction and depletion in AIDS: the programmed cell death hypothesis. *Immunol. Today* **12**:102-105.

Banda, N.K., Bernier, J., Kurahara, D.K., Kurrle, R., Haigwood, N., Sekaly, R.P., Finkel, T.H. (1992) Crosslinking CD4 by human immunodeficiency virus gp120 primes T cells for activation-induced apoptosis. *J. Exp. Med.* **176**:1099-1106.

Carbonari, M., Cibati, M., Cherchi, M., Sbarigia, D., Pesce, A.M., Dell'Anna, L., Modica, A., and Fiorilli, M. (1994) Detection and characterization of apoptotic peripheral blood lymphocytes in HIV infection and cancer chemotherapy by a novel flow immunocytometric method. *Blood* **83**:1268-1277.

Clem, R.J., Fecheimer, M. and Miller, L.K. (1991) Prevention of apoptosis by a baculovirus gene during infection of insect cells. *Science* **254**:1388-1390.

Crook, N.E., Clem, R.J., Miller, L.K. (1993) An apoptosis-inhibiting baculovirus gene with a zinc finger-like motif. *J. Virol.* 67: 2168-2174.

Duvall, E. and Wyllie, A.H. (1986) Death and the cell. *Immunol. Today* **7**:115-119.

Evans C.A., Owen-Lynch, P.J., Whetton, A.D., Dive, C. (1993) Activation of the Abelson tyrosine kinase activity is associated with suppression of apoptosis in hematopoietic cells. *Cancer Res.* **53**:1735-1738.

Evans, C.A., Owen-Lynch, P.J., Whetton, A.D., Dive, C. (1993) Activation of the Abelson tyrosine kinase activity is associated with suppression of apoptosis in hemopoietic cells. *Cancer Res.* **53**:1735-1738.

Gagliardini, V., Fernandez, P.A., Lee, R.K.K., Drexler, H.C.A., Rotello, R.J., Fishman, M.C., and Yuan, J. (1994) Prevention of vertebrate neuronal death by the *crm A* gene. *Science* **263**:826-828.

Gougeon, M.L. and Montagnier, L. (1992) New concepts in the mechanisms of CD4 lymphocyte depletion in AIDS, and the influence of opportunistic infections. *Res. in Microbiol.* **143**:362-368.

Gougeon, M.L., Garcia, S., Heeney, J., Tschopp, R., Lecoeur, H., Guetard, D., Rame, V., Dauguet, C., and Montagnier, L. (1993) Programmed cell death in AIDS-related HIV and SIV infections. *AIDS Res. Hum. Retrovir.* **9**:553-563.

Gregory, C.D., Dive, C., Henderson, S., Smith, C.A., Williams, G.T., Gordon, J., and Rickinson, A.B. (1991) Activation of Epstein-Barr Virus latent genes protects human B cells from death by apoptosis. *Nature* **349**:612-614.

Groux, H., Torpier, G., Monte, D., Mouton, Y., Capron, A., Ameisen, J.C. (1992) Activation-induced death by apoptosis in CD4+ T cells from human immunodeficiency virus-infected asymptomatic individuals. *J. Exp. Med.* **175**:331-340.

Henderson S., Huen D., Rowe M., Dawson C., Johnson G., and Rickinson A. (1993) Epstein-Barr virus-coded BHRF1 protein, a viral homologue of Bcl-2, protects human B cells from programmed cell death. *Proc Natl Acad Sci USA* **90**:8479-8483.

Henderson, S., Rowe, M., Gregory, C., Croom-Carter, D., Wang, F., Longnecker, R., Kieff, E., and Rickinson, A.B. (1991) Induction of bcl-2 expression by Epstein-Barr virus latent membrane protein 1 protects infected B cells from programmed cell death. *Cell* **65**:1107-1115.

Kagi, D., Vignaux, F., Ledermann, B., Burki, K., Depraetere, V., Nagata, S., Hengartner, H., and Goldstein, P. (1994) Fas and perforin as major mechanisms of T-cell mediated cytotoxixity. *Science* **265**:528-530.

Kerr, J.F.R., Wyllie, A.H. and Currie, A.R. (1972) Apoptosis: a basic biological phenomenon with wide-ranging implications in tissue kinetics. *Br. J. Can.* **26**:239-257.

Korsmeyer, S.J. (1992) Bcl-2: a repressor of lymphocyte death. *Immunol. Today* **13**:285-287.

Laster, S.M., Wood, J.G. and Gooding, L.R. (1988) Tumor necrosis factor can induce both apoptotic and necrotic forms of cell lysis. *J. Immunol.* **141**:2629-2634.

Laurent-Crawford, A.G., Krust, B., Muller, S., Riviere, Y., Rey-Cuille, M.A., Bechet, J.M., Montagnier, L., Hovanessian, A.G. (1991) The cytopathic effect of HIV is asscoiated with apoptosis. *Virology* **185**:829-839.

Lerch, R.A, Friesen, P.D. (1993) The 35-kilodalton protein gene (p35) of Autographa california nuclear polyhedrosis virus and the neomycin resistance gene provide dominant selection of recombinant baculoviruses. *Nuc. Acids Res.* **21**:1753-1760.

Liegler, T.J., and Stites, D.P. (1994) HIV-1 gp120 and anti-gp120 induce reversible unresponsiveness in peripheral CD4T lymphocytes. *J. AIDS* **7**:340-348.

Lifson, J.D., Feinberg, M.B., Reyes, G.R., Rabin, L., Banapour, B., Chakrabarti, S., Moss, B., Wong-Stall, F., Steimer, K.S., and Engelman, E.G. (1986a) Induction of CD4-dependent cell fusion by the HTLV-III/LAV envelope in syncytium formation and cytopathicity. *Nature* **323**:725-728.

Lifson, J.D., Reyes, G.R., McGrath, M.S., Stein, B.S., and Engelman, E.G. (1986b) AIDS retrovirus induced cytopathology: giant cell formation and involvement of the CD4 antigen. *Science* **232**:1123-1127.

Martin, S.J. (1993a) Programmed cell death and AIDS. *Science* **262**:1355-1356.

Martin, S.J. (1993b) Protein or RNA synthesis inhibition induces apoptosis of mature CD4+ T cell blasts. *Immunol. Letts.* **35**:125-131.

Martin, S.J., Green, D.R., and Cotter T.G. (1994a) Dicing with death; dissecting the components of the apoptosis machinery. *Trends in Biochemical Sci.*, **19**:26-30.

Martin, S.J., Matear, P. and Vyakarnam, A. (1994b) HIV-1 infection of CD4+ T cells *in vitro*: differential induction of apoptosis in these cells. *J. Immunol.*, **152**:330-342.

McGahon A., Bissonnette R., Schmitt M., Cotter K.M., Green D.R., Cotter T.G. (1994) BCR-ABL maintains resistance of chronic myelogenous leukemia cells to apoptotic cell death. *Blood* **83**: 1179-1187.

Meyaard, L., Otto, S.A., Jonker, R.R., Mijnster, M.J., Keet, R.P., Miedema, F. (1992) Programmed death of T cells in HIV infection. *Science* **257**:217-219.

Midema, F., Tersmette, M. and van Lier R.A.W. (1990) AIDS pathogenesis: a dynamic interaction between HIV and the immune system. *Immunol. Today* **11**:293-297.

Moore, J.P., McKeating, J.A., Weiss, R.A. and Sattentau, Q.S. (1990) *Science* **250**:1139-1142.

Neilan, J.G., Lu, Z., Afonso, C.L., Kutish, G.F., Sussman, M.D., Rock, D.L. (1993) An African swine fever virus gene with similarity to the proto-oncogene bcl-2 and the Epstein barr Virus gene BHRF-1. *J. Virol.* **67**:4391-4394.

Newell, M.K., Haughn, L.J., Maroun, C.R. and Julius, M.H. (1990) Death of mature T cells by separate ligation of CD4 and the T cell receptor for antigen. *Nature* **347**:286-289.

Nixon, D.F., Townsend, A.R.M., Elvin, J.G., Rizza, C.R., Gallwey, J., McMichael, A.J. (1988) HIV-1 gag specific cytotoxic T lymphocytes defined with recombinant vaccinia virus and synthetic peptides. *Nature* **336**:484-487.

Oyaizy, N., McCloskey, T.W., Coronesi, M., Chirmule, N., Kalyanaraman, V.S., and Pahwa, S. (1993) Accelerated apoptosis in peripheral blood mononuclear cells (PBMCs) from human immunodeficiency virus type-1 infected patients and in CD4 cross-linked PBMCs from normal individuals. *Blood* **82**:3392-3400.

Pantaleo, G., Graziosi, C., Demarest, J.F., Butini, L., montroni, M., Fox, C.H., Orenstein, J.M., Kotler, D.P., and Fauci, A.S. (1993) HIV infection is active and progresive in lymphoid tissue during the clinically latent stage of disease. *Nature* **362**:355-358.

Salmon, M., Pilling, D., Borthwick, N.J., Viner, N., Janossy, G., Bacon, P.A., Akbar, A.N. (1994) The progressive differentiation of primed T cells is associated with apoptosis. *Eur. J. Immunol.* **24**:892-899.

Savill, J.S., Fadok, V., Henson, P., Haslett, C. (1993) Phagocyte recognition of cells undergoing apoptosis. *Immunol Today* **14**:131-136.

Terai, C., Kornbluth, R., Pauza, C., Richman, D.D., and Carson, D.A. (1991) Apoptosis as a mechanism of cell death in cultured T lymphoblasts acutely infected with HIV-1. *J. Clin. Invest.* **87**:1710-1715.

Vyakarnam, A., Matear, P., Meager, A., kelly, G., Stanley, B., Weller, I., Beverly, P.C.L. (1991) Altered production of TNFα,β and IFNγ by HIV-infected individuals. *Clin. Exp. Immunol.* **84**:109-115.

White, E., Cipriani, R., Sabbatini, P., Denton, A. (1991) Adenovirus E1B 19-kilodalton protein overcomes the cytoxicity of E1A proteins. *J Virol* . **65**:2968-2978.

Wyllie, A.H., Kerr, J.F.R. and Currie, A.R. (1980) Cell death: the significance of apoptosis. *Int. Rev. Cytol.* **68**:251-306.

Yamada, T., Yamaoka, S., Nakai, M., Tsujimoto, Y., Hatanaka, M. (1994) The human T cell leukemia virus type 1 Tax protein induces apoptosis which is blocked by bcl-2 protein. *J. Virol.* **68**:3374-3379.

Zauli, G., Gibellini, D., Milani, D., Mazzoni, M., Borgatti, P., La Placa, M., Capitani S. (1993) Human immunodeficiency virus type 1 Tat protein protects lymphoid, epithelial, and neuronal cell lines from death by apoptosis. *Cancer Res.* **53**:4481-4485.

Zinkernagel, R.M. (1988) Virus triggered AIDS: a T cell-mediated immunopathology? *Immunol. Today* **9**:370-372.

Zychlinsky, A., Zheng, L-M., Liu, C-C. and Ding-E Young, J. (1991) Cytolytic lymphocytes induce both apoptosis and necrosis in target cells. *J. Immunol.* **146**:393-400.

13

FROM CELL ACTIVATION TO CELL DEPLETION

The Programmed Cell Death Hypothesis of AIDS Pathogenesis

Jean Claude Ameisen

INSERM U 415 Pathogenèse du sida et des infections à tropisme
   immunitaire et nerveux
Institut Pasteur
1 rue du Pr. A. Calmette
59019 Lille and
Faculté de Médecine
Université Lille II
Lille, France

THE HYPOTHESIS

Acquired immunodeficiency syndrom (AIDS) provides a spectacular illustration of the capacity of a pathogen, the human immunodeficiency virus (HIV), to induce in about ten years a progressive and complete loss of immune competence in the infected host by causing the loss of the lymphocyte population that plays a central role in the control of the immune response, the CD4[+] T helper cells[1,2].

The major pathological features of AIDS are the progressive collapse of the two most complex regulatory networks of the human body, the immune system, leading to immune incompetence, and the central nervous system, leading to brain atrophy and dementia[1-3]. In both organs, AIDS induces the loss of a major cell population: the CD4[+] T cell in the immune system[1], and the neuron in the brain[3].

After the identification of HIV as the causative agent of AIDS, the observations of the tropism of HIV for CD4[+] T cells and of its cytopathic effect on CD4[+] T cells *in vitro* have initially suggested that the pathogenesis of AIDS is solely related to direct virus-mediated cell destruction of HIV-infected cells. However, this concept has been progressively challenged by a series of observations. First, a global CD4[+] T-cell dysfunction is observed long before cell depletion is detected, at a time when few peripheral blood CD4[+] T cells are infected[4,5]. CD4[+] T-helper cells present early and profound functional defects that are characterized by a selective loss of memory function. These qualitative defects include *in vivo* a failure of CD4[+] T cells to mediate delayed-type hypersensitivity reactions to self-major histocompatibility complex-class II-restricted recall antigens, and *in vitro* a selective loss of the ability of T cells to proliferate in response to T-cell receptor stimulation by these recall antigens and by antibodies directed to the CD3/T-cell receptor complex, as well as to defined polyclonal activators such as pokeweed mitogen[6-11]. These findings therefore suggested that HIV can also affect the behaviour of uninfected CD4$^+$ T cells. Second, neuronal loss is observed in the brain[3] while neurons, in contrast to CD4$^+$ T cells, are not targets for HIV infection; HIV in the central nervous system being expressed primarily in cells of the macrophage lineage[12,13]. These observations suggested that HIV can also cause the death of uninfected cells. Finally, the study of primate models of chronic lentiviral infection with the human (HIV) and the closely related simian (SIV) immunodeficiency viruses have raised important and paradoxical questions about the pathogenesis of AIDS. Chimpanzees, the only primates that can be productively and chronically infected with HIV-1, do not, in contrast to HIV-1-infected humans, develop any AIDS-related disease[14], even when infected with HIV-1 isolates that are, *in vitro*, cytopathic for chimpanzee CD4$^+$ T cells[15]. Natural SIV infection of primates of African origin such as African green monkeys and sooty mangabey monkeys results in a stable nonpathogenic viral-host interaction with high viral loads and does not lead to disease[16], indicating that lentiviruses do not need to destroy the immune system to persist in the infected host and to spread in a wide proportion of the infected species. Experimental infection of primate species of Asian origin with lentiviral strains that do not infect them naturally has led to two opposite outcomes: an absence of disease in chimpanzees experimentally infected with HIV-1, as mentioned above, and AIDS development in rhesus macaques experimentally infected with SIV[17]. The rhesus macaque model has provided very important insights into lentiviral pathogenesis by showing that a given primate species can be experimentally infected either with pathogenic viral strains or recombinant molecular clones of SIVmac that induce AIDS, or with viral recombinant molecular clones of SIVmac whose sequences differ by less than 2% from those of pathogenic clones and that do not induce disease[17,18]. In summary, these primate models of chronic lentiviral infection indicate that pathogenesis does not result solely from the ability of a lentivirus to infect CD4$^+$ T cells, a property shared by all these viruses. Rather, they strongly suggest that pathogenesis involves an additional and complex interplay between defined retroviral gene sequences (as indicated by the opposite outcome of rhesus macaque infection with different SIVmac molecular clones) and defined genes of the host species (as shown by the opposite outcome of HIV-1 infection in humans and in chimpanzees).

There are two major groups of retroviruses that have been shown to be pathogenic in the human and non human primate species: oncoretroviruses, that can cause cancers, and lentiviruses, including HIV, that can cause AIDS. Oncoviruses cause cancer by inducing the inappropriate expression in adult cells of genes that play an essential role, during normal development, in cell proliferation, differentiation and migration. In a paper submitted in May 1990, we proposed that lentiviruses may cause cell depletion and tissue atrophy in the immune system and the brain by an inverse capacity to dysregulate the expression in adult cells of genes that play an essential role, during normal development, in the induction of programmed cell death[19,20]. A long prevailing view in cell biology has been that all forms of premature cell death, in particular pathological cell death caused by infectious agents, are a passive consequence of cell injury or degeneration leading to cell destruction by necrosis. The study of embryonic development, however, has led to the identification of a different form of premature cell death that occurs in the absence of disease, is physiologically regulated, and has been termed programmed cell death or apoptosis[21-25]. Programmed cell death plays an essential role in the functional maturation of the developing nervous and immune systems, in particular in the negative selection of the T-cell repertoire and the establishment of self-tolerance. More recently, programmed cell death has also been shown to occur in adult tissues and in mature T cells. Unlike cell degeneration or necrosis, programmed cell death is an active cell suicide process regulated by signals provided by the environment[26-31]. Our theoritical model of AIDS pathogenesis proposed that most immunological and nonimmunological defects in HIV-infected persons, including CD4[+] T-cell depletion, brain atrophy and dementia, could be related to the inappropriate induction in various infected and uninfected cell populations of an activation-induced cell-suicide process by programmed cell death, caused by indirect interference of HIV with intercellular and intracellular signalling. This hypothesis made several testable predictions and proposed that modulation of cell signalling may have therapeutic implications by preventing premature cell death and restoring normal cell functions[19].

There are two major ways in which cells are known to die. The first recognized form of cell death, necrosis, is always associated with disease and is a consequence of cell destruction by several agents, including infectious pathogens, complement, antibodies plus complement, toxins, or hypoxemia. During necrosis, cell swelling and rupture of the cell membrane lead to the release of proteases and other intracellular toxic enzymes, causing the death of bystander cells, an inflammatory reaction and a scarring process that disorganize the architecture of the tissue or the organ in which necrosis is occurring[23,28].

The observation that the massive episodes of cell death that occur during development do not harm the tissue and organs in which they take place led to the suggestion that the process of programmed cell death must be radically different from necrosis[21]. There are many morphological and biochemical differences between programmed cell death and pathological forms of cell death such as cell degeneration or necrosis. In most instances, programmed cell death involves an orderly process of morphological disintegration that has been termed apoptosis[22], and includes shrinkage of the cell and the nucleus; condensation and fragmentation of the nuclear chromatin; maintenance of organelle and plasma membrane integrity despite membrane blebbing; and the segmentation of the cell into apoptotic bodies that are rapidly ingested by neighboring epithelial or phagocytic cells. One of the spectacular features frequently associated with apoptosis, the regular fragmentation of the entire cellular DNA due to the activation of an endogenous endonuclease into regular multiples of an oligonucleosome-length unit of 180 base pairs, may not, however, represent an essential component of the process[28,29]. In contrast to necrosis, programmed cell death does not induce bystander-cell death or inflammation, or tissue disorganization, and therefore remains most often undetected if not thoroughly investigated[23,26,28,29].

The most important difference between programmed cell death and necrosis, however, is of a functional nature. Programmed cell death is an active cell-suicide process that requires activation signals, signal transduction and in several instances gene expression, and protein synthesis in the dying cell[26,28,29,32,33]. Therefore, programmed cell death is regulated by signals provided by the local environment. Unlike cell degeneration or necrosis, programmed cell death can be induced or suppressed in most cell populations by the withdrawal or addition of defined activation signals[26,28,32,33] and its induction or prevention depends on the expression of defined genes, that have been characterized in primitive invertebrates and begin to be identified in mammals and humans[24,26-30]. When a cell undergoes necrosis, the only way to prevent death is to remove the causative agent; when a cell undergoes programmed cell death, death can be prevented, in most cases, by the modulation of cell signalling (for a review, see Ref. 31).

The programmed cell death hypothesis of AIDS pathogenesis provided a potentially unifying explanation for most pathological features of the disease by relating them to programmed cell death dysregulation[19]. Such a mechanism could account in particular for the two major defects of CD4[+] T cells from HIV-infected persons: their early *in vitro* dysfunction and their progressive and late *in vivo* depletion, leading to immune incompetence. In this model, the reason that these cells do not proliferate *in vitro* to stimuli, including recall antigens, would be that these stimuli induce cell-suicide. *In vivo*, CD4[+] T-cell suicide after activation would be an ongoing process that would progressively overwhelm the renewal capacity of the immune system and lead to the progressive disappearance of this cell population. In contrast to the normal generation and maintenance of immune memory, stimulation of both naive and memory mature CD4+ T cells would lead in HIV-infected persons to a form of inappropriate and continuous tolerance, as a consequence of negative selection of the repertoire in response to non-self antigens expressed by various pathogens and the environment.

The hypothesis also provided a possible explanation for two paradoxical features that were observed in HIV-infected people. The first was the existence and persistence of B-cell and CD8+ T-cell hyperactivation in spite of an apparent lack of CD4+ T-cell function[1]; programmed cell death, as an active process associated with transient lymphokine secretion[34] and with release of nucleosomes that can activate B cells[35], could account for a truncated and inappropriate form of helper function provided by the dying CD4+ T cells[19]. The second paradoxical feature was the persistence, before the last stages of the disease, of a low percentage only of peripheral blood CD4+ T cells which are productively infected by HIV and which express viral RNA[4,5]. Since HIV proviral expression requires activation of infected CD4+ T-cells, a rapid CD4+ T-cell suicide process in response to activation could have a beneficial effect on the control of viral replication[19]. Such a prediction was consistent with a previous hypothesis of a beneficial role for apoptosis induction by specialized cytotoxic lymphocyte and natural killer cells in containing the spreading of various viral infections[36] and with the subsequent findings that beyond any involvement of immune effector cells, programmed cell death induction represents an evolutionary conserved mechanism that may be very efficient in limiting viral spreading in insect[37], plant[38] and mammalian[39] tissues. Although it has now been realized that the viral burden in HIV-infected persons is much higher than initially described[40], it is still generally assumed that the spreading of HIV infection is restrained until the last stages of the disease by some immune effector mechanisms, and it is possible that programmed cell death induction participates in such a control of viral spreading.

Beyond the scope of AIDS pathogenesis, the hypothesis also questionned the validity of two concepts that prevailed at that time. The first one was that programmed cell death always represents a beneficial and physiological form of cell death. Our model model predicted, however, that cell suicide in response to inappropriate activation signals could lead to disease. The second prevailing concept was that the outcome of T-cell receptor occupancy strictly depends on the developmental stage of the T cell, and that T-cell receptor stimulation can lead in mature T cells to either proliferation or clonal anergy, but not, as in immature thymocytes, to clonal deletion[41]. Our model predicted, however, that a cell-death program could remain functional in mature CD4+ T cells, and be expressed in response to inappropriate T-cell activation. After this hypothesis was first submitted for publication, two *in vitro* experimental observations from murine models were published that indicated that T-cell receptor stimulation could indeed lead to programmed death in mature T cells. The first observation showed that antibody-mediated ligation of the CD4 molecule from resting mature CD4+ T cells primed them for programmed cell death upon further stimulation of the T-cell receptor[42]; the second one indicated that T-cell receptor restimulation of a mature murine CD4+ T-cell clone in the absence of cosignal provided by accessory cells induced programmed cell death[43]. These findings led us to include in our hypothesis two candidate mechanisms for the induction of CD4+ T-cell programmed death in HIV-1-infected persons: a direct negative signalling to CD4+ T cells due to the ligation of the CD4 molecule by the gp120 HIV envelope, gp 120-anti-gp120 antibody immune complexes or by crossreactive anti-CD4 autoantibodies; or an indirect mechanism related to a possible inhibitory effect of HIV on accessory-cell function, leading to a lack of appropriate cosignal delivery by accessory cells to activated CD4+ T cells[19].

In addition to providing a possible explanation for many features of AIDS, the hypothesis made several experimentally testable predictions. The first prediction was that polyclonal T-cell activators that failed to induce proper *in vitro* proliferation of T cells from HIV-infected persons should lead to detectable activation-induced CD4[+] T-cell death, with characteristic features of apoptosis, including regular cellular DNA fragmentation and ultrastructural aspects of chromatin condensation. The second one was that, as in immature thymocytes[32], such T-cell death could be expected to be prevented either by inhibitors of gene expression and protein synthesis or of signal transduction such as cyclosporin A or by the addition of activation cosignals, such as cytokines, that may also restore CD4[+] T-cell proliferation to stimuli. The third one was that investigation of the *in vitro* programmed death of CD4[+] T cells from HIV-infected persons in response to T-cell receptor stimulation by self major histocompatibility complex-II-restricted antigens would raise a potential problem; since memory CD4[+] T cells specific for any given antigen are rare (around 1/10,000) and since apoptosis is a process that spares bystander cells, memory CD4[+] T-cell death in response to self-major histocompatibility complex-II-restricted recall antigens should not be expected to be detectable, provided it occurred; accordingly, it would not be possible to assess whether impaired *in vitro* proliferation to recall antigens is related to an abnormal *in vitro* T-cell death induction or to the fact that the antigen-specific memory CD4[+] T cells have already been deleted *in vivo*. In order to investigate whether T-cell death may occur in response to T-cell receptor mobilization by self-major histocompatibility complex-II-dependent ligands, it was therefore proposed the use of bacterial superantigens[44], which at that time had not been used to explore the response of T cells from HIV-infected individuals. Superantigens were thought to mimic in an enhanced way, the normal CD4[+] T-cell response to recall antigens by directly binding to major histocompatibility complex-II molecules and interacting with defined Vβ T-cell receptor molecules expressed by up to 30% of human T cells, inducing *in vitro* proliferation in both memory and naive normal mature human CD4[+] T cells and programmed death in normal human immature thymocytes[44,45]. It was predicted that in CD4[+] T cells from HIV-infected persons, T-cell receptor stimulation by superantigens would induce abnormal programmed death in a percentage of cells high enough to allow detection. Fourth, activation cosignals that would prevent CD4[+] T-cell programmed death and restore proliferation to polyclonal activators should also be expected to restore proliferation to specific recall antigens of memory-CD4[+] T cells that have not already been deleted *in vivo*. Finally, if CD4[+] T-cell programmed death were to represent a crucial event in the pathogenesis of AIDS, it should be detected in HIV-infected humans, but not in HIV-infected chimpanzees that do not develop any AIDS-related disease[19].

THE EXPERIMENTAL EVIDENCE

Since publication of our hypothesis in April 1991, experimental reports from about twenty laboratories, including ours, have indicated the validity of several of its predictions, by showing the existence of a relationship between HIV infection, AIDS, and programmed death induction in both HIV-infected and uninfected cells, including mature T cells, thymocytes, and haematopoietic progenitor cells[20]. First, the *in vitro* dysfunction of peripheral blood T cells from HIV-1-infected persons has been found to be indeed related to a process of abnormal induction of programmed cell death, and this process has been shown to be prevented *in vitro* by the modulation of cell activation, including the addition of protein synthesis inhibitors, of cyclosporin A, of protease inhibitors or the addition of activation cosignals, such as cytokines[46-56]. Second, the *in vitro* cytopathogenic effect of HIV-1 in cultures of HIV-1-infected CD4[+] T cells has been found to be due to programmed cell death induction[57-60]. Third, the crosslinking of the CD4 molecule by anti-CD4 antibodies[51,61] or by the HIV-1 envelope protein, either expressed at the surface of infected cells[62-64], or in the form of antibody bound immune complexes[61] has been shown to trigger programmed death in uninfected human CD4$^+$ T cells as well as in uninfected human bone marrow haematopoietic progenitor cells that express the CD4 molecule[65]. Fourth, HIV-1 infection of severe combined immunodeficiency (SCID)-hu mice reconstituted with adult human T cells has been found to lead to rapid CD4$^+$ T-cell depletion through *in vivo* induction of programmed death[66,67]. Fifth, HIV-1-mediated programmed cell death may also impair the renewal of CD4$^+$ T cells, as indicated by experiments of HIV-1 infection of SCID-hu mice reconstituted with human fetal thymuses, leading *in vivo* to thymocyte programmed death, thymic involution and a complete depletion of CD4$^+$ thymocytes[68], and by experiments mentioned above in which HIV was shown to induce programmed death *in vitro* in uninfected human bone marrow haematopoietic progenitor cells[65]. Finally, the relevance of these findings to AIDS pathogenesis has been further extended by the observations of abnormal levels of *in vitro* programmed death of peripheral blood T cells in primate models[20,50,54,69] and in feline models[70] of pathogenic lentiviral infections that induce AIDS-related diseases, but not in HIV-1-infected chimpanzees that do not develop disease[20,50,71]; and by the recent observation that abnormal levels of programmed T-cell death also occur *in vivo* in lymph nodes from HIV-1-infected persons[72].

While testing the experimental validity of our hypothesis, Groux and coworkers in our laboratory found that abnormal levels of programmed death in peripheral blood T cells from HIV-1-infected persons involved only the CD4$^+$ T-cell subset, and not the CD8$^+$ T cells[47,48]. Subsequent work performed in our laboratory by other investigators, using four different assays to measure apoptosis[54], has shown, in accordance with findings from other laboratories[46,49,50,52,53], that abnormal programmed cell death induction also involves CD8$^+$ T cells.

The finding that both CD4$^+$ and CD8$^+$ T cells from HIV-infected persons undergo abnormal programmed death, whereas selective CD4$^+$ T-cell depletion is an *in vivo* feature of progression to AIDS, has raised the question of the significance of these *in vitro* findings. A first possibility is that *in vitro* programmed T-cell death does not reflect the *in vivo* fate of the T cells. This seems unlikely, however, in the view of recent preliminary evidence that abnormally high levels of programmed death, involving both CD4$^+$ and CD8$^+$ T cells, are observed in lymph nodes from HIV-1-infected persons, at various stages of the disease[73]. Another possible explanation is that both CD4$^+$ and CD8$^+$ T cells undergo excessive programmed death *in vivo*, but that, in such conditions, renewal of CD4$^+$ T cells is selectively impaired. Such a possibility is supported by two series of recent findings. The first one, involving whole-body irradiation in primates; indeed, whole body irradiation induces an identical profound depletion of CD4$^+$ and CD8$^+$ T cells, that is followed by a rapid reappearance of normal numbers of CD8$^+$ T cells in the peripheral blood, but by a very prolonged state of CD4$^+$ T-cell depletion[74]. The second observation suggests an additional potential effect of pathogenic lentiviruses on the renewal capacity of CD4$^+$ T cells, since, as mentioned above, HIV-1 infection of SCIDhu mice reconstituted with human fetal thymuses leads to a profound thymocyte depletion, related to massive *in vivo* programmed cell death induction, that affects CD4$^+$ thymocytes more profoundly than CD8$^+$ thymocytes[68] and involves both infected and uninfected CD4$^+$ thymocytes. This latter finding is consistent with the idea that any mechanism that could induce abnormal apoptosis in uninfected mature T cells should be at least as effective in inducing programmed death in their uninfected immature precursors, and therefore in interfering with T-cell renewal. This idea is further supported by the observation that thymic depletion is observed *in vivo* in rhesus macaques infected with a pathogenic strain of SIVmac[75] that also leads to depletion of mature CD4$^+$ T cells and AIDS, but not in macaques infected with a nonpathogenic molecular clone of SIVmac[76] although the thymus, as the mature CD4$^+$ T cells, are targets of viral infection in both models of SIV infection[76].

A central question in AIDS pathogenesis is whether excessive death of mature CD4$^+$ T cells is sufficient to account for CD4$^+$ T-cell depletion *in vivo*, or if impairment of renewal of CD4[+] T cells is also required in order for HIV infection to lead to AIDS. If this were the case, and if depletion of progenitor cells were a process that begins early after HIV infection, effective antiviral therapy might not be sufficient to prevent disease progression in the absence of effective immune reconstitution strategies.

The programmed cell death hypothesis of AIDS pathogenesis proposed that abnormal programmed death induction in mature peripheral T cells may neither be pathogenic *per se* nor unique to HIV-1 infection, and may even have a beneficial inhibitory effect on viral production, but that the induction in HIV-1-infected persons of a prolonged and ongoing process of programmed T-cell death may lead to disease by interfering with the maintenance of memory T cells and the renewal of effector T cells[19,20]. Subsequent experimental findings have been consistent with such a prediction, by showing that transient abnormal priming of activated T cells for *in vitro* programmed death can be observed during several acute viral infections that lead to transient immunosuppression[77-80]. Therefore, an essential question that has remained unresolved for most abnormal features identified so far in HIV-1-infected persons, is whether programmed T-cell death plays a central role in AIDS pathogenesis, or is merely a consequence of an ongoing and ineffective stimulation of the immune system in a chronic lentiviral infection. In order to address this question, we have compared *in vitro* programmed T-cell death induction in HIV-1-infected persons and in various primate models that allow one to discriminate between biological features associated with pathogenic or nonpathogenic chronic lentiviral infections

The infected and uninfected primates that we explored included chimpanzees experimentally infected with HIV-1, that do not develop disease; african green monkeys naturally infected by SIVagm, that do not develop disease; and rhesus macaques experimentally infected either with a viral strain of SIVmac that induces AIDS, or with a recombinant molecular clone of SIVmac that does not lead to disease. Abnormal levels of activation-induced programmed death of the CD8[+] T-cell-depleted peripheral blood mononuclear cells (containing the CD4[+] T cells) were only observed in the two models leading to AIDS: HIV-1-infected humans and rhesus macaques infected with a pathogenic strain of SIVmac. In contrast, enhanced *in vitro* levels of activation-induced programmed death in CD4[+] T-cell-depleted peripheral blood mononuclear cells (containing the CD8[+] T cells) could be detected after *in vitro* stimulation in both pathogenic and nonpathogenic models of chronic lentiviral infections, as well as in some uninfected primate controls[54].

Together, these data suggest that the abnormal priming of CD4[+] and CD8[+] T cells for programmed death that occurs in HIV-1-infected humans may be due to two different processes, with distinct significance. The one involving CD4[+] T cells seems closely related to AIDS pathogenesis; the other, involving CD8[+] T cells, could be an indirect consequence of immune stimulation that may occur during both pathogenic and nonpathogenic lentiviral infections, as well as in other circumstances. Such a possibility is further suggested by our preliminary finding of a pattern of a similar abnormal *in vitro* programmed T-cell death restricted to the CD8[+] T cells in some HIV-1-infected persons (J. Estaquier et al., unpublished), characterized as long-term nonprogressors or long-term survivors[81], who are infected for more than six years and have retained normal CD4[+] T-cell counts and CD4[+] T-cell functions.

CANDIDATE MECHANISMS FOR PROGRAMMED CELL DEATH IN AIDS

In HIV-infected persons, the percentage of CD4[+] T cells in the peripheral blood that are abnormally prone to undergo apoptosis in response to activation of the T-cell receptor greatly exceeds the percentage of HIV-infected CD4[+] T cells[40,48,50,51,53], raising the question of the mechanisms through which HIV induces apoptosis in uninfected CD4+ T cells. We initially proposed two candidate mechanisms that were not mutually exclusive[19], one involving HIV envelope-mediated signalling through the CD4 molecule, and the other HIV-mediated impaired monocyte/macrophage function.

The HIV Envelope

As mentioned above, HIV strains that are cytopathic *in vitro* have been shown to kill CD4+ T cells by inducing apoptosis[57,58]. After initial infection of the culture, the addition of an antibody against the HIV envelope glycoprotein (env) that blocks further CD4+ T-cell superinfection was also found to block apoptosis induction and to allow HIV-infected CD4+ T cells to produce virus *in vitro* without CD4+ T-cell death[57].

The interpretation proposed for this finding was that HIV-1-mediated programmed cell death induction was a consequence of the cellular accumulation of unintegrated proviral DNA that occurs during the multiple cycles of superinfection[57] and therefore only involved the infected cells. An alternative possible interpretation, however, was that the preventive effect of the anti-HIV env antibody on programmed cell death was not due to an inhibition of CD4+ T-cell superinfection, but rather to the blocking of the interaction between the HIV env expressed by the infected cells, and the CD4 molecule expressed by neighboring uninfected or infected CD4+ T cells[20]. This alternative interpretation was supported by subsequent findings[62-64] showing that an interaction between the HIV env expressed by infected or transfected cells and the CD4 molecule expressed by uninfected CD4+ T cells induces programmed death of the uninfected CD4+ T cells; a process that can be prevented either by selective inhibitors of T-cell activation[62,63], or by CD4 antibodies that do not inhibit binding of HIV env to the CD4 molecule but may act by modifying CD4-mediated signal transduction[64]. Other experimental findings, extending previous *in vitro* observations in murine T cells[42], indicated that crosslinking of the CD4 molecule by anti-CD4 antibodies or by HIV env plus anti-env antibodies primed purified normal human CD4+ T cells for programmed death in response to subsequent T-cell receptor stimulation[61], or induced programmed death in normal resting human CD4+ T cells, in the absence of T-cell receptor stimulation, provided that accessory cells were present in the culture[51]. More recently, crosslinking of the CD4 molecule by injection of anti-CD4 antibodies was also found to lead to CD4+ T-cell depletion through programmed death induction *in vivo* in mice[82,83].

An extreme interpretation of this series of findings is that there is no such a thing as an HIV-mediated cytopathic effect at the level of a single infected cell, and that programmed cell death induction requires, in all cases, an interaction between "effector" infected cells, expressing the HIV env, and neighboring infected or uninfected "target" cells. It has even been recently proposed that chronically infected CD4+ T cells may represent long lived cells that induce programmed cell death in uninfected CD4+ T cells while at the same time escaping programmed cell death induction by downregulating their CD4 molecules[84]. Whatever the fate of an HIV-infected CD4+ T cell may be, it should be remembered that HIV infection is noncytopathic in the monocyte/macrophage cell population; therefore, HIV-infected monocytes/macrophages may represent good candidates for a long-lived effector-cell population able to induce programmed cell death in the CD4+ T cells. *In vitro* experiments of limiting dilutions of HIV-infected CD4+ T cells remain to be performed in order to assess whether HIV infection can or cannot induce cell death at the level of a single infected CD4+ T cell.

It is possible that some level of cytopathic effect is induced by all lentiviruses in infected CD4+ T cells *in vivo*, regardless of whether they induce AIDS or not, but that cytopathicity alone does not suffice to induce CD4+ T-cell depletion and disease in the absence of additional indirect mechanisms of HIV envelope-mediated programmed cell death induction in uninfected CD4⁺ T cells. Whatever the answer may be, the findings mentioned above suggest that the HIV envelope glycoprotein and the immune response to it may participate in CD4⁺ T-cell apoptosis induction in HIV-infected persons by at least two distinct means: in uninfected CD4⁺ T cells that are in close vicinity to HIV-infected cells - a situation that is likely to occur in the lymph nodes, in particular through contacts between CD4⁺ T cells and HIV-infected accessory cells - but also in uninfected CD4⁺ T cells that are at a distance from any HIV-infected cell, through the binding to the CD4 molecule of HIV envelope-anti-envelope immune complexes. Possible molecular mechanisms involved in CD4⁺ T-cell programmed death induction through HIV envelope-mediated CD4 signalling have been discussed elsewhere[85]. They could include the uncoordinated activation (or sequestration) of the src-family tyrosine kinase-p56^{lck}, that is associated with the cytoplasmic domain of the CD4 molecule[61], or the premature activation of the p34^{cdc2} kinase[86], which plays a crucial role in the regulation of the cell cycle, and has been shown to participate in serine protease-mediated apoptosis induction[87]. The possibility that HIV env-mediated CD4 signalling leads to programmed cell death by inducing the expression of molecules such as Fas-APO1 and the Fas ligand is suggested by the finding that injection of anti-CD4 antibodies in the lpr mice in which the fas gene is mutated fails to induce CD4⁺ T-cell apoptosis and CD4⁺ T-cell depletion[83].

Although the HIV envelope glycoprotein is a tempting candidate for programmed death induction in CD4⁺ T cells from HIV-infected persons, such a possibility has to be considered in the broader context of the primate models of pathogenic and nonpathogenic lentiviral infection discussed above. In these models, the binding of the viral envelope to the CD4 molecule is a feature that is required for CD4⁺ T-cell infection and is shared by all these lentiviruses. Therefore, one is forced to postulate that subtle differences in the CD4 molecules (in human and chimpanzee) or in the lentiviral envelope (in pathogenic and nonpathogenic molecular clones of SIVmac) are sufficient to account for radical differences in the capacity of envelope-CD4 interaction to induce programmed cell death. Such a mechanism awaits to be addressed experimentally in an *in vitro* system using envelopes from these lentiviruses and CD4⁺ T cells from different primate species.

Finally, another possibility is that HIV envelope-mediated CD4 signalling in uninfected CD4⁺ T cells occurs during both pathogenic and nonpathogenic primate lentiviral infections and represents a mechanism that is necessary but not sufficient for the induction of apoptosis of uninfected CD4⁺ T cells.

HIV-Mediated Accessory-Cell Dysfunction

The second mechanism that we originally proposed as a candidate for the priming of CD4⁺ T cells for programmed death in HIV-1-infected persons was related to a general property of lentiviruses, their tropism for accessory cells such as monocytes/macrophages[19]. If lentiviral infection of monocytes/macrophages induced a defect in their accessory-cell function, this could lead to T-cell programmed death through inappropriate delivery of the activation cosignals that are required for appropriate T-cell activation[19]. The two-signal model of T-cell activation, a paradigm in cellular immunology, implies that T-cell differentiation and proliferation requires both T-cell receptor stimulation by antigen, and appropriate cosignalling provided by antigen-presenting accessory cells, such as monocytes, dendritic cells or B cells in the form of membrane costimulatory molecules, such as B7.1, B7.2, or heat stable antigen[88-91]. Mature T-cell receptor stimulation in the absence of appropriate accessory-cell cosignalling was shown to lead to a state of T-cell desensitization that has been termed anergy[89]. During the last four years, however, it has been found that T-cell receptor stimulation in the presence of inappropriate cosignalling can also induce T-cell death by apoptosis, a finding that has led to a blurring of the frontiers between anergy and programmed cell death induction, and to a progressive reassessment of the outcome of T-cell activation (anergy or death) in conditions that do not lead to T-cell proliferation[92].

Programmed death of mature T cells has been shown to occur *in vitro* when T-cell receptor stimulation is performed in resting T cells after antibody-mediated ligation of CD4[42] and in preactivated T cells that have received a prior stimulation by IL-2 alone[93] or in which consecutive T-cell receptor stimulation is performed under different conditions[94]. Concerning the role of accessory cells, findings by several laboratories including ours have shown that programmed death is induced in preactivated mature T cells that are restimulated in the absence of accessory cells[43]; that cytokines secreted by accessory cells regulate programmed T-cell death induction in response to T-cell receptor stimulation[56,95]; and that cytokine-mediated modification of accessory-cell function can affect the capacity of the accessory cell to prevent programmed T-cell death induction in response to a given level of T-cell receptor stimulation[96].

In vivo, bacterial superantigens that bind to MHC-II molecules were found to induce, in apparent contrast with conventional antigens, the deletion of mature peripheral T cells expressing the corresponding TCR Vβ molecules, through an activation process that leads first to cell proliferation, then to PCD[97]. A murine oncoretrovirus, the mouse mammary tumor virus (MMTV), was subsequently found to encode a superantigen[98] and to induce deletion of mature T-cell subsets through a similar process[99] Finally, recent findings have shown that a massive CD8[+] T-cell activation during an acute murine infection with the lymphochoriomeningitis virus can lead to the complete and permanent deletion of the antigen-specific mature CD8[+] T-cell population[100].

Together, these findings suggest that a death program is functional in mature T cells and that its expression may depend both on the degree of T-cell activation and on the nature of the environmental cosignals provided to the T cell by the accessory cell. Such a death program might have a physiological role in both the maintenance of extrathymic self-tolerance and the ending of a normal immune response to foreign antigens. In the latter case, it is expected that programmed death involves bystander-activated T cells as well as terminally differentiated effector T cells, and it is obvious that memory T cells are spared. During development, many cell types have been shown to require signals from other cells in order to prevent programmed cell death and to survive. More recently, adult cell types have also been found to require signals from other cells to survive, deprivation of such signals leading to premature deletion by programmed cell death[101,102]. The recent observation that all mammalian nucleated-cell types studied so far, with the exception of embryonic blastomeres, undergo programmed death *in vitro* when cultured in the absence of exogenous signals and/or at low cell density, supports the concept that the fate of each cell may depend on the presence and activity of other cells and may require an active and constant repression of programmed cell death induction[26]. Accordingly, a possible representation of T-cell survival regulation is that any activation of the T-cell receptor will lead to programmed cell death induction, unless environmental cosignals adapted to the activation state of the T cell are provided that will prevent programmed cell death, and allow differentiation and proliferation to proceed. The two-signal model of T-cell activation would then only represent a particularly well-studied example of the general control exerted on cell survival by the environment[20,26]. T-cell anergy may represent a particular case, in which the initial T-cell receptor activating signal is not strong enough to induce programmed cell death, and therefore does not require additional cosignalling in order to allow T-cell survival. The possibility, however, that T-cell anergy may represent a state of priming for programmed death that will lead to T-cell death upon further restimulation is consistent with the recent finding that anergic T and B cells have a reduced lifespan *in vivo*[92,103].

Provided that pathogenic lentiviruses have the capacity to modify accessory-cell function, they may lead to programmed T-cell death "by default", simply by altering the balance required to prevent programmed death induction in activated T cells; such an inbalance could be achieved in two opposite ways that are not mutually exclusive: a reduction in the availability of the accessory-cell cosignals required to prevent T-cell death in response to a given activation signal; or alternatively an increase in the intensity or duration of the initial T-cell activation signal that will render inoperative the normal amount of preventive accessory-cell cosignals that are present in the T-cell environment. The molecular mechanisms that may participate in CD4+ T-cell programmed death induction as a consequence of accessory-cell dysfunction have been discussed elsewhere[85]. These include the activation of the Ca++/calmodulin-dependent phosphatase calcineurin of proteases such as IL-1β converting enzyme (ICE) or calpain, and the expression of genes such as *c-myc* or *nur77* and may involve expression of the Fas and Fas ligand molecules.

Recent findings suggest that HIV-1 infection of accessory cells may indeed play a role in programmed T-cell death induction. The first observation concerns HIV-1-infected chimpanzees and suggest that the lack of *in vivo* pathogenesis of HIV-1 as well as the lack of priming of peripheral blood T cells for *in vitro* programmed death induction in this model is not related to a lack of cytopathic properties of these viruses (since some of these HIV-1 strains are cytopathic *in vitro* for chimpanzee CD4+ T cells) but to a lack in the capacity of all these HIV strains to infect chimpanzee monocytes[71]; the validity of this observation remains however to be confirmed[104]. Another finding concerns SCID-hu mice reconstituted with adult human T cells and monocytes and infected with various molecular clones of HIV-1; infection with molecular clones of HIV-1, that infect monocytes and are noncytopathic *in vitro* for CD4+ T cells, leads in this model to a more rapid and profound *in vivo* depletion of CD4+ T cells than infection with clones of HIV-1 that are highly cytopathic *in vitro* for CD4+ T cells, but poorly infect monocytes[66]. *In vivo* CD4+ T-cell depletion in this model seems to be related to *in vivo* programmed death induction in both infected and uninfected CD4+ T cells that are in the vicinity of HIV-1-infected monocytes[67].

Another possibility of defective accessory-cell cosignalling related to HIV infection is suggested by the observation that HIV-1 viral particles, when grown in human cells, bear major histocompatibility complex-class-II molecules on their surface[105], that are able to bind bacterial superantigens, and to induce T-cell programmed death in the absence of any accessory cell[106]. It is therefore possible that major histocompatibility complex-class-II-mediated presentation by the viral particle to the T-cell receptor of various self and foreign peptides, in the absence of any accessory cell, may play a role in programmed T-cell death induction.

Finally, recent findings by our laboratory[55,56] and another[107] indicate that two cytokines secreted by accessory cells may participate in the regulation of programmed death in T cells from HIV-1-infected persons: IL-10, by inducing programmed T-cell death; and IL-12, by preventing programmed T-cell death. These data suggest that the progressive loss of *in vivo* and *in vitro* CD4+ T helper (Th)1-cell-mediated response that characterizes progression to AIDS could involve cytokine-mediated CD4+ T-cell programmed death as a consequence of accessory-cell dysfunction.

Th1/Th2 Cytokines and Accessory-Cell Dysfunction

Cytokines play a critical role in the immune response to pathogens[108]. Differentiated CD4+ T helper cells have been shown in mice and humans to segregate in two functional subsets, based on their cytokine secretion pattern; Th1 cells secrete IL-2 and gamma-interferon (IFN-γ), promote macrophage activation, and induce cell-mediated immunity and delayed-type hypersensitivity reactions; Th2 cells secrete IL-4, IL-5 and IL-10, which favor optimal activation of B cells to secrete antibody, in particular certain types of antibody such as immunoglobulin E (IgE), and promote mast-cell and eosinophil activation[109-113]. Therefore, differentiation of CD4[+] T cells in Th1 or Th2 cells in response to invasion by an infectious pathogen represents a crucial event in determining the nature and outcome of the immune response, i.e. persistance of the pathogen, protection of the host or immunopatho-genesis.

Importantly, some of the Th1 and Th2 cytokines can also be produced by cells other than CD4[+] T cells, including differentiated CD8[+] T cells and activated acessory cells such as activated macrophages, B cells, natural killer cells, basophils and mast cells[109,110,112,114]. Cytokines secreted by accessory cells activated by the invading pathogen play an essential role in the decision of naive CD4[+] T helper precursor cells to differentiate into Th1 or Th2 cells[112]. In particular, IL-12, secreted by activated macrophages, will favor Th1-cell induction[115], whereas IL-4, secreted by activated B cells, basophils or mast cells, together with IL-10, secreted by activated B cells or macrophages, will favor Th2 induction[113,116].

Several studies have suggested that the pathogenesis and persistence of various chronic bacterial, viral or parasite infections involve a Th1 to Th2 cytokine switch[117-121].

In HIV-1-infected persons, the early functional defects of cell-mediated immunity that precede CD4[+] T-cell depletion, involve the CD4[+] Th1-cell population, and lead to a downregulation of delayed-type hypersensitivity reactions[1,40]. Recently the idea was proposed that this loss of CD4[+] Th1 cell-function, may be due to a progressive shift of CD4[+] T cells from Th1 to Th2, leading to a loss of IL-2 and IFN-γ production, concomitant with increases in IL-4 and IL-10 secretion[122,123]; and it was subsequently suggested that such a process may involve accessory-cell dysfunction in HIV-infected persons[124]. In keeping with the idea that costimulatory signals expressed by accessory cells play a key role in the control of T-cell survival and T-cell death, we have explored the possibility that HIV-mediated downregulation of Th1 cell-reponse may involve programmed T-cell death induction. We have investigated the Th1/Th2 cytokine secretion profile in HIV-infected persons, and the possible role these cytokines may play in programmed T-cell death. Our results indicate that stimuli that induce programmed death in T cells from HIV-infected persons lead to *in vitro* levels of IL-2 and IFN-γ secretion that are similar in HIV-infected persons and healthy controls. No significant IL-4 or IL-5 secretion was detected in most HIV-infected persons up to several days after *in vitro* stimulation, and IL-10 secretion was similar in activated T cells from HIV-infected persons and controls. In HIV-infected persons, IL-2 was secreted exclusively by the CD4[+] T cells, and IFN-γ mainly by the CD8[+] T cells. Rather than the existence of an increased proportion of CD4[+] Th2 cells, this cytokine secretion pattern suggests the sole presence, in HIV-infected persons, of CD4[+] Th1 cells, or maybe of T helper precursor CD4[+] cells, that only secrete IL-2[55,56]. Our findings of a lack of Th2-cell expansion and a lack of increased Th2 cytokine production are consistent with recent results from cytokine messenger RNA analysis *in vivo* in the lymph nodes of HIV-infected persons[125]. Therefore, we favour the interpretation that the progressive loss of sustained *in vitro* and *in vivo* Th1 cell response that characterize AIDS progression is not related to an absence of Th1 CD4[+] cells (nor to a downregulation of Th1 cells by an expanding Th2 cell population) but to the fact that the stimulation of Th1 cells from HIV-infected persons induces their rapid death by apoptosis.

The addition of antibodies against theTh2 cytokines IL-10 or IL-4, or the addition of the Th1 cytokine IL-12 has been reported to restore the early defective *in vitro* proliferative response of T cells from HIV-infected persons to stimuli[122]. Recent results also indicate that the addition of antibodies to IL-10 or the addition of IL-12 have a preventive effect on abnormal programmed T-cell death induction in response to *in vitro* stimulation in HIV-infected persons[55,56,107], further supporting the idea that the early T-cell functional defects in HIV-infected persons are related to abnormal programmed T-cell death induction. Together, these results imply that T cells from HIV-infected persons may have an abnormal response to IL-10; the preventive effect of IL-12 on programmed T-cell death suggests the possibility that this abnormal response to IL-10 may be related to the reported defect of IL-12 secretion by accessory cells from HIV-infected persons[126].

It has been shown that Th1 and Th2 cytokines regulate the Th1/Th2 cell ratio by two different effects; first, cytokines such as IL-2 and IL-4 act as growth factors inducing the expansion of the Th1 and Th2 CD4[+] cell population, respectively; second, other cytokines, that can be secreted by accessory cells play an indirect role in Th1 or Th2 expansion by downregulating the converse T helper-cell population: the Th2 cytokine IL-10 by inhibiting Th1 cell expansion, and the Th1 cytokine IFN-γ by inhibiting Th2 cell expansion[109,110,112,113]. In this context, our findings have several implications. First, they suggest that cytokine-mediated regulation of the Th1/Th2 cell ratio also operates through the control of programmed T-cell death induction, and that cytokine-mediated Th1-cell programmed death may represent a general mechanism of Th1-cell downregulation. Among cytokines secreted by accessory cells, IL-12 and IL-10 could play an essential role in controlling the decision of CD4[+] T helper cells to expand or to die. A general model of cytokine-mediated regulation of programmed CD4[+] Th-cell death has been discussed elsewhere[56].

If accessory cell dysfunction represents, as we initially proposed, a major pathological feature in HIV-infected persons, it is tempting to speculate that accessory cells from HIV-1-infected persons may secrete the cytokines or express the cell surface molecules that normally play an essential role in Th1-cell programmed death induction during an efficient process of Th1 to Th2 switch, in the absence of the cytokines that normally allow the concomitant expansion of the Th2 CD4[+] cells. Accordingly, in contrast to other infectious diseases, a progressive loss of Th1 CD4[+] cells would occur in HIV-infected persons in the absence of a compensatory expansion of Th2 CD4[+] cells, leading to a form of abortive Th1/Th2 switch that could at least partly account for both the progressive CD4[+] T-cell dysfunction and depletion that lead to AIDS[55].

An obvious implication is that therapeutic strategies designed to prevent Th1 CD4[+] cell programmed death and to allow Th1 CD4[+] cell expansion may have beneficial effects. But our findings also have a paradoxical implication. In contrast to the infectious and parasitic diseases in which a Th1 to Th2 switch has been shown to be involved in pathogenesis, it is important to considere that immunodeficiency and disease in HIV-infected persons is primarily a direct consequence of CD4[+] T-cell depletion. If an ineffective abortive Th1/Th2 switch is involved in AIDS pathogenesis, one may not exclude the provocative possibility that therapeutic strategies designed to allow an efficient Th2 CD4[+] cells switch and to induce Th2 CD4[+] cell expansion may have beneficial effects during the course of CD4[+] T-cell depletion and AIDS[55]. The recent finding, however, that HIV-1 may preferentially replicate in Th2 and Th0 CD4[+] T-cell clones, and not in Th1-cell clones[127], provides a possible mechanism for the absence of a detectable Th1/Th2 switch in AIDS and raises the question of the possible consequences of such strategy on the viral growth in HIV-1-infected persons. Analysis of the cytokine profile in the various primate models of non pathogenic HIV and SIV infection models that do not lead to AIDS may be required to assess whether the absence of CD4[+] T cell programmed death *in vitro* [54] and the absence of CD4[+] T-cell depletion *in vivo* in these models are always correlated with the presence of a Th1 CD4[+] cell response, or may also involve, at least in some cases, a non pathogenic CD4[+] Th2-cell expansion. Investigating the role of Th1 and Th2 cytokines in both pathogenic and non pathogenic primate models of lentiviral infection may represent an essential step prior to the design of cytokine-based therapy in AIDS.

Programmed Cell Death by Deprivation, by Exhaustion, or by Fratricidal Cell Killing

An important implication of our hypothesis was that if programmed cell death were to represent a central event in AIDS pathogenesis, modulation of cell signalling may constitute a therapeutic approach able to prevent CD4+ T-cell depletion in HIV-infected persons. It is however important to remember that programmed cell death induction in T cells can result from several different mechanisms and that the possibility for intervention may therefore greatly vary depending on the nature of the mechanisms involved.

It is generally assumed that programmed T-cell death represents an autonomous cell-suicide process related to an inbalance of environmental signals, leading, as discussed above, to deprivation from survival factors. Observations of programmed T-cell death in murine models of viral infection with the lymphocytic choriomeningitis virus and the murine mammary tumor virus have suggested the alternative possibility that programmed death of mature peripheral T cells could be a consequence of overactivation leading to their "clonal exhaustion" and "clonal abortion" through a process of terminal differentiation[128,129]. This idea has potential important implications for T-cell death in AIDS, since it implies that signal modulation may fail to prevent such a process. However, other findings suggest that even in these murine models of viral infection, the outcome of T-cell stimulation (death or survival) may not only result from the intensity of T-cell activation achieved through T-cell receptor signalling, but also on the nature of cosignals provided by accessory cells[99,130].

Finally, it is important to remember that some T-lymphocyte subsets have evolved defence mechanisms that involve programmed death induction in target cells as a killing mechanism[33]. In particular, CD4+ T cells have been recently shown to be able to induce, through the expression of the Fas ligand molecule, programmed death in other activated lymphocytes that express the Fas molecule[131-133]. It has recently been proposed that the perforin-granule exocytosis-pathway of CD8+ cytotoxic T-cell killing may ensure the classical defence responses against infected cells, whereas Fas-mediated apoptosis, that can be induced by both CD4+ and CD8+ T cells, may be directed against uninfected activated syngeneic lymphocytes, and play a role in immunoregulation[132]. These findings raise the important possibility that the broad notion of activation-induced T-cell suicide may, in several circumstances, involve a process of activation-induced Fas-mediated fratricidal T-cell killing. Such a process may render inoperative strategies aimed at enhancing the expression of death repressor genes such as *bcl-2,* that prevent programmed cell death in response to deprivation from survival factors[134], but have a poor protective effect against programmed cell death mediated by T-cell killing[135-137].

Therefore, investigating the nature of the programmed T-cell death mechanisms that may be involved in AIDS (induction of cell autonomous suicide, terminal differentiation, or T-cell/T-cell killing) will have major implications for determining both the possibility of intervention, and the choice of potential therapeutical strategies.

FURTHER QUESTIONS

Accessory-Cell Dysfunction as a Candidate for Programmed Cell Death Induction in Immunological and Nonimmunological Organs

When discussing the possible role of HIV-infected accessory cells in programmed T-cell death, it is important to consider that until the late stage of the disease, most of the virus is trapped in the lymphoid organs and associated with accessory cells[138,139]. It is also important to note that the T cells that are recirculating in the peripheral blood represent, at any given time, less than 2% of the total lymphocyte pool in the body, that is essentially present in the lymphoid organs[140]. Therefore, the presence of T cells primed for programmed death in the peripheral blood of HIV-infected persons, that does not appear to increase with progression to disease[141], could only represent a very indirect consequence of two major additive events that may play an essential role in AIDS pathogenesis and occur outside the peripheral blood: mature T-cell deletion following programmed cell death induction in the lymph nodes; and impairment of T-cell renewal by programmed cell death induction in progenitor cells in both the thymus and the bone marrow. The progressive depletion of accessory cells such as the follicular dendritic cells in the lymph nodes[40] could lead, at a late stage of the disease, to irreversible programmed T-cell death due to a complete absence of appropriate accessory-cell cosignal delivery. Mechanisms involved in the death of follicular dendritic cells in HIV-infected persons remain unknown. Since these cells appear not to be targets for HIV infection[40], the possibility that follicular dendritic cells are destroyed by HIV-specific cytotoxic CD8[+] T lymphocytes seems unlikely[142]. Another possibility is that activated accessory cells also require signals from activated CD4[+] T cells in order to survive. Recent findings support this possibility, by showing that the proliferation of follicular dendritic cells depends on the presence of activated T cells[143]. Therefore, continuous CD4[+] T-cell programmed death induction, as a consequence of HIV-mediated accessory-cell dysfunction could, in turn, lead to the death of follicular dendritic cells[143], and participate in the progressive collapse of lymphoid organs that occur at the late stage of the disease[40].

Whether cell loss and tissue atrophy that occur in nonimmunological organs from HIV-infected persons, such as neuronal loss and muscle atrophy, are also related to inappropriate induction of programmed cell death remains to be investigated. The ultrastructural observation of abnormal levels of epithelial cell apoptosis in rectal crypts of AIDS patients[144] support the possibility that abnormal programmed cell death induction in AIDS involves a wide range of cell populations. Concerning the brain, several HIV-related factors have been shown to be potential candidates for neuronal death induction. These include viral or nonviral factors released by HIV-infected monocytes, and various HIV proteins, such as the HIV envelope, or the regulatory gene products Nef, Tat, and Rev. The *in vivo* relevance of these findings, and the nature of the mechanisms of neuronal cell death induced, remain however, to be investigated.

In the immune system, both CD4[+] T cells and accessory cells are targets for HIV infection. HIV-infected accessory cells include macrophages in the lymph nodes and in the bone marrow, and epithelial cells in the thymus[2,40]. Therefore, it is difficult to assess whether deletion of CD4[+] T cells, thymocytes and haematopoietic progenitor cells are due to direct HIV-mediated death of infected cells, or to death of both infected and uninfected cells as an indirect consequence of accessory-cell infection. When considering the brain, however, a very different situation emerges. In the brain, neuronal loss[3] is observed while neurons, in contrast to CD4[+] T cells, do not seem to be targets for HIV-1 infection. HIV-1 in the central nervous system is expressed primarily in cells of the macrophage lineage[12,13], and HIV-infected macrophages have been shown to be able to induce neuronal cell death through yet unclear mechanisms[145]. Similar to T cells, neurons normally depend on signals provided by other cell-populations in order to prevent programmed cell death induction[101]. It is tempting to propose that abnormal delivery of survival signals by infected accessory cells represents a unifying mechanism by which HIV- or SIV-infection of macrophages could induce programmed death in CD4[+] T cells, haematopoietic progenitors and neurons, and therefore play a crucial role in the pathogenesis of both immunological and nonimmunological defects leading to AIDS. A prediction of this hypothesis is that the tropism of a given lentivirus for accessory cells and the nature of the functional changes that this virus induces in the infected accessory cells would represent the critical features that distinguish lentiviral infections leading to AIDS from nonpathogenic lentiviral infections.

Programmed T-Cell Death, T-Cell Renewal and T-Cell Depletion

Although several observations are now consistent with our hypothesis, no experimental findings have yet confirmed, or contradicted, the potential role of programmed cell death as a causative event in AIDS. Therefore, the idea that an infectious pathogen could cause the death of both infected and uninfected cell populations by dysregulating a physiological cell suicide process that plays an essential role in the homeostasis of the infected host still remains of a speculative nature. During the last four years, the potential relevance of this idea to AIDS pathogenesis has been questionned in two successive and opposite ways. Initially, the importance of programmed cell death in the regulation of adult tissues, and in particular of the adult immune system, was not recognized. Since the differentiated adult T-cell population was considered as having lost its capacity to undergo negative selection, and therefore its propensity to undergo suicide in response to activation signals, any situation leading to T-cell death and T-cell depletion was attributed to a process of T-cell destruction. Accordingly, T-cell death in AIDS was expected to only result from particular destructive properties of the infectious pathogen in the infected cell, and/or from destruction of the infected cell by killing immune effector mechanisms. When speculating about the existence of alternate indirect mechanisms that may achieve depletion of uninfected cells, destruction by killing immune effector mechanisms was again proposed, involving either the targeting by soluble viral proteins of uninfected bystander cells, or the existence of molecular mimicry between viral and self proteins leading to autoimmune responses. The progressive realization that programmed cell death may indeed represent an essential component of the regulation of the adult T-cell responses generated a new and different form of skepticism about its potential role in AIDS. It became difficult to accept the idea that such a common feature of T-cell regulation in both physiological and pathological situations could play a major and specific causative role in a disease with such unique feature as AIDS. Therefore, it was proposed that the abnormal levels of programmed T-cell death that were indeed observed in HIV-infected persons only represented a consequence, and not a part of the specific pathogenic events leading to AIDS[124]. In summary, the initial view that it was highly unlikely that a virus causes cell depletion by triggering a cell suicide process that may not be operational in adult cells was progressively replaced by the converse view that it is unlikely that dysregulation of such a common and widely used cell suicide process may be sufficient to account for the pathogenesis of shuch a dramatic disease as AIDS.

The importance of programmed cell death regulation as a mechanism for the survival of adult T cells is supported, however, by a recent finding in mice. In this model, the targeted disruption of the programmed cell death suppressor gene *bcl-2* leads to a rapid postnatal involution of all lymphoid organs through the massive induction of adult T- and B-cell programmed death[146]. This finding indicates that the lack of a single gene whose expression is normally regulated by extracellular signals provided by the environment leads to the death of the entire T-cell population. Dysregulation of programmed cell death is therefore a mechanism sufficient to cause T-cell depletion and immune incompetence in the absence of any additional mechanism of T-cell aggression and destruction. This finding provides support to the concept that interference of HIV with the intercellular signals that regulate the expression of such genes could in theory represent a pathogenic mechanism potent enough to cause the depletion of both infected and uninfected cell populations in AIDS.

It is obvious however, that extensive induction of programmed cell death in a cell population is not obligatorily sufficient to induce its depletion, such outcome depending on the extent of the cell renewal processs. The CD8[+] T cells in HIV-infected persons provide, as discussed above, a relevant example. Despite the fact that they undergo extensive programmed cell death, as observed *in vitro*[46,49,50,52-54] and *in vivo*[73], absolute numbers of CD8+ T cells are maintained until the last stages of the disease.

Therefore, beyond the nature of the cell death mechanism that is responsible for CD4+ T-cell depletion (activation-induced cell suicide, viral cytopathic effects, or CD8+ cytotoxic effector T cells), a central question in AIDS pathogenesis that remains yet to be addressed, concerns both the lifespan and renewal potential of CD4+ T cells in HIV-infected persons. Although such questions have been difficult to address in general, recent findings suggest that naive and memory CD4+ T cells are normally long-lived cell populations[92,147]. *Ex vivo* labeling and reinjection of CD4 T cells could allow one to compare the lifespan of resting and activated CD4+ T cells in HIV-infected persons and in controls. Experiments performed in the primate models of lentiviral infection could allow one to compare the *in vivo* fate of uninfected CD4+ T cells and of *in vitro* infected CD4+ T cells, and therefore to assess whether infected cells are selectively destroyed as a consequence of viral cytopathic effects or of immune recognition by effector cells, or are in contrast long-lived in the infected host, as recently suggested[84]. Furthermore, comparative experiments of *in vivo* lifespan of injected labeled CD4+ T cells and of *in situ* assessment of the extent of apoptosis in the lymphoid organs in both pathogenic and nonpathogenic primate models of SIV infection, such as rhesus macaques infected with different viral clones, would allow one to explore, in an indirect way, the potential importance of central and peripheral CD4+ T-cell renewal in AIDS pathogenesis. Obviously, it is possible that nonpathogenic models are characterized by both a normal lifespan of CD4+ T cells and an absence of abnormal induction of programmed CD4+ T-cell death in the lymphoid tissues. On the other hand, if CD4+ T-cell lifespan *in vivo* were found not to be reduced in the nonpathogenic primate models and associated with abnormal levels of apoptosis in the lymphoid organs, this would suggest that it is the interruption of the peripheral renewal capacity of the CD4+ T cells that plays a central role in AIDS.

In fact, the slow and constant decrease in absolute CD4+ T-cell numbers in HIV-infected persons could be the consequence of two very different processes. The first possibility is that the capacity of the immune system to regenerate itself is impaired very early on after infection, and that therefore the loss in CD4+ T-cell numbers is a direct reflection of the number of CD4+ T cells that die *in vivo* each day. Another possibility, however, is that a very high rate of daily CD4+ T-cell death is partially compensated, during a very long period, by the continuous differentiation of progenitor cells. If this were the case, the excessive production of newly differentiated CD4+ T cells may lead to an impairment of their fitness, a mechanism that could play a role in the enhanced susceptibility of the mature CD4+ T cells for programmed cell death induction. In the adult, the capacity of the immune system to renew itself, as well as the mechanisms and location of this renewal process (thymic remnants, bone marrow) are still poorly known. In the newborn, however, it is known that the thymus plays a major role in T-cell renewal. Therefore, experiments of neonatal thymectomy performed in newborn primates could provide a way to address the question of the role of T-cell renewal, by comparing the course of both pathogenic and nonpathogenic SIV infections in euthymic and thymectomized primates.

Spatial Heterogeneity of Viral Sequences in the Lymphoid Organs and the Spatial Distribution of CD4+ T-Cell Death

Independently of the nature of the mechanism that may cause CD4+ T-cell death *in vivo*, there are reasons for speculating that, at any given time, the spatial distribution of cell-death induction in the lymphoid organs may be heterogeneous. Indeed, on the one hand, recent analysis of viral sequences in the spleen of HIV-infected patients has shown a spatial compartimentalization of viral genotypes throughout the organ[148]. On the other hand, studies in the macaque models of SIV infection have revealed that pathogenic SIV viral isolates are a mixture of viral genotypes that are either nonpathogenic or pathogenic when injected individually in a macaque. Therefore, it is possible that infection with an SIV (or HIV) isolate will result in the concomitant expansion of pathogenic and nonpathogenic viral clones. It would be important to assess whether the extent of CD4+ T-cell death that is observed in a given location of a lymphoid organ is always proportional to the extent of cellular viral RNA expressed, and therefore, to the extent of local viral replication. If this were not the case, it would suggest the possibility that the extent of CD4+ T-cell death is related to the genotype of the viral clone, and not directly to the extent of virus produced by the infected cells.

Cell Activation, Programmed Cell Death, Viral Replication, and Oncogenesis

Several recent findings are consistent with the view that subversion of programmed cell death regulation may represent an important component of the interaction between infectious pathogens and their host (for a review, see Ref. 31).

Induction of programmed death in infected cells may represent an evolutionary conserved efficient host protective mechanism limiting the spread of infectious pathogens[37-39]. Conversely, inhibition of programmed death in the infected cell can provide a selective advantage to the pathogen by extending the survival of infected cells (reviewed in Refs. 29,30,149,150). Finally, the induction of a shortening in the lifespan of neighboring cells may be beneficial to the pathogen when neighboring cells are deleterious to the infected cell, or when activation-induced programmed death of neighboring cells lead to the release of growth factors that will enhance survival or migration of the infected cell, such as occurs during murine mammary tumor virus infection[151]. Therefore, therapeutic strategies aimed at preventing the premature induction of programmed CD4+ T-cell death could have a profound influence on the viral load in HIV infected persons. Since an increase in both viral production and numbers of infected cells is a possible outcome of such strategies, combining immuno-therapy and anti-viral therapy may represent an optimal approach in order to extend T-cell survival without raising the viral load. The great dependance of HIV on host proteins and T-cell activation for most aspects of their replication cycle raises however the fascinating possibility that unique therapeutic approaches may be found that will interfere both with programmed T-cell death induction and viral replication. Cyclosporin A, whose clinical use in AIDS has led todate to contradictory results[152-154], presents several *in vitro* properties that may provide an example for the design of such therapeutic approaches. First, cyclosporin A prevents viral replication in HIV-infected CD4+ T-cell cultures by two different effects, the selective inhibition of T-cell receptor-induced CD4+ T-cell activation that is required for proviral integration and expression[155], and the prevention of the incorporation of cyclophilin A in the viral particle that has been recently shown to be required for the formation of infectious virions[156,157]; second, cyclosporin A prevents programmed cell death induction in response to T-cell receptor stimulation in CD4+ T cells from HIV-infected persons[48,50].

Another intrinsic risk in any attempt to prevent programmed cell death in a cell population that can undergo mitosis is the possibility of favouring the development of tumors. Recent findings have indicated that aberrant cell survival resulting from inhibition of programmed cell death can represent an essential step in oncogenesis[30,134]. However, expression of a gene that prevents in a given cell population programmed cell death induction in response to a given signal, does not prevent programmed cell death in response to all signals, and therefore does not obligatorily lead to cell immortalization. For example, the permanent expression of the *bcl-2* gene in the B-cell population of transgenic mice favours the development of B-cell lymphomas, but the permanent expression of the same gene in the T-cell population does not appear to favour the development of cancers[134]. It is therefore possible that the extension of CD4$^+$ T-cell survival may be achieved by therapeutic strategies that will not lead to T-cell lymphomas. Finally, it is important to consider that the pathology induced by HIV infection is not only related to excessive cell loss. In particular cell populations, indirect mechanisms favours the development of tumors, such as Kaposi's sarcoma. The Kaposi's sarcoma cells of fibroblast or endothelial origin are not infected by HIV, and depend, in order to proliferate and to survive, on inflammatory cytokines secreted by HIV-infected CD4$^+$ T cells and macrophages and the uptake of an HIV regulatory gene product, Tat, that is released by the HIV-infected cells[158]. It is tempting to speculate that AIDS represents a disease in which retroviral-mediated interference with cell signalling has important and widespread indirect effects on the regulation of programmed cell death, leading in different cell populations, either to cell loss by excessive programmed cell death induction, or to cell immortalization by excessive programmed cell death prevention. Consistent with this idea are the observations that the HIV envelope gene product is able, as discussed above, to induce programmed cell death in the CD4$^+$ T-cell population, while another HIV gene product, tat, has been shown to have a preventive effect on programmed cell death induction in several transformed cell lines[159]. Also consistent with this idea is the finding that another retrovirus, the murine mammary tumor virus, has been found to induce programmed cell death in one cell population (a subset of uninfected T cells) while inducing cancer in another cell population (the infected mammary gland epithelial cells)[151]. Understanding the nature of the mechanisms involved in retroviral-mediated modulation of cell survival and cell death may have wide ranging implications for therapy.

ACKNOWLEDGMENTS

Our work is supported by INSERM, ANRS, Pasteur Institute of Lille, Lille II University School of Medicine.

REFERENCES

1. Fauci A. S., 1988. The human immunodeficiency virus: infectivity and mechanisms of pathogenesis. *Science* 239: 617-620.
2. Levy J. A., 1993. Pathogenesis of HIV infection. *Microbiol. Rev.* 57: 183-289.
3. Everall I. P., Luthert P. J. and Lantos P. L., 1991. Neuronal loss in the frontal cortex in HIV-infection. *Lancet* 337: 1119-1121.
4. Schnittman S. M., Psallidopoulos M. C., Lane H. C., Thompson L., Baseler M., Massari F., Fox C. H., Salzman N. P. and Fauci A. S., 1989. The reservoir for HIV-1 in human peripheral blood is a cell that maintains expression of CD4. *Science* 245: 305-308.
5. Brinchman J. E., Albert J. and Vartdal F., 1991. Few infected CD4+ T cells but a high proportion of replication-competent provirus copies in asymptomatic HIV-1 infection. *J. Virol.* 65: 2019-2023.
6. Lane H. C., Depper J. M., Greene W. C., Whalen G., Waldmann T. A. and Fauci A. S., 1985. Qualitative analysis of immune function in patients with the acquired immunodeficiency syndrome. *N. Engl. J. Med.* 313: 79-84.
7. Shearer G. M., Bernstein D. C., Tung K. S. K., Via C. S., Redfield R., Salahuddin S. Z. and Gallo R. C., 1986. A model for the selective loss of major histocompatibility complex self-restricted T cell immune responses during the development of AIDS. *J. Immunol.* 137: 2514-2521.
8. Hofmann B., Jakobsen K. D., Odum N., Dickmeiss E., Platz P., Ryder L. P., Pedersen C., Mathiesen L., Bygbjerg I., Faber V. and Svejgaard A., 1989. HIV-induced immunodeficiency relatively preserved PHA as opposed to decreased PWM responses via CD2/PHA pathway. *J. Immunol.* 142: 1874-1880.

9. Miedema F., Petit A. J. C., Terpestra F. G., Eeftinck Schattenkerk J. K. M., Dewolf F., Al B. J. M., Roos M., Lange J. M. A., Danner S. A., Goudsmit J. and Schellekens P. T. A., 1988. Immunological abnormalities in HIV-infected asymptomatic homosexual men. *J. Clin. Invest.* 82: 1908-1914.

10. Clerici M., Stocks N. I., Zajac R. A., Boswell R. N., Lucey D. R., Via C. S. and Shearer G. M., 1989. Detection of three distinct patterns of T helper cell dysfunction in asymptomatic, HIV-seropositive patients. *J. Clin. Invest.* 84: 1892-1899.

11. Clerici M., Stocks N. I., Zajac R. A., Boswell R. N., Bernstein D. C., Mann D. L., Shearer G. M. and Berzofsky J. A., 1989. Interleukin-2 production used to detect antigenic peptide recognition by T-helper lymphocytes from asymptomatic HIV-seropositive individuals. *Nature* 339: 383-385.

12. Koenig S., Gendelman H. E., Orenstein J. M., Dal Canto M. C., Pezeshkpour G. H., Yungbluth M., Janotta F., Aksamit A., Martin M. A. and Fauci A. S., 1986. Detection of AIDS virus in macrophages in brain tissue from AIDS patients with encephalopathy. *Science* 233: 1089-1093.

13. Michaels J., Sharer L. R. and Epstein L. G., 1988. HIV-1 infection of the nervous system: a review. *Immunodeficiency Rev.* 1: 71-104.

14. Johnson B. K., Stone G. A., Godec M. S., Asher D. M., Gajdusek D. C. and Gibbs Jr C. J., 1993. Long-term observations of HIV-infected chimpanzees. *AIDS Res. Hum. Retrovir.* 9: 375-378.

15. Watanabe M., Ringler D. J., Fultz P. N., MacKey J. J., Boyson J. E., Levine C. G. and Letvin N. L., 1991. A Chimpanzee-passaged HIV isolate is cytopathic for chimpanzee cells but does not induce disease. *J. Virol.* 65: 3344-3348.

16. Müller M. C., Saksena N. K., Nerrienet E., Chappey C., Hervé V. M. A., Durand J. P., Legal-Campodonico P., Lang M. C., Digoutte J. P., Georges A. G., Georges-Courbot M. C., Sonigo P. and Barré-Sinoussi F., 1993. Simian immunodeficiency viruses from Central and Western Africa: evidence for a new species-specific lentivirus in tantalus monkeys. *J. Virol.* 67: 1227-1235.

17. Desrosiers R. C., 1990. The simian immunodeficiency viruses. *Annu. Rev. Immunol.* 8: 557-578.

18. Kestler H., Kodama T., Ringler D., Marthas M., Pedersen N., Lackner A., Regier D., Sehgal P., Daniel M., King N. and Desrosiers R., 1990. Induction of AIDS in rhesus monkeys by molecularly cloned SIV. *Science* 248: 1109-1112.

19. Ameisen J. C. and Capron A., 1991. Cell dysfunction and depletion in AIDS: the programmed cell death hypothesis. *Immunol. Today* 12: 102-105.

20. Ameisen J. C., 1992. Programmed cell death and AIDS: from hypothesis to experiment. *Immunol. Today* 13: 388-391.

21. Saunders J. W. J., 1966. Death in the embryonic systems. *Science* 154: 604-612.

22. Kerr J. F. R., Willie A. H. and Currie A. R., 1972. Apoptosis: a basic biological phenomenon with wide-ranging implications in tissue kinetics. *Br. J. Cancer.* 26: 239-257.

23. Duvall E. and Wyllie A. H., 1986. Death and the cell. *Immunol. Today* 7: 115-119.

24. Ellis R. E., Yuan J. and Horvitz H. R., 1991. Mechanisms and functions of cell death. *Annual Review of Cell Biology* 7: 663-698.

25. Oppenheim R. W., 1991. Cell death during development of the nervous system. *Annu. Rev. Neurosci.* 14: 453-501.

26. Raff M., 1992. Social controls on cell survival and cell death. *Nature* 356: 397-400.

27. Vaux D. L., 1993. Towards an understanding of the molecular mechanisms of physiological cell death. *Proc. Natl. Acad. Sci. USA* 90: 786-789.

28. Cohen J. J., 1993. Apoptosis. *Immunol. Today* 14: 126-130.

29. Schwartz L. M. and Osborne B. A., 1993. Programmed cell death, apoptosis, and killer genes. *Immunol. Today* 14: 582-590.

30. Williams G. T. and Smith C. T., 1993. Molecular regulation of apoptosis: genetic controls on cell death. *Cell* 74: 777-779.

31. Ameisen J. C., 1994. Programmed cell death (apoptosis) and cell survival regulation: relevance to AIDS and cancer. *AIDS* 8: 1197-1213.

32. Mc Conkey D. J., Orrenius S. and Jondal M., 1990. Cellular signaling in programmed cell death (apoptosis). *Immunol. Today* 11: 120-121.

33. Golstein P., Ojcius D. M. and Young J. D. E., 1991. Cell death mechanism and the immune system. *Immunological Reviews* 121: 29-65.

34. Odaka C., Hizaki H. and Tadakuma T., 1990. T-cell receptor-mediated DNA fragmentation and cell death in T-cell hybridoma. *J. Immunol.* 144: 2096-2101.

35. Bell D. A., Morrison B. and Vandenbygaart P., 1990. Immunogenic DNA-related factors: Nucleosomes spontaneously released from normal murine lymphoid cells stimulate proliferation and immunoglobulin synthesis of normal mouse lymphocytes. *J. Clin. Invest.* 85: 1437-1496.

36. Clouston W. M. and Kerr J. F. R., 1985. Apoptosis, lymphocytotoxicity and the containment of viral infections. *Medical Hypothesis* 18: 399-404.

37. Clem R. J., Fechheimer M. and Miller L. K., 1991. Prevention of apoptosis by a baculovirus gene during infection of insect cells. *Science* 254: 1388-1390.

38. Greenberg J., Guo A., Klessig D. and Ausubel F., 1994. Programmed cell death in plants: a pathogen-triggered response activated coordinately with multiple defence functions. *Cell* 77: 551.

39. Levine B., Huang Q., Isaacs J., Reed J., Griffin D. and Hardwick J., 1993. Conversion of lytic to persistent alphavirus infection by the *bcl-2* oncogene. *Nature* 361: 739-742.

40. Fauci A. S., 1993. Multifactorial nature of HIV disease: implications for therapy. *Science* 262: 1011-1018.

41. Blackman M., Kappler J. and Marrack P., 1990. The role of T-cell receptor in positive and negative selection of developing T cells. *Science* 248: 1335-1341.

42. Newell M. K., Haughn L. J., Maroun C. R. and Julius M. H., 1990. Death of mature T cells by separate ligation of CD4 and the T-cell receptor for antigen. *Nature* 347: 286-289.

43. Liu Y. and Janeway C. A., 1990. INFγ plays a crucial role in induced cell death of effector T cell: a possible third mechanism of self tolerance. *J. Exp. Med.* 172: 1735-1741.

44. Marrack P. and Kappler J., 1990. The staphylococcal enterotoxins and their relatives. *Science* 248: 705-711.

45. Jenkinson E. J., Kingston R., Smith C. A., Williams G. T. and Owen J. J. T., 1989. Antigen-induced apoptosis in developing T cells: a mechanism for negative selection of the T-cell repertoire. *Eur. J. Immunol.* 19: 2175-2177.

46. Gougeon M.-L., Olivier R., Garcia S., Guétard D., Dragic T., Dauguet C. and Montagnier L., 1991. Mise en évidence d'un processus d'engagement vers la mort cellulaire par apoptose dans les lymphocytes de patients infectés par le VIH. *C. R. Acad. Sci. Paris* 312: 529-537.

47. Groux H., Monté D., Bourez J. M., Capron A. and Ameisen J. C., 1991. L'activation des lymphocytes TCD4+ de sujets asymptomatiques infectés par le VIH entraîne le déclenchement d'un programme de mort lymphocytaire par apoptose. *C. R. Acad. Sci. Paris* 312: 599-606.

48. Groux H., Torpier G., Monté D., Mouton Y., Capron A. and Ameisen J. C., 1992. Activation-induced death by apoptosis in CD4+ T Cells from HIV-infected asymptomatic individuals. *J. Exp. Med.* 175: 331-340.

49. Meyaard L., Otto S. A., Jonker R. R., Mijnster M. J., Keet I. P. M. and Miedema F., 1992. Programmed cell death of T cells in HIV-1 infection. *Science* 257: 217-219.

50. Gougeon M.-L., Garcia S., Heeney J., Tschopp R., Lecoeur H., Guétard D., Rame V., Dauguet C. and Montagnier L., 1993. Programmed cell death in AIDS-related HIV and SIV infections. *AIDS Res. Hum. Retrovir.* 9: 553-563.

51. Oyaizu N., McCloskey T. W., Coronesi M., Chirmule N. and Pahwa S., 1993. Accelerated apoptosis in PBMCs from HIV-1 infected patients and in CD4 cross-linked PBMCs from normal individuals. *Blood* 82: 3392-3400.

52. Lewis D. E., Ng Tang D. S., Adu-Oppong A., Schober W. and Rodgers J. R., 1994. Anergy and apoptosis in CD8+ T cells from HIV-infected persons. *J. Immunol.* 153: 412-420.

53. Sarin A., Clerici M., Blatt S. P., Hendrix C. W., Shearer G. M. and Henkart P. A., 1994. Inhibition of activation-induced programmed cell death and restoration of defective immune responses of HIV+ donors by cysteine protease inhibitors. *J. Immunol.* 153: 862-872.

54. Estaquier J., Idziorek T., De Bels F., Barré-Sinoussi F., Hurtrel B., Aubertin A. M., Venet A., Mehtali M., Muchmore E., Michel P., Mouton Y., Girard M. and Ameisen J. C., 1994. Programmed cell death and AIDS: the significance of T-cell apoptosis in pathogenic and non pathogenic primate lentiviral infections. *Proc. Natl Acad. Sci. USA* 91: 9431-9435.

55. Estaquier J. and Ameisen J. C., 1994. Programmed cell death (apoptosis) and AIDS: Is Th1 dysfunction and deletion related to an abortive Th1/Th2 switch process? In *Challenges of Modern Medicine. Cytokines: Basic Principles and Practical Applications.* (Edited by Romagnani S., Del Prete G. and Abbas K.), ARES SERONO Symposia, Rome. pp. 195-201.

56. Ameisen J. C., Estaquier J. and Idziorek T., 1994. From AIDS to parasite infection: pathogen-mediated subversion of programmed cell death as a mechanism for immune dysregulation. *Immunological Reviews* 142: in press.

57. Terai C., Kornbluth R. S., Pauza C. D., Richman D. D. and Carson D. A., 1991. Apoptosis as a mechanism of cell death in cultured T lymphoblasts acutely infected with HIV-1. *J. Clin. Invest.* 87: 1710-1715.

58. Laurent-Crawford A. G., Krust B., Muller S., Rivière Y., Rey-Cuillé M. A., Béchet J. M., Montagnier L. and Hovanessian A. G., 1991. The cytopathic effect of HIV is associated with apoptosis. *Virology* 185: 829-839.

59. Martin S. J., Matear P. and Vyakarnam A., 1994. HIV-1 infection of human CD4 T cells in vitro. Differential induction of apoptosis in these cells. *J. Immunol.* 152: 330-342.

60. Cameron P. U., Pope M., Gezelter S. and Steinman R. M., 1994. Infection and apoptotic cell death of CD4 T cells during an immune response to HIV-1-pulsed dendritic cells. *AIDS Res. Hum. Retrovir.* 10: 61-71.

61. Banda N. K., Bernier J., Kurahara D. K., Kurrle R., Haigwood N., Sekaly R. P. and Finkel T. H., 1992. Crosslinking CD4 by HIV gp120 primes T cells for activation-induced apoptosis. *J. Exp. Med.* 176: 1099-1106.

62. Cohen D. I., Tani Y., Tian H., Boone E., Samelson L. and Lane H. C., 1992. Participation of tyrosine phosphorylation in the cytopathic effect of HIV-1. *Science* 256: 542-545.

63. Tian H., Kolesnitchenko V., Donoghue E., Shaw G., Lane C. and Cohen D., 1993. HIV envelope-directed CD4 T-cell degeneration represents a novel cell death program. In *The first national conference on human retroviruses and related infections*; Washington DC (Edited by American Society for Microbiology. Abstr. 275.

64. Laurent-Crawford A. G., Krust B., Rivière Y., Desgranges C., Muller S., Kiény M. P., Dauguet C. and Hovanessian A. G., 1993. Membrane expression of HIV envelope glycoproteins triggers apoptosis in CD4 cells. *AIDS Res. Hum. Retrovir.* 9: 761-773.

65. Zauli G., Vitale M., Re M. C., Furlini G., Zamai L., Falcieri E., Gibellini D., Visani G., Davis B. R., Capitani S. and La Placa M., 1994. *In vitro* exposure to HIV-1 induces apoptotic cell death of the factor-dependent TF-1 hematopoietic cell line. *Blood* 83: 167-175.

66. Mosier D. E., Gulizia R. J., MacIsaac P. D., Torbett B. E. and Levy J. A., 1993. Rapid loss of CD4+ T cells in human-PBL-SCID mice by noncytopathic HIV isolates. *Science* 260: 689-692.

67. Mosier D. and Sieburg H., 1994. Macrophage-tropic HIV: critical for AIDS pathogenesis? *Immunol. Today* 15: 332-339.

68. Bonyhadi M. L., Rabin L., Salimi S., Brown D. A., Kosek J., McCune J. M. and Kaneshima H., 1993. HIV induces thymus depletion *in vivo*. *Nature* 363: 728-732.

69. Del Llano A. M., Amieiro-Puig J. P., Kraiselburd E. N., Kessler M. J., Malaga C. A. and Lavergne J. A., 1993. The combined assessment of cellular apoptosis, mitochondrial function and proliferative response to pokeweed mitogen has prognostic value in SIV infection. *J. Med. Primatol.* 22: 194-200.

70. Bishop S. A., Gruffydd-Jones T. J., Harbour D. A. and Stokes C. R., 1993. Programmed cell death (apoptosis) as a mechanism of cell death in PBMC from cats infected with feline immunodeficiency virus (FIV). *Clin. Exp. Immunol.* 93: 65-71.

71. Schuitemaker H., Meyaard L., Kootstra N. A., Otto S. A., Dubbes R., Tersmette M., Heeney J. L. and Miedema F., 1993. Lack of T-cell dysfunction and programmed cell death correlates with inability of HIV-1 to infect chimpanzee monocytes. *J. Inf. Dis.* 168: 1140-1147.

72. Fauci A. S., 1994. Multifactorial and multiphasic components of the immunopathogenic mechanisms of HIV disease. In *Retroviruses of Human AIDS and Related Animal Diseases (VIII Colloque des Cent Gardes, 1993)* (Edited by Girard M. and Valette L.), Fondation M. Mérieux, Lyon. pp. 81-85.

73. Pantaleo G., Graziosi C., Demarest J. F., Cohen O. J., Vaccarezza M., Gantt K., Muro-Cacho C. and Fauci A. S., 1994. Role of lymphoid organs in the pathogenesis of HIV infection. *Immunological Reviews* 140: 105-130.

74. Fultz P. N., Schwiebert R. S., Su L. Y. and Salter M. M., 1994. Total lymphoid irradiation as a novel therapeutic approach for treatment of HIV-induced disease. In *Retroviruses of Human AIDS and Related Animal Diseases (VIII Colloque des Cent Gardes, 1993)* (Edited by Girard M. and Valette L.), Fondation M. Mérieux, Lyon. pp. 245-249.

75. Baskin G. B., Murphey-Corb M., Martin L. N., Davison-Fairburn B., Hu F. S. and Kuebler D., 1991. Thymus in simian immunodeficiency virus infected rhesus monkeys. *Lab. Invest.* 65: 400-407.

76. Lackner A. A., Vogel P., Hoogenboom E., Luge J. D. and Marthas M., 1994. Pathogenic (SIVmac-239) and nonpathogenic (SIVmac-1A11) molecular clones of SIV have distinct tissue distributions that vary with length of infection. In *Retroviruses of Human AIDS and Related Animal Diseases (VIII Colloque des Cent Gardes, 1993)* (Edited by Girard M. and Valette L.), Fondation M. Mérieux, Lyon. pp. 27-34.

77. Uehara T., Miyawaki T., Ohta K., Tamaru Y., Yokoi T., Nakamura S. and Taniguchi N., 1992. Apoptotic cell death of primed CD45RO+ T lymphocytes in Epstein-Barr virus-induced infectious mononucleosis. *Blood* 80: 452-458.

78. Akbar A. N., Borthwick N., Salmon M., Gombert W., Bofill M., Shamsadeen N., Pilling D., Pett S., Grundy J. E. and Janossy G., 1993. The significance of low *bcl-2* expression by CD45RO+ T cells in normal individuals and patients with acute viral infections. The role of apoptosis in T cell memory. *J. Exp. Med.* 178: 427-438.

79. Razvi E. S. and Welsh R. M., 1993. Programmed cell death of T lymphocytes during acute viral infection: a mechanism for virus-induced immunodeficiency. *J. Virol.* 67: 5754-5765.

80. Tamaru Y., Miyawaki T., Iwai T., Nibu R., Yachie A., Koizumi S. and Taniguchi N., 1993. Absence of *bcl-2* expression by activated CD45RO+ T lymphocytes in acute infectious mononucleosis supporting their susceptibility to programmed cell death. *Blood* 82: 521-527.

81. Levy J. A., 1993. HIV pathogenesis and long-term survival. *AIDS* 7: 1401-1410.

82. Howie S., Sommerfield A. J., Gray E. and Harrison D. J., 1994. Peripheral T lymphocyte depletion by apoptosis after CD4 ligation *in vivo*: selective loss of CD44-negative and 'activating' memory T cells. *Clin. Exp. Immunol.* 95: 195-200.

83. Wang Z. Q., Dudhane A., Orlikowski T., Clarke K., Li X., Darzynkiewicz Z. and Hoffmann M. K., 1994. CD4 engagement induces Fas antigen-dependent apoptosis of T cells *in vivo*. *Eur. J. Immunol.* 24: 1549-1552.

84. Finkel T. H. and Banda N. K., 1994. Indirect mechanisms of HIV pathogenesis: how does HIV kill T cells? *Current Opinion in Immunology* 6: 605-615.

85. Ameisen J. C., Estaquier J., Idziorek T. and De Bels F., 1995. The relevance of apoptosis to AIDS pathogenesis. *Trends in Cell Biology* 5: 27-32.

86. Tian H., Donoghue E. T., Fang F., Newport J. W. and Cohen D. I., 1994. Cells expressing CDC2 kinase undergo programmed cell death with striking similarities to HIV-directed cytopathicity. *J. Cell. Biochem.* Sup. 18B: Abst. J275.

87. Shi L., Nishioka W. K., Th'ng J., Bradbury E. M., Litchfield D. W. and Greenberg A. H., 1994. Premature p34^{cdc2} activation required for apoptosis. *Science* 263: 1143-1145.

88. Bretscher P. and Cohn M., 1970. A theory of self-nonself discrimination. *Science* 169: 1042-1049.

89. Jenkins M., 1992. The role of cell division in the induction of clonal anergy. *Immunol. Today* 13: 69-73.

90. Janeway C. A., 1992. The immune system evolved to dicriminate infectious nonself from non infectious self. *Immunol. Today* 13: 11-16.

91. Janeway C. A. and Bottomly K., 1994. Signals and signs for lymphocyte responses. *Cell* 76: 275-285.

92. Sprent J., 1994. T and B memory cells. *Cell* 76: 315-322.

93. Lenardo M. J., 1991. IL-2 programs mouse αβ T-lymphocytes for apoptosis. *Nature* 353: 858-861.

94. Russell J. H., White C. L., Loh D. Y. and Meleedy-Rey P., 1991. Receptor stimulated death pathway is opened by antigen in mature T cells. *Proc. Natl Acad. Sci. USA* 88: 2151-2155.

95. Groux H., Monté D., Plouvier B., Capron A. and Ameisen J. C., 1993. CD3-mediated apoptosis of human medullary thymocytes and activated peripheral T cells: respective roles of IL-1, IL-2, IFNγ and accessory cells. *Eur. J. Immunol.* 23: 1623-1629.

96. Wang R., Murphy K., Loh D., Weaver C. and Russell J., 1993. Differential activation of antigen-stimulated suicide and cytokine production pathways in CD4 T cells is regulated by the antigen-presenting cell. *J. Immunol.* 150: 3832-3842.

97. Kawabe Y. and Yoshi A., 1991. Programmed cell death and extrathymic reduction of Vβ8+ CD4+ T cells in mice tolerant to staphylococcus aureus enterotoxin B. *Nature* 349: 245-247.

98. Choi Y. W., Kappler J. W. and Marrack P., 1991. A superantigen encoded in the open reading frame of the 3' long terminal repeat of MMTV. *Nature* 350: 203-207.

99. Mc Cormack J. E., Callahan J. E., Kappler J. and Marrack P. C., 1993. Profound deletion of mature T cells in vivo by chronic exposure to exogenous superantigen. *J. Immunol.* 150: 3785-3792.

100. Moskophidis D., Lechner F., Pircher H. and Zinkernagel R. M., 1993. Virus persistence in acutely infected immunocompetent mice by exhaustion of antiviral cytotoxic effector T cells. *Nature* 362: 758-761.

101. Raff M. C., Barres B. A., Burne J. F., Coles H. S., Ishizaki Y. and Jacobson M. D., 1993. Programmed cell death and the control of cell survival: lessons from the nervous system. *Science* 262. 695-700.

102. Ruoslahti E. and Reed J. C., 1994. Anchorage dependence, integrins, and apoptosis. *Cell* 77: 477-478.

103. Fulcher D. A. and Basten A., 1994. Reduced life span of anergic self-reactive B cells in a double-transgenic model. *J. Exp. Med.* 179: 125-134.

104. Mannhalter J. W., Husch B., Küpcü Z. and Eibl M. M., 1994. Capacity of HIV-1 to infect chimpanzee monocyte in vitro. *The Journal of Infectious Diseases* 169: 1407-1409.

105. Arthur L. O., Bess J. W., Sowder II R. C., Benveniste R. E., Mann D. L., Chermann J. C. and Henderson L. E., 1992. Cellular proteins bound to immunodeficiency viruses: Implications for pathogenesis and vaccines. *Science* 258: 1935-1941.

106. Rossio J. L., Bess Jr J., Henderson L. E. and Arthur L. O., 1994. Consequences of HIV-mediated superantigen stimulation of human T lymphocytes. *J. Cell. Biochem.* Sup. 18B: Abst. J267.

107. Clerici M. and Shearer G. M., 1994. The Th1-Th2 hypothesis of HIV infection: new insights. *Immunol. Today* 15: 575-581.

108. Marrack P. and Kappler J., 1994. Subversion of the immune system by pathogens. *Cell* 76: 323-332.

109. Coffman R. L., Varkila K., Scott P. and Chatelain R., 1991. Role of cytokines in the differentiation of CD4 T-cell subsets in vivo. *Immunological Reviews* 123: 189-207.

110. Mosmann T. R., Schumacher J. H., Street N. F., Budd R., O'Garra A., Fong T. A. T., Bond M. W., Moore K. W. M., Sher A. and Fiorentino D. F., 1991. Diversity of cytokine synthesis and function of mouse CD4 T cells. *Immunological Reviews* 123: 209-229.

111. Romagnani S., 1991. Human TH1 and TH2 subsets: doubt no more. *Immunol. Today* 12: 256-257.

112. Romagnani S., 1992. Induction of Th1 and Th2 responses: a key role for the 'natural' immune response? *Immunol. Today* 13: 379-381.

113. Powrie F. and Coffman R. L., 1993. Cytokine regulation of T-cell function: potential for therapeutic intervention. *Immunol. Today* 14: 270-274.

114. Erard F., Wild M. T., Garcia-Sanz J. A. and Le Gros G., 1993. Switch of CD8 T cells to noncytolytic CD8-negative/CD4-negative cells that make Th2 cytokines and help B cells. *Science* 260: 1802-1805.

115. Scott P., 1993. IL-12: initiation cytokine for cell-mediated immunity. *Science* 260: 496-497.

116. deWaal Malefyt R., Yssel H. and De Vries J. E., 1993. Direct effects of IL-10 on subsets of human CD4 T cell clones and resting T cells. Specific inhibition of IL-2 production and proliferation. *J. Immunol.* 150: 4754-4765.

117. Heinzel F., Sadick S., Mutha S. and Locksley M., 1991. Production of IFNγ, IL-2, IL-4 and IL-10 by CD4+ lymphocytes *in vivo* during healing and progressive leishmaniasis. *Proc. Natl. Acad. Sci. USA* 88: 7011-7015.

118. Salgame P., Abrams J. S., Clayberger C., Goldstein H., Convit J., Modlin R. L. and Bloom B. R., 1991. Differing lymphokine profiles of functional subsets of human CD4 and CD8 T-cell clones. *Science* 254: 279-282.

119. Yamamura M., Uyemura K., Deans R. J., Weinberg K., Rea T. H., Bloom B. R. and Modlin R. L., 1991. Defining protective responses to pathogens: cytokine profiles in leprosy lesions. *Science* 25: 277-279.

120. Gazzinelli R. T., Makino M., Chattopadhyay S. K., Snapper C. M., Sher A., Hügin A. W. and Morse III H. C., 1992. CD4 subset regulation in viral infection. Preferential activation of Th2 cells during progression of retrovirus-induced immunodeficiency in mice. *J. Immunol.* 148: 182-188.

121. Sher A. and Coffman R. L., 1992. Regulation of immunity to parasites by T cells and T cell-derived cytokines. *Annu. Rev. Immunol.* 10: 385-409.

122. Clerici M., Lucey D. R., Berzofsky J. A., Pinto L. A., Wynn T. A., Blatt S. P., Dolan M. J., Hendrix C. W., Wolf S. F. and Shearer G. M., 1993. Restoration of HIV-specific cell-mediated immune response by IL-12 in vitro. *Science* 262: 1721-1724.

123. Clerici M. and Shearer G. M., 1993. A TH1/TH2 switch is a critical step in the etiology of HIV infection. *Immunol. Today* 14: 107-111.

124. Meyaard L., Otto S. A., Schuitemaker H. and Miedema F., 1993. T-cell dysfunction in HIV infection: anergy due to defective antigen-presenting cell function? *Immunol. Today* 14: 161-164.

125. Graziosi C., Pantaleo G., Gantt K. R., Fortin J. P., Demarest J. F., Cohen O. J., Sékaly R. and Fauci A. S., 1994. Lack of evidence for the dichotomy of TH1 and TH2 predominance in HIV-infected individuals. *Science* 265: 248-252.

126. Chehimi J., Starr S. E., Frank I., D'Andrea A., Ma X., MacGregor R. R., Sennelier J. and Trinchieri G., 1994. Impaired IL-12 production in HIV-infected patients. *J. Exp. Med.* 179: 1361-1366.

127. Maggi E., Mazzetti M., Ravina A., Annunziato F., De Carli M., Piccinni M. P., Manetti R., Carbonari M., Pesce A. M., Del Prete G. and Romagnani S., 1994. Ability of HIV to promote a TH1 to TH0 shift and to replicate preferentially in TH2 and TH0 cells. *Science* 265: 244-248.

128. Webb S., Morris C. and Sprent J., 1990. Extrathymic tolerance of mature T cells: clonal elimination as a consequence of immunity. *Cell* 63: 1249.

129. Zinkernagel R. M., Moskophidis D., Kündig T., Oehen S., Pircher H. and Hengartner H., 1993. Effector T-cell induction and T-cell memory *versus* peripheral deletion of T cells. *Immunological Reviews* 131: 199-223.

130. Marrack P., Hugo P., McCormack J. and Kappler J., 1993. Death and T cells. *Immunological Reviews* 133: 119-129.

131. Rouvier E., Luciani M.-F. and Golstein P., 1993. Fas involvement in Ca++-independent T cell-mediated cytotoxocity. *J. Exp. Med.* 177: 195-200.

132. Kägi D., Vignaux F., Lederman B., Bürki K., Depraetere V., Nagata S., Hengartner H. and Golstein P., 1994. Fas and perforin pathways as major mechanisms of T-cell-mediated cytotoxicity. *Science* 265: 528-530.

133. Ju S. T., Cui H. L., Panka D. J., Ettinger R. and Marshak-Rothstein A., 1994. Participation of target Fas protein in apoptosis pathway induced by CD4+ TH1 and CD8+ cytotoxic T cells. *Proc. Natl. Acad. Sci. USA* 91: 4185-4189.

134. Korsmeyer S., 1992. *Bcl-2*: a repressor of lymphocyte death. *Immunol. Today* 13: 285-288.

135. Vaux D. L., Aguila H. L. and Weissman I. L., 1992. *Bcl-2* prevents death of factor-deprived cells but fails to prevent apoptosis in targets of cell mediated killing. *International Immunology* 4: 821-824.

136. Cory S., 1994. Fascinating death factor. *Nature* 367: 317-318.

137. Itoh N., Tsujimoto Y. and Nagata S., 1993. Effect of Bcl-2 on Fas antigen-mediated cell death. *J. Immunol.* 151: 621-627.

138. Embretson J., Zupancic M., Ribas J. L., Burke A., Racz P., Tenner-Racz K. and Haase A. T., 1993. Massive covert infection of helper T lymphocytes and macrophages by HIV during the incubation period of AIDS. *Nature* 362: 359-362.

139. Pantaleo G., Graziosi C., Demarest J. F., Butini L., Montroni M., Fox C. H., Orenstein J. M., Kotler D. P. and Fauci A. S., 1993. HIV infection is active and progressive in lymphoid tissue during the clinically latent stage of disease. *Nature* 362: 355-358.

140. Westermann J. and Pabst R., 1990. Lymphocyte subsets in the blood: a diagnostic window on the lymphoïd system? *Immunol. Today* 11: 406-410.

141. Meyaard L., Otto S. A., Keet I. P. M., Roos M. T. L. and Miedema F., 1994. Programmed cell death of T cells in HIV infection. No correlation with progression to disease. *J. Clin. Invest.* 93: 982-988.

142. Zinkernagel R. M. and Hengartner H., 1994. T-cell mediated immunopathology *versus* direct cytolysis by virus: implications for HIV and AIDS. *Immunol. Today* 15: 262-268.

143. Kim H. S., Zhang X. and Choi Y. S., 1994. Activation and proliferation of follicular dendritic cell-like cells by activated T lymphocytes. *J. Immunol.* 153: 2951-2961.

144. Kotler D. P., Weaver S. C. and Terzakis J. A., 1986. Ultrastructural features of epithelial cell degeneration in rectal crypts of patients with AIDS. *Am. J. Surg. Pathol.* 10: 531-538.

145. Genis P., Jett M., Bernton E. W., Boyle T., Gelbard H. A., Dzenko K., Keane R. W., Resnick L., Mizrachi Y., Volsky D. J., Epstein L. G. and Gendelman H. E., 1992. Cytokines and arachidonic metabolites produced during HIV-infected macrophage-astroglia interactions: implications for the neuropathogenesis of HIV disease. *J. Exp. Med.* 176: 1703-1718.

146. Veis D. J., Sorenson C. M., Shutter J. R. and Korsmeyer S. J., 1993. *Bcl-2*-deficient mice demonstrate fulminant lymphoid apoptosis, polycystic kidneys, and hypopigmented hair. *Cell* 75: 229-240.

147. Swain S. L., 1994. Generation and in vivo persistence of polarized Th1 and Th2 memory cells. *Immunity* 1: 543-552.

148. Cheynier R., Henrichwark S., Hadida F., Pelletier E., Oksenhendler E., Autran B. and Wain-Hobson S., 1994. Clonal expansion of T cells and HIV genotypes in microdissected splenic white pulps, indicate viral replication in situ and infiltration of HIV-specific cytotoxic T lymphocytes. *Cell* 78: 373-385.

149. Williams G. T., 1991. Programmed cell death: apoptosis and oncogenesis. *Cell* 65: 1097-1098.

150. Vaux D. L., Haeker G. and Strasser A., 1994. An evolutionary perspective on apoptosis. *Cell* 76: 777-779.

151. Held W., Acha-Orbea H., McDonals H. R. and Waanders G. A., 1994. Superantigens and retroviral infection: insights from MMTV. *Immunol. Today* 15: 184-190.

152. Andrieu J. M., Even P., Venet A., Tourani J. M., Stern M., Lowenstein W. *et al.*, 1988. Effects of cyclosporin on T-cell subsets in HIV disease. *Clin. Immunol. Immunopathol.* 46: 181-.

153. Phillips A., Wainberg M. A., Coates R., Klein M., Rachlis A., Read S. *et al.*, 1989. Cyclosporin-induced deterioration in patients with AIDS. *C.M.A.J.* 140: 1456-.

154. Schwartz A., Offermann G., Keller F., Bennhold I., L'Age-Stehr J., Krause P. H. *et al.*, 1993. The effect of cyclosporine on the progression of HIV-1 infection transmitted by transplantation - data on 4 cases and review of the literature. *Transplantation* 55: 95-.

155. Bell K. D., Ramilo O. and Vitetta E. S., 1993. Combined use of an immunotoxin and cyclosporine to prevent both activated and quiescent peripheral blood T cells from producing HIV-1. *Proc. Natl. Acad. Sci. USA* 90: 1411 .

156. Franke E. K., Yuan H. E. H. and Luban J., 1994. Specific incorporation of cyclophilin A into HIV-1 virions. *Nature* 372: 359-362.

157. Thali M., Bukovsky A., Kondo E., Rosenwirth B., Walsh C. T., Sodroski J. and Göttlinger H. G., 1994. Functional association of cyclophilin A with HIV-1 virions. *Nature* 372: 363-365.

158. Ensoli B., Gendelman R., Markham P., Fiorelli V., Colombini S., Raffeld M., Cafaro A., Chang H. K., Brady J. N. and Gallo R. C., 1994. Synergy between basic fibroblast growth factor and HIV-1 Tat protein in induction of Kaposi's sarcoma. *Nature* 371: 674-680.

159. Zauli G., Gibellini D. and Milani D., 1993. *Cancer Research* 53: 4481-4485.

IMMUNOSUPPRESSION BY A NONCYTOLYTIC VIRUS VIA T CELL MEDIATED IMMUNOPATHOLOGY

Implication for AIDS

Rolf M. Zinkernagel

University of Zurich
Institute of Experimental Immunology
Switzerland

ABSTRACT

HIV is basically a non- or poorly cytocidal virus. Therefore, HIV infections in humans represent an apparent perversity in the balance between the host immune system and infectious agent: This noncytopathic virus infects macrophages, antigen presenting cells, helper T cells and other host cells which are then destroyed by the CD8[+] T cell immune response. Thus, HIV infects some of the key cells involved in immune reactions and therefore induces the immune system to destroy itself and thereby enables the virus to persist. Accordingly, immunosuppression is not a cause of HIV cytopathogenicity but a consequence of conventional T cell mediated immunopathology that destroys macrophages antigen presenting cells, T helper cells and facilitates infection by trivial intracellular parasites which eventually cause fatal disease. This immunopathological view of AIDS is testable and, if correct, impinges on rationales for AIDS prevention and treatment.

INTRODUCTION

HIV infection with HIV in man has launched intensive research efforts to understand both virus and disease. While the virus is being analysed and understood in ever greater detail, the complexities of the disease are still poorly understood[1-5] explanations for pathogenesis of AIDS therefore tend to be complex, if not emotional or political[6-8]. The most commonly invoked pathogenetic mechanisms of HIV infection leading to AIDS are: HIV is cytopathic i.e. destroys cells it infects,[9-13], causes cells to fuse and form syncytia,[14,15], induces auto-antibodies that attack the host's immune cells[1,3,16-20] stimulates T cells overwhelmingly so that they undergo apoptosis[21,22] cause dysregulation of interleukins[23-25]. Nevertheless, the clinical findings can not be readily explained so far by these mechanisms and two main questions remain unresolved: First, is HIV really a cytopathic virus or not in the host, and if it is not cytopathic, how does it cause immunosuppression? Second, why do CD4+ T cells decrease?

We have argued for several years[26-31] that HIV is noncytopathic in vivo and immunosuppression is a consequence of conventional anti-viral CD8+ T cells protecting against HIV but also mediating immunopathology. According to this proposal, HIV does not directly destroy cells it infects; instead conventional cytotoxic T cells specific for HIV destroy infected cells, mainly HIV-infected antigen presenting cells and macrophages, some CD4+ T cells and others, thereby causing immunodeficiency and disease via T cell mediated immunopathology. Understanding the pathogenesis of AIDS has suffered from two major problems: First, HIV has been assumed to be cytopathic and second, for obvious practical reasons, in general peripheral blood has been analysed and therefore CD4+ T cell counts have cought too much attention. However, there is no convinicing evidence that HIV is cytopathic in vivo[9,32]; we argue that host cell damage and decrease of CD4 T cells is not a direct consequence of HIV infection but a result of HIV specific CD8+ T cells destroying HIV-infected host cells; therefore, pathology is a consequence of the relative balance between the host's immune response and spread of HIV. Thus if there is little HIV it is eliminated or well controlled by potent HIV-specific CD8+ T[33,34] and we predict that, if there is no immune response to HIV there will be no disease in an infected host; therefore, more or less HIV with much, more or less CD8+ T cell anti-HIV response causes more or less disease[31].

The consequences of this hypothesis will be discussed below, suffice it to remind here, that although some of the clinically most important human virus infections cause disease because the viruses involved are usually cytopathic, there are many more, some of great importance, that are noncytopathic. For example, Hepatitis B viruses cause no liver cell damage directly as demonstrated by healthy virus carriers. Liver cell damage is a result of CD8 T cell mediated destruction of infected host cells[35,36]. Extensive histopathological analysis[37-42] of lymphnodes of HIV-infected patients may therefore similarly reflect immunopathological damage triggered by HIV but mediated by T cells rather than direct lysis by HIV.

Why Do CD4+ T Cells Decrease If HIV Is Noncytopathic?

Our proposal of an immunopathological nature of AIDS is based mainly on results obtained from studies on immunodeficiency in adult mice infected with lymphocytic choriomeningits virus (LCMV). Although only few CD4+ T cells are infected by LCMV in carriers and < 0.1% in acutely infected mice[43-46], T helper cell function is drastically suppressed in the LCMV infected host[26,28,29,47-49]. This immunosuppression is apparently due to the fact that LCMV, like HIV, replicates predominantly in monocytes-macrophages, and antigen presenting cells, but also in T helper cells; since LCMV is noncytopathic in vivo (as postulated here for HIV), these cells are not destroyed by infection directly but by LCMV-specific CD8+ T cells; in fact in the LCMV-model infection, elimination of CD8+ T cells prevents immunosuppression despite virus persistence[26,49]. By analogy, if HIV is noncytopathic, impairment of CD4+ T cells and their eventual decline in HIV infected patients is not easily explained by direct effects of the virus but is compatible with the view that CTL mediated lysis of infected CD4+ T cells and decrease of antigen presenting cells and macrophages deprives T helper cells of relevant stimuli and some of the essential lymphokines/cytokines[50-52]. Therefore, their expansion is hampered, their life span is shortened and this eventually causes their decrease and disappearance[53,54]. In fact detailed histopathological analysis of lymphnodes from HIV infected patients reveal pictures similar to those seen in immunosuppressive LCMV infections that are compatible with the immunopathological view of AIDS[37,38,41,42,55,56].

Predictions by the "Immunopathological" Versus the "HIV-Is-Cytopathic" View?

What are the consequences of HIV infection of T cell incompetent hosts: HIV infection in newborn babies suffering from a genetic form of severe T cell immunodeficiency, or alternatively in embryos transplacentally infected before 7 weeks of gestation, at a time when T cell competence has not developed yet[57-60] should reveal distinct clinical courses of disease.

The following consequences of modulating CD8+ T cell responses may be expected on HIV infection and disease development: From several points of view it has been argued that it makes no difference whether HIV lyses infected cells or whther specific CD8+ T cells do it but the consequences for prevention or curative measures are fundamentally different. For the cytopathic-virus and the immunopathological view, reducing virus spread by virustatic drugs will be beneficial[61,62]. But the two views predict opposite results in several situations: Modulation of anti-CD8+ T cell immunity may be beneficial or harmful dependent upon extent of spread of virus and the stage of infection. Whenever, HIV can spread more widely, blocking of CD8+ T cell responses will enhance virus spread further; according to the cytopathic virus view, this enhances cytopathic damage and severeness of disease, whereas, the immunopathological hypothesis predicts less or no immunopathology and therefore less disease.

Significance of High HIV Titers Late in Disease and of Increased Susceptibility to Intracellular Parasites

The late surge of HIV titers in AIDS patients may again parallel findings with the noncytopathic LCMV in mice[63], where it has been shown that overwhelming rapid virus spread may rapidly induce all available specific CD8+ T cells; these enddifferentiated cells dye within a few days and leave the host depleted of this T cell specificity. Thus high HIV titers may reflect exhaustive differentiation of HIV controlling CD8+ T cells. According to the "cytopathogenic HIV view" this late surge of HIV titers should cause (and seemingly fits the symptoms of) rapid lethal AIDS. This late phenotype of disease needs explanations from the immunopathological point of view as outlined above: It is readily envisaged that the immunosuppressive immunopathology enhances exhaustion of the antiviral CD8+ T cell response because it deprives the hosts immune system of T help and of interleukins ("second signals")[50,64,65] and of macrophages. The immunopathological impairment and destruction of macrophages and antigen-presenting cells and T helper cells causes a increase of susceptibility to superinfections with various mostly intracellular parasites including toxoplasma, pneumocystis carinii, tuberculosis etc. are the likely cause of death[66-68]. Since the two important consequences of HIV infection i.e. immunosuppression by immunopathology and subsequent superinfections causing severe life-threatening disease most often cannot be separated either clinically or therapeutically this explanation remains hypothetical, but no more so than does the view that high titer of cytopathic HIV causes direct death of infected cells. Survival of high titer HIV carriers lacking anti-HIV CD8+ T responses whose superinfections are well controlled therapeutically and who remain well, should be formal proof of the immunopathological pathogenesis of AIDS triggered by HIV.

Practical Consequences

If T cell mediated immunopathology is the crucial pathogenetic principle of AIDS it follows that impairment of virus spread reduces the target size for immunopathological attack and if virus has spread widely, elimination of anti-HIV CD8[+] T cells should be beneficial therapeutically. Therefore, pre- or post-exposure-vaccination[4,69,70], if efficient and applied early enough may be able to limit immunopathological damage and keep further virus spread and consequental immunopathology under control. Thus, potentiation of neutralizing antibody and of HIV specific CD8[+] T cell responses by vaccination may be very beneficial and reduce pathology, if present early during infection. Therefore, vaccination is an important strategy to reduce immunopathology, despite the fact that HIV usually cannot be eliminated or controlled completely because of its retroviral nature[4,69-71].

If postexposure vaccination is applied at a time where virus has spread too far, it may prove to be harmful. In the latter case, immunosuppression by anti-CD8 antibody treatment or by cyclosporin A[72-74] or cytostatic drugs,[75] to drastically reduce CD8[+] T cells should enhance exhaustion of the severely immunopathological T cell response. Although this is beneficial for the patient the latter will become a virus carrier, and this poses new problems epidemiologically. Also, if immunosuppressive treatment is incomplete, sufficient anti-HIV CD8[+] T cells may remain to eventually cause even more severe immunopathology because during such treatment, the virus has spread more widely.

For these reasons it seems still somewhat risky to propose anti CD8 treatment to prove the view that AIDS is an immunopathological disease[26,28,31]. However, the recent demonstration of exhaustion of specific T cell responses under conditions where stimulation by virus effector cells is overwhelming for the relatively few precursors, such an approach seems both feasible[72,74-77] and reasonable under certain conditions. Formal proof of our view would be patients depleated of specific CD8[+] T cells who become HIV carriers and exhibit attenuated, slowing down of, eventually possibly even recovery from disease. The problem is that immunopathological damage once established and chronically perpetuated, may not be repaired rapidly and therefore leaves the patient susceptible to superinfections for some time. Relatively early cytostatic or anti-CD8[+] treatment or lethal irradiation and the reconstitution with the patient's virus-free bone marrow stem cell[74,78] may therefore be beneficial; complete protection from infections of so treated AIDS patients by isolation may be necessary to permit recovery from immunopathological damage and leave time for immunological reconstitution which may take more than 12 months as revealed by kintecis of therapeutic bone marrow reconstitution protocols.

In conclusion the example of HIV infection in humans may in a way represent an ultimate perversity in the balance between the host immune system and infectious agent: HIV infects some of the key cells involved in immune reactions and therefore induces the immune system to destroy itself and thereby enables the virus to persist. Accordingly immunosuppression is not a direct cause of HIV cytopathogenicity but a consequence of conventional T cell mediated protection and immunopathology that destroys macrophages and antigen presenting cells, reduces T helper cells and thereby facilitates infection by intracellular parasites which eventually cause fatal disease.

ACKNOWLEDGMENTS

This work was supported by the Swiss National Fonds (# 31-32195.91) and the Kanton of Zurich.

REFERENCES

1. Rosenberg ZF, Fauci AS. The immunopathogenesis of HIV infection. **Adv Immunol** 1989; **47**: 377-431.
2. Levy GA. Mysteries of HIV: challenges of therapy and prevention. **Nature** 1988; **333**: 519-522.

3. Ho DD, Pomerantz RJ, Kaplan JC. Pathogenesis of infection with human immunodeficiency virus. **N Engl J Med** 1987; **317**: 278-286.
4. Salk J. Prospects for the controls of AIDS by immunizing seropositive individuals. **Nature** 1987; **327**: 473-476.
5. Köhler G, Fischer Lindahl K, Heusser C. The Immune System. Karger, Basel, 1981; 20 Vol.2.
6. Duesberg PH. Human immunodeficiency virus and acquired immunodeficiency syndrome: Correlation but not causation. **Proc Natl Acad Sci USA** 1989; **86**: 755-764.
7. Duesberg PH. AIDS epidemiology: Inconsistencies with human immunodeficiency virus and with infectious disease. **Proc Natl Acad Sci USA** 1991; **88**: 1575-1579.
8. Maddox J. AIDS research turned upside down. **Nature** 1991; **353**: 297.
9. Clark SJ, Saag MS, Decker WD, et al. High titers of cytopathic virus in plasma of patients with symptomatic primary HIV-1 infection. **N Engl J Med** 1991; **324**: 954-960.
10. Balter M. Montagnier pursues the mycoplasma-AIDS link. **Science** 1991; **251**: 271.
11. Lemaitre M, Guérard D, Hénin Y, Montagnier L, Zerial A. Protective activity of tetracycline analogs against the cytopathic effect of the human immunodeficiency virus in CEM cells. **Res Virol** 1990; **141**: 5-13.
12. Tersmette M, Schuitemaker H. Virulent HIV strains? **Aids** 1993; **7**: 1123-1125.
13. Schwarz A, Offermann G, Keller F, et al. The effect of cyclosporine on the progression of human immunodeficiency virus type 1 infection transmitted by transplantation - data on four cases and review of the literature. **Transplantation** 1993; **55**: 95-103.
14. Sodroski J, Goh WC, Rosen C, Campbell K, Haseltine WA. Role of the HTLV-III/LAV envelope in syncytium formation and cytopathicity. **Nature** 1986; **322**: 470-474.
15. Lifson JD, Feinberg MB, Reyes GR, et al. Induction of CD4-dependent cell fusion by the HTLV-III/LAV envelope glycoprotein. **Nature** 1986; **323**: 725-728.
16. Stricker RB, McHugh TM, Moody DJ, et al. An AIDS-related cytotoxic autoantibody reacts with a specific antigen on stimulated CD4+ T cells. **Nature** 1987; **327**: 710-713.
17. Via CS, Morse III HC, Shearer GM. Altered immunoregulation and autoimmune aspects of HIV infection: relevant murine models. **Immunol Today** 1990; **11**: 250-255.
18. Bangham CRM, McMichael AJ. Why the long latent period? **Nature** 1990; **348**: 388.
19. Levy JA. Mysteries of HIV: challenges for therapy and prevention. **Nature** 1988; **333**: 519-522.
20. Süsal C, Kröpelin M, Daniel V, Opelz G. Molecular mimicry between HIV-1 and antigen receptor molecules: A clue to the pathogenesis of AIDS. **Vox Sang** 1993; **65**: 10-17.
21. Gougeon M-L, Montagnier L. Apoptosis in AIDS. **Science** 1993; **260**: 1269-1270.
22. Groux H, Torpier G, Monté D, Mouton Y, Capron A, Ameisen JC. Activation-induced death by apoptosis in CD4+ T cells from human immunodeficiency virus-infected asymptomatic individuals. **J Exp Med** 1992; **175**: 331-330.
23. Shearer GM, Clerici M. Early T-helper cell defects in HIV infection. **Aids** 1991; **5**: 245-253.
24. Miedema F. Immunological abnormalities in the natural history of HIV infection: Mechanisms and clinical relevance. **Immunodef Rev** 1992; **3**: 173-193.
25. Meyaard L, Schuitemaker H, Miedema F. T-cell dysfunction in HIV infection: anergy due to defective antigen-presenting cell function? **Immunol Today** 1993; **14**: 161-164.
26. Leist TP, Rüedi E, Zinkernagel RM. Virus-triggered immune suppression in mice caused by virus-specific cytotoxic T cells. **J Exp Med** 1988; **167**: 1749-1754.
27. Zinkernagel RM. Virus triggered AIDS is a T cell mediated immunopathology. Prevention by tolerance or by treatment with anti-CD8 antibodies. **Immunol Today** 1988; **9**: 370-371.
28. Odermatt B, Eppler M, Leist TP, Hengartner H, Zinkernagel RM. Virus-triggered acquired immunodeficiency by cytotoxic T-cell dependent destruction of antigen-presenting cells and lymph follicle structure. **Proc Natl Acad Sci USA** 1991; **88**: 8252-8256.
29. Althage A, Odermatt B, Moskophidis D, Kündig Th, Hengartner H, Zinkernagel RM. Immunosuppression by lymphocytic choriomeningitis virus infection: competent effector T and B cells but impaired antigen presentation. **Eur J Immunol** 1992; **22**: 1803-1812.
30. Battegay M, Moskophidis D, Waldner H, et al. Impairment and delay of neutralizing antiviral antibody responses by virus specific cytotoxic T cells. **J Immunol** 1993; **151**: 5408-5415.
31. Zinkernagel RM, Hengartner H. T cell mediated immunopathology versus direct cytolysis by virus: implications for HIV and AIDS. **Immunol Today** 1994; **15**: 262-268.
32. Lo S-C, Tsai S, Benish JR, Shih JW-K, Wear DJ, Wong DM. Enhancement of HIV-1 cytocidal effects in CD4+ lymphocytes by the AIDS-associated mycoplasma. **Science** 1991; **251**: 1074-1075.
33. Clerici M, Giorgi JV, Chou C-C, et al. Cell mediated immune response to HIV Type 1 in seronegative homosexual men with recent sexual exposure to HIV-1. **J Infect Dis** 1992; **165**: 1012-1019.

34. Walker CM, Moody DJ, Stites DP, Levy JA. CD8[+] lymphocytes can control HIV infection in vitro by suppressing virus replication. **Science** 1986; **234**: 1563-1566.

35. Peters M, Vierling J, Gershwin ME, Milich D, Chisari FV, Hoofnagle JH. Immunology and the Liver. **Hepatology** 1991; **13**: 977-994.

36. Mondelli M, Eddleston ALWF. Mechanisms of liver cell injury in acute and chronic hepatitis B. **Semin Liver Dis** 1984; **4**: 47-58.

37. Racz P, Tenner-Racz K, Kahl C, Feller AC, Kern P, Dietrich M. Spectrum of morphologic changes of lymph nodes from patients with AIDS or AIDS-related complexes. In: Karger S, ed. Progress in Allergy: AIDS. Basel: Karger,S., 1986: 81-181.

38. Biberfeld P, Ost A, Porwit A, Sandstedt B, Pallesen G, Bottiger B. Histopathology and immunohistology of HTLV-III/LAV related disease. **Acta Pathol Microbiol Scand** 1987; **95**: 47-65.

39. Tenner-Racz K, Racz P, Dietrich M, Kern P. Altered follicular dendritic cells and virus-like particles in AIDS and AIDS-related lymphadenopathy. **Lancet** 1985; **1**: 105-106.

40. Gartner S, Markovits P, Markovitz DM, Kaplan MH, Gallo R, Popovic M. The role of mononuclear phagocytes in HTLV III/LAV infection. **Science** 1986; **233**: 215-219.

41. Pantaleo G, Graziosi C, Demarest JF, et al. HIV infection is active and progressive in lymphoid tissue during the clinically latent stage of disease. **Nature** 1993; **362**: 355-358.

42. Embretson J, Zupancic M, Ribas JL, et al. Massive covert infection of helper T lymphocytes and macrophages by HIV during the incubation period of AIDS. **Nature** 1993; **362**: 359-362.

43. Doyle MV, Oldstone MBA. Interactions between viruses and lymphocytes. I. In vivo replication of lymphocytic choriomeningitis virus during both chronic and acute viral infections. **J Immunol** 1978; **121**: 1262-1269.

44. Cihak J, Lehmann-Grube F. Immunological tolerance to lymphocytic choriomeningitis virus in neo-natally infected carrier mice: Evidence supporting a clonal inactivation mechanism. **Immunology** 1978; **34**: 265.

45. Borrow P, Tishon A, Oldstone MBA. Infection of lymphocytes by a virus that aborts cytotoxic T lymphocyte activity and establishes persistent infection. **J Exp Med** 1991; **174**: 203-212.

46. Tishon A, Southern PJ, Oldstone MBA. Virus-lymphocyte interactions. II. Expression of viral sequences during the course of persistent lymphocytic choriomeningitis virus infection and their localization to the L3T4 lymphocyte subset. **J Immunol** 1988; **140**: 1280-1284.

47. Mims CA, Wainwright S. The immunodepressive action of lymphocytic choriomeningitis virus in mice. **J Immunol** 1968; **101**: 717-724.

48. Jacobs RP, Cole GA. Lymphocytic choriomeningitis virus-induced immunosuppression: A virus-induced macrophage defect. **J Immunol** 1976; **117**: 1004-1009.

49. Moskophidis D, Pircher HP, Ciernik I, Odermatt B, Hengartner H, Zinkernagel RM. Suppression of virus specific antibody production by CD8+ class I-restricted antiviral cytotoxic T cells in vivo. **J Virol** 1992; **66**: 3661-3668.

50. Schwartz RH. A cell culture model for T lymphocyte clonal anergy. **Science** 1990; **248**: 1349-1356.

51. Saron MF, Shidani B, Nahori MA, Guillon JC, Truffa Bachi P. Lymphocytic choriomeningitis virus-in-duced immunodepression: inherent defect of B and T lymphocytes. **J Virol** 1990; **64**: 4076-4083.

52. Campbell IL, Lepay DA, Oldstone MBA. Differential regulation of cytokine gene product expression in macrophages infected with wild type versus an immunosuppressive variant lymphocytic choriomeningitis virus (LCMV). **J Cell Biochem** 1992; **16c**: 141.

53. Cheynier R, Langlade-Demoyen P, Marescot M-R, et al. Cytotoxic T lymphocyte responses in the peripheral blood of children born to human immunodeficiency virus-1-infected mothers. **Eur J Immunol** 1992; **22**: 2211-2217.

54. Pantaleo G, Koenig S, Baseler M, Lane HC, Fauci AS. Defective clonogenic potential of CD8+ T lymphocytes in patients with AIDS. Expansion in vivo of a nonclonogenic CD3+CD8+DR+CD25-T cell population. **J Immunol** 1990; **144**: 1696-1704.

55. Fox CH, Cottler-Fox M. The pathobiology of HIV infection. **Immunol Today** 1992; **13**: 353-356.

56. Spiegel H, Herbst H, Niedobitek G, Foss H-D, Stein H. Rapid communication. Follicular dendritic cells are a major reservoir for human immunodeficiency virus type 1 in lymphoid tissues facilitating infection of CD4+ T helper cells. **American Journal of Pathology** 1992; **140**: 15-22.

57. Courgnaud V, Laure F, Broussard A, et al. Frequency and early in utero HIV-1 infection. **AIDS Res Hum Retroviruses** 1991; **7**: 337-341.

58. Mano H, Chermann JC. Fetal human immunodeficiency virus type 1 infection of different organs in the second trimester. **AIDS Res Hum Retroviruses** 1991; **7**: 83-88.

59. Turner BJ, Denison M, Eppes SC, Houchens R, Fanning T, Markson LE. Survival experience of 789 children with the acquired immunodeficiency syndrome. **Pediatr Infect Dis J** 1993; **12**: 310-320.

60. Blanche S, Tardieu M, Duliege A-M, et al. Longitudinal study of 94 symptomatic infants with perinatally acquired human immunodeficiency virus infection. **AJDC** 1990; **144**: 1210-1215.
61. Volberding PA, Lagakos SW, Koch MA, et al. Zidovudine in asymptomatic human immunodeficiency virus infection. **N Engl J Med** 1990; **322**: 941-949.
62. Portnoi D, Stall AM, Schwartz D, Merigan TC, Herzenberg LA, Basham T. AZT inhibits characteristic early alteration of lymphoid cell populations in retrovirus-induced murine AIDS. **J Immunol** 1990; **144**: 1705.
63. Moskophidis D, Lechner F, Pircher HP, Zinkernagel RM. Virus persistence in acutely infected immuno-competent mice by exhaustion of antiviral cytotoxic effector T cells. **Nature** 1993; **362**: 758-761.
64. Bretscher P, Cohn M. A theory of self-nonself discrimination. **Science** 1970; **169**: 1042-1049.
65. Lafferty KJ, Cunningham AJ. A new analysis of allogeneic interactions. **Aust J Exp Biol Med Sci** 1975; **53**: 27-42.
66. Guarda LA, Stein SA, Cleary KA, Ordonez NG. Human cryptosporidiosis in the acquired immune deficiency syndrome. **Arch Pathol** 1983; **107**: 562-566.
67. Daley CL, Small PM. An outbreak of tuberculosis with accelerated progression among persons infected with the human immunodeficiency virus. **N Engl J Med** 1992; **326**: 231-235.
68. Phair J, Munoz A. The risk of pneumocystis carinii pneumonia among men infected with human immunodeficiency virus type 1. **N Engl J Med** 1990; **322**: 161-165.
69. Sabin AB. Improbability of effective vaccination against human immunodeficiency virus because of its intracellular transmission and rectal portal of entry. **Proc Natl Acad Sci USA** 1992; **89**: 8852-8855.
70. Ada GL. Prospects for HIV vaccines. **J Acquir Immune Defic Syndr** 1988; **1**: 295-303.
71. Fauci AS, Gallo RC, Koenig S, Salk J, Purcell RH. NIH conference. Development and evaluation of a vaccine for human immunodeficiency virus (HIV) infection. **Ann Intern Med** 1989; **110**: 373-385.
72. Stitz L. Induction of antigen-specific tolerance by cyclosporin A. **Eur J Immunol** 1992; **22**: 1995-2001.
73. Klinman DM, Krieg A, Conover J, Ussery MA, Black PL. Effect of cyclophosphamide, total body irradiation, and Zidovudine on retrovirus proliferation and disease progression in murine AIDS. **AIDS Res Hum Retroviruses** 1992; **8**: 101-106.
74. Holland HK, Saral R, Rossi JJ. Allogeneic bone marrow transplantation, zidovudine, and HIV-1 infection. **Ann Intern Med** 1989; **111**: 973-981.
75. Gilden DH, Cole GA, Monjan AA, Nathanson N. Immunopathogenesis of acute central nervous system disease produced by lymphocytic choriomeningitis virus. I. Cyclophosphamide-mediated induction of the virus-carrier state in adult mice. **J Exp Med** 1972; **135**: 860-873.
76. Vilmer E, Rhoses A, Rabian C. Clinical and immunological restoration in patients with AIDS after marrow transplantation, using lymphocyte transfusion from the marrow donor. **Transplantation** 1987; **44**: 25.
77. Deng G, Podack ER. Suppression of apoptosis in a cytotoxic T-cell line by interleukin 2- mediated gene transcription and deregulated expression of the protooncogene bcl-2. **Proc Natl Acad Sci USA** 1993; **90**: 2189-2193.
78. Cerny A, Merino R, Makino M, Waldvogel FA, Morse HCIII, Izui S. Protective effect of cyclosporin A on immune abnormalities observed in the murine acquired immunodeficiency syndrome. **Eur J Immunol** 1991; **21**: 1747-1750.

CLONAL EXPANSION OF T CELLS AND HIV GENOTYPES IN MICRODISSECTED SPLENIC WHITE PULPS INDICATES VIRAL REPLICATION IN SITU AND INFILTRATION OF HIV-SPECIFIC CYTOTOXIC T LYMPHOCYTES

Rémi Cheynier,[1] Sven Henrichwark,[1] Fabienne Hadida,[2] Eric Pelletier,[1] Eric Oksenhendler,[3] Brigitte Autran,[2] and Simon Wain-Hobson[1]

[1] Unité de Rétrovirologie Moléculaire
Institut Pasteur
Paris, France
[2] Laboratoire d'Immunologie Cellulaire et Tissulaire
Hôpital La Pitié-Salpétrière
Paris, France
[3] Service d'Immunopathologie et d'Hématologie
Hôpital Saint Louis
Paris, France

ABSTRACT

Human immunodeficiency virus (HIV) replication and T cell proliferation was investigated in situ by a PCR based analysis of individual microdissected splenic white pulps. Founder effects, revealed by an exquisite compartmentalization of HIV genotypes and T cells, indicated the recruitment of latently infected CD4+ T cells through highly localized antigen presentation, rather than the infection of CD4+ T lymphoblasts by blood borne virus or immune complexes. HIV infected white pulps could be infiltrated by HIV specific cytotoxic T lymphocytes, so implicating them in CD4+ T cell destruction in vivo. Together these data describe an iterative and deleterious mechanism of antigen driven T cell recruitment and activation, HIV replication and spread, with consequent destruction of the newly infected cells.

INTRODUCTION

The genetic variation exhibited by the HIV is an inevitable consequence of massive replication and clearance of infected cells and virions by the immune system. Infection is probably initiated by a single infectious virion or infected cell which results in a near homogenous population of genomes during primary infection (Wolfs et al., 1991; Zhu et al., 1993). From this point on, viral variants are remorselessly accumulated over time, giving rise to a population of viral genotypes, or quasispecies (Holland et al., 1992). HIV quasispecies fluctuate in as little as three months to three days in peripheral blood (Meyerhans et al., 1989; Pelletier et al., unpublished data), may vary between different organs (Epstein et al., 1991) and even within an organ (Delassus et al., 1992; Sala et al., 1994). All data point to a rapid genetic radiation of HIV coincident with the AIDS pandemic.

HIV replication in vivo occurs mainly within CD4+ T lymphocytes. However only a small fraction (~2%) of lymphocytes are found in peripheral blood. Secondary lymphoid organs are heavily infected by HIV (Armstrong et al., 1984; Tenner-Racz et al., 1985; Racz et al., 1986; Biberfeld et al., 1986; Le Tourneau et al., 1986; Embretson et al., 1993; Pantaleo et al., 1993). Occasionally HIV infection may be associated with immune thrombocytopenia purpura (ITP). While approximately 2/3rds of ITP cases can be successfully managed by immunosuppressive or anti-retroviral therapy, the remaining third prove refractory and requires splenectomy. HIV infection may also be associated with an intense diffuse proliferation of B and T cells with histological features of Castleman's disease or of pseudotumoral lymphoid hyperplasia (Oksenhendler et al., 1992). In such conditions splenectomy may be warranted because of massive splenomegaly, subsequent pancytopenia or clinical suspicion of non-Hodgkin's lymphoma. The discrete organization of the splenic white pulps allows easy microdissection.

White Pulps Are Heavily Infected by HIV

PCR amplification of the HIV-1 V1V2 env region sequence was performed on 134 white pulps for four spleens. Most white pulps (54/54, 18/20 and 19/20 from 4 spleens) were infected by HIV as evidenced by nested PCR. In just one spleen a minority (4/40) were infected. Interestingly these four positive white pulps were all dissected from the same larger $1 cm^3$ block of spleen. Yet the same block contained 6 white pulps negative for proviral DNA, indicating an extraordinary spatial distribution of HIV infected cells within the spleen.

Extraordinary sequence heterogeneity was apparent in many white pulps. The sequence complexity within each of the 4 white pulps from spleen S was probably the greatest with up to 15-20 distinct amino acid sequences per white pulp. The data for white pulp B6 from spleen I again revealed a complex structure (15 different sequences, $\leq 16\%$ internal amino acid sequence variation). In order to appreciate such complexity it may be noted that while intra-white pulp amino acid sequence variation ranged from 11-20% for the V1V2 region, interpatient variation is typically 13-50% for the same region (Pedroza Martins et al., 1992; Myers et al., 1993). For the two white pulps P-B1 and P-B2 derived from spleen P, each harboured a major protein sequence, respectively 01 and 04, the variants being derived from the major form by one or two substitutions (Figure 1). Strikingly sequences 01 and 04 differed by 16 amino acid residues (17%). These clusters would appear to reflect multiple founder effects within each white pulp.

Restricted Distribution of T Cells Within Individual White Pulps

The remarkable compartmentalization of HIV proviruses within individual white pulps suggested that CD4+ T cells, the preferred host cell for HIV, might also be highly

```
            10        20        30        40        50        60        70        80        90
01  KLTPLCVTLBCTDDLGNTTNANRSNISISSNGTMETGEIKNCSFNITTVIRDKKKESALFYRLDIVPIDNDNTSYRLINCNTSTITQACPKVS  80%
03  ..........A..................................................................................
16  ............D................................................................................
14  .............................................................................................
12  .................................................L...........R...............................

04  ............N.I.Y...A...T.KDN.S..GR.........E.............V.....................S.V.........I   50%
03  ............N.I.Y...A...T.KDN.S..GR.........AE............V.....................S.V.........H   15%
02  ............N.I.Y...A...T.KDN.S..GR.........E.G..........V.....................S.V.........I
07  ..........IN.I.Y...A...T.KDN.S..GR.........E.............V.....................S.V.........I
10  ............N.I.Y...A...T.KDN.S..GR.........E.............V..............H......S.V.........I
11  ............N.I.Y...A...T.KDN.S..GR.........E.............V.....................S.VV........I
01  ............NRI.Y...A...T.KDN.S..GR.........AE............V.....................S.V.........I
14  ............N.I.Y...A...T.KDN.S..-GR........AE............V.....................S.V.........I
19  ............N.I.Y...A...T.KGN.S..GR.........AE............V.....................S.V.........I
```

Figure 1. Microscopic HIV quasispecies for the V1V2 region derived from individual white pulps. Sequences were either derived from two white pulps of spleen P. A sequence identifier code is given on the left while the proportion of the total number of clones _10% is shown on the right. The frequency of all other clones was 5%. The amino acid sequences, given in the one letter code, are aligned to that of the predominant sequence in each white pulp. Only differences were noted. A dot (.) indicates sequence identity.

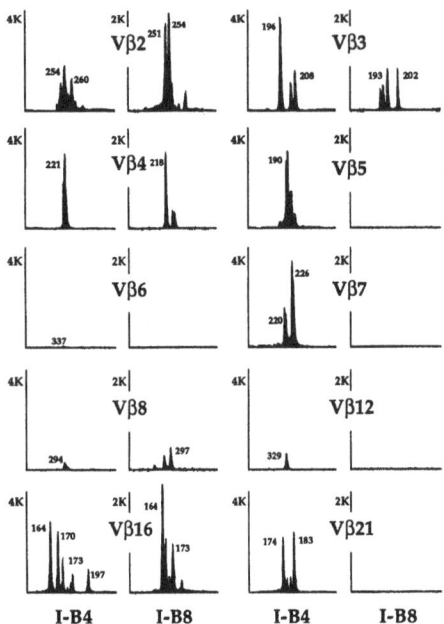

Figure 2. Ten Vβ repertoires derived from two white pulps, B4 and B8, of spleen I. A further 18 white pulps were analyzed and yielded qualitatively similar profiles (data not shown). The ordinate reveals the peak intensity in arbitrary units which are the same for a single white pulp. The abscissa depicts the length (molecular weight) of the run-off product, and hence CDR3 length polymorphisms. Peaks may appear as doublets, differing by a single nucleotide. This is due to non-templated addition of a single adenosine at the 3' end of the strands. The ratio of the two peaks reflects the proportion of PCR products with the extra A. The numbers surrounding peaks refers to the molecular weight in base pairs. The Vβ6 amplification primer does not efficiently amplify all genes of this large family.

localized. Accordingly the repertoires of 10 Vβ segments rearranged with the Jβ1.6 segment were analyzed. Ten TCR Vβ chain repertoires within two representative HIV positive white pulps (I-B4 and I-B8) from spleen I are shown in Fig. 2. As can be seen they harboured very different populations of T cells. Some specificities were virtually absent (Vβ6) while others (Vβ5, 7, 12 and 21) were present in one but not the other. However Vβ6 specificities were found in some of the 23 other white pulps analyzed (data not shown). There were no systematically negative data for any Vβ family, arguing against a HIV encoded superantigen-like depletion of T cells.

The peaks were usually separated by 3bps, indicative of functionally rearranged V, D and J segments. Both the number (0-5) and amplitude of peaks varied for a given Vβ family. While it may not be prudent to compare peak intensities between different white pulps due to the non-quantitative PCR amplification, relative intensities for a set of related sequences from the same sample were reliable. Thus certain specificities were found expanded over and above others. Occasionally a few peaks common to two or more white pulps could be found, i.e. a peak at 254bp for Vβ2 and peaks at 164 and 173 for Vβ16 (Fig. 2).

Controls

To find out whether such exquisite distribution of T cells was typical of a "normal" spleen a comparable analysis was undertaken of a spleen taken from a graft donor after an intracranial hemorrhage secondary to an arterial aneurysm. The donor was otherwise healthy and seronegative for HIV-1, HIV-2, hepatitis B and C viruses, human T cell leukemia viruses 1 and 2 and cytomegalovirus. Analyses of 10 Vβ families from two white pulps from the HIV negative spleen D revealed qualitatively similar features, i.e. extensive differences between individual white pulps and a limited number of VDJ specificities with the expansion of some. Just occasionally a Gaussian-like distribution, characteristic of an unbiased distribution of Vβ chains (Cochet et al., 1992; Pannetier et al., 1993), was observed (D-A5, Vβ2,

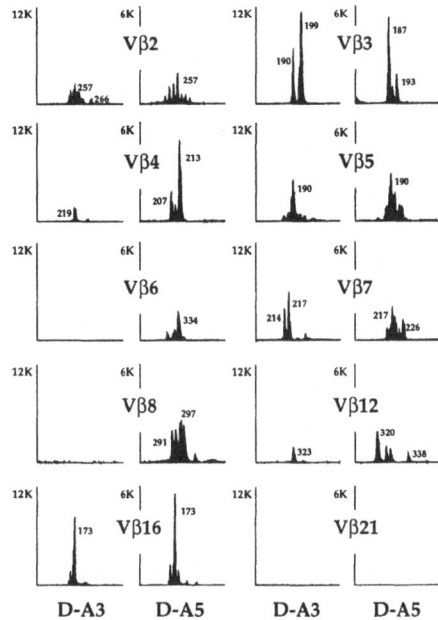

Figure 3. Ten Vβ repertoires of two white pulps, A3 and A5, derived from the spleen of a seronegative patient, D. In total 10 white pulps were studied in this manner. Qualitatively similar results were obtained (data not shown).

Fig. 3). These findings, confirmed by the analysis of a further 8 white pulps from the same spleen (data not shown), suggest that an exquisite compartmentalization of T cells within white pulps is the norm.

HIV-Specific CTL Infiltrate White Pulps

In the absence of viral infection, other than HIV, it is likely that within the white pulp recruited T cells would be mainly HLA class II-restricted CD4+ helper cells. This is presumably the case for spleen D (Fig. 3). However due to HIV replication, infected cells must be presenting HIV epitopes via HLA class I antigens which should recruit HIV specific, HLA class I restricted, CD8+ cytotoxic T lymphocytes (CTL). Classical CTL analyses did indeed show that the splenocytes harboured HIV-specific CTL to HIV-1 gag, pol, env or nef proteins.

Rarely, in fact only twice (Vβ5 for spleen I and Vβ2 for spleen P), could a peak common to a majority of white pulps be identified. In the case of patient I a peak of 190bp was present in 22/25 white pulps, some of which are shown in Fig. 4. Such a peak is indicative of either a common antigen specific CD4+ T lymphocyte clone or infiltration of an anti-HIV specific CTL clone. In order to distinguish between the two possibilities the Vβ5 signature was determined for the HIV specific bulk CTL line established from SMC of patient I (Fig. 4). A single peak at 190bp dominated the Vβ5 signature (CTL-1, Fig. 4). In order to prove that the 190bp peak in both the CTL line and the white pulps was the same, the Vβ5 PCR products from the bulk CTL and white pulps E1, E2 and E4 were molecularly cloned and sequenced. The CDR3 amino acid sequence CASS **YGGSG** SPLH, where bold type indicates the clonotypic residues flanked by those of Vβ5 and Jβ1.6, was identified in the 4 samples (65% in bulk CTL, 30% in E1, 40% E2 and 5% in E4). This Vβ5 sequences corresponded to the Vβ5.3 subset (Kimura et al., 1986). These and other data suggest that HIV specific CTL may infiltrate infected white pulps.

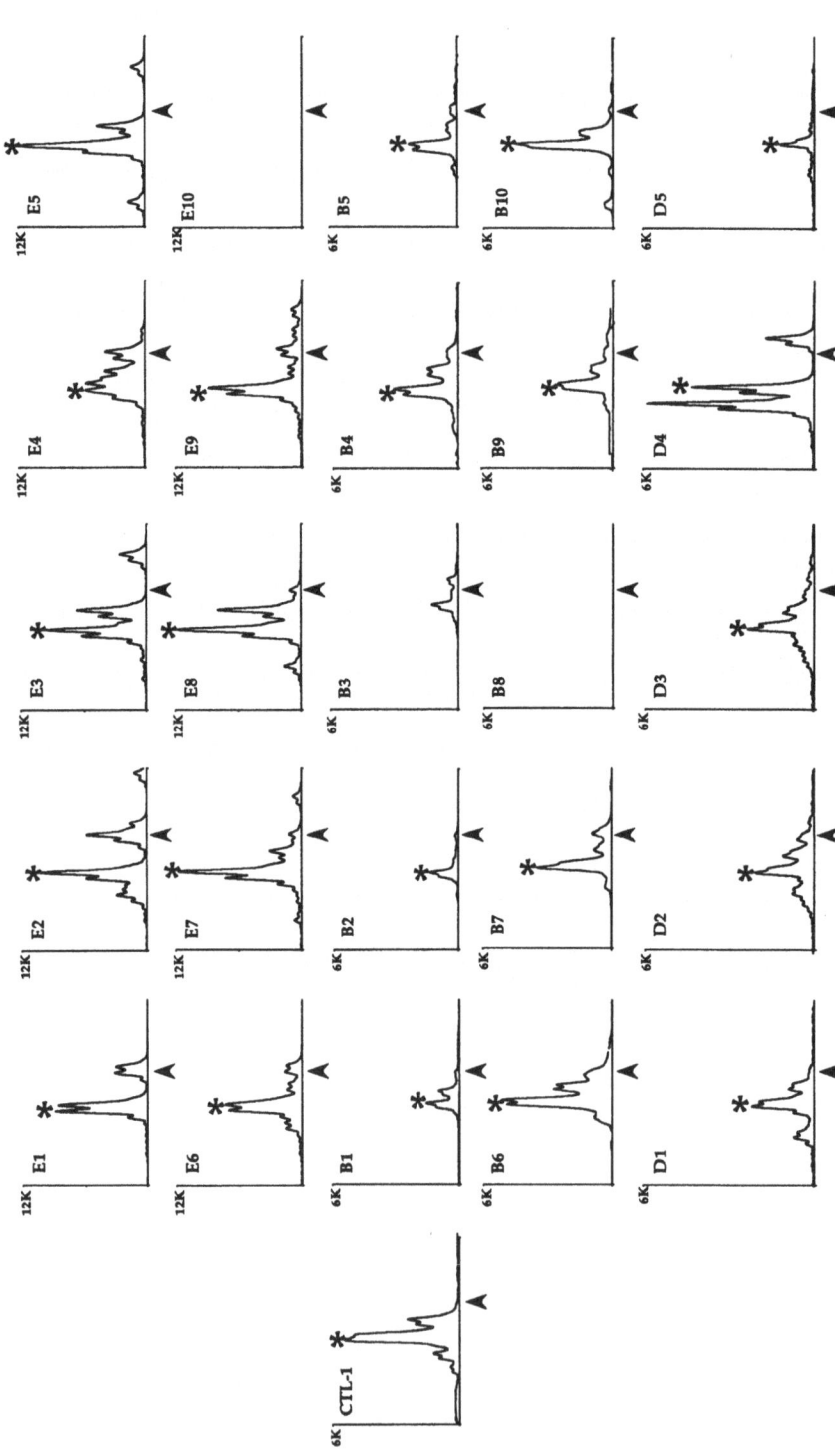

Figure 4. CTL infiltration of splenic white pulps. (A): Common Vβ5 peak in 22 out of 25 white pulps (E1-25) from a 1cm³ block of spleen I. The peak at 190bp, denoted by (*), corresponds to a functionally rearranged Vβ gene. The arrow head represents a 196bp internal standard. To the left the Vβ5 repertoire from a HIV specific CTL cell lines (CTL-1) from spleen I. The clonotypic CDR3 sequence was CASS YGGSG SPLH, where bold type indicates the clonotypic residues flanked by those of Vβ5 and Jβ1.6.

DISCUSSION

The current data show that HIV quasispecies are organized at a microscopic scale, the tremendous spatial discontinuities reflecting the architecture of secondary lymphoid organs. The distribution of HIV sequences within a white pulp was indicative of founder effects whereby one or a few proviruses became amplified locally. This was most clear for P-B1 and P-B2 (Fig. 1) where each white pulp harboured a single founder sequence along with a number of highly related variants. Progeny derived from a founder genome would reinfect neighbouring activated T cells and, due to error prone reverse transcription, generate variants of the founder sequence.

An equally exquisite compartmentalization of T cells characterized individual splenic white pulps from HIV positive individuals. However this proved to be the case whether they were uninfected or infected, normal or pathological spleens. The Vβ repertoire data showed that white pulps represented islands of restricted and specialized T cell function which effectively did not communicate with each other. This is hardly surprising given the immunological nature of splenic white pulps. Blood borne pathogens or antigens enter the marginal zone where most is destroyed by marginal zone macrophages (Van den Eertwegh et al., 1992). Within the PALS, a small proportion of antigen is presented by FDC to CD4+ T lymphocytes. Those bearing specific TCR will be retained and activated in situ. FDC are among the most efficient antigen presenting cells in the body being capable of activating both memory and naive CD4+ T cells (Steinman, 1991). In contrast, GC antigen presentation is very different. Antigen, in the context of immunoglobulin and complement, is presented on the surface of FDC to B cells, which in turn may process antigen and present it to CD4+ T cells via HLA class II molecules. Within GC, selection for high-affinity immunoglobulin results in relatively few antigen specific B cell clones, perhaps no more than 1-6 per GCs (Jacob et al., 1991; Liu et al., 1991). Although few in GC, T cells are antigen specific and presumably recruited and retained to allow B-T cell interactions (Fuller et al., 1993).

The singular compartmentalization of both HIV and T cells is indicative of little or no trafficking between adjacent white pulps. Therefore the crucial question becomes how did HIV get into the white pulps? It is likely that HIV enters the white pulps by a Trojan horse mechanism (Peluso et al., 1985; Sonigo et al., 1985; Embretson et al., 1993) i.e. via the recruitment of latently infected CD4+ lymphocytes in response to antigen presentation. Were a small fraction of the newly recruited lymphocytes, perhaps just one, to harbour a non defective HIV provirus, antigen presentation would result in T cell activation. There is a wealth of data indicating that T cell activation results in HIV replication (Tong-Starksen et al., 1987; Brinchmann et al., 1992; Janoff et al. 1993; Wallis et al. 1993). Indeed this is how HIV is isolated. Within the white pulp viral progeny would find themselves juxtaposed to large numbers of uninfected CD4+ T lymphoblasts recruited by the same antigen; and CD4+ T lymphoblasts are ideal targets for HIV. Thus the discrete immunological structures, such as the T cell dominated PALS, allow the induction and maintenance of HIV replication. The observed founder effects as well as the cluster of attendant variants are in keeping with this possibility.

That antigen presentation may induce HIV replication is also suggested by the finding of augmented plasma viremia following influenza A vaccination (Ho, 1993) or increased viral titres in bronchial alveolar lavages of patients with Pneumocystis carinii pneumonia (Lu et al., 1993). However the opportunistic infections typical of AIDS are only a part of the antigenic world in which humans live. Consequently the immune system is constantly at work, as evidenced by the oligoclonal expansion of T cells in the white pulps of patient D, a HIV negative individual. Furthermore Peyer's patches in the gut show well developed germinal centers (Butcher et al., 1982; Weinstein et al., 1991), demonstrating that there is sufficient antigen (food, bacteria, etc.) in the gut environment to ensure activation of immune responses.

HIV infected cells may be cleared by a variety of mechanisms among which cytotoxic T lymphocytes make up an important part of the anti-HIV immunity both in the periphery (Plata et al., 1987; Walker et al., 1987) and in lymphoid organs (Hadida et al., 1992). The dominant role of the immune system, as opposed to HIV cytopathicity, in the destruction of HIV infected cells has come from an appreciation of longitudinal sequence variation (Wain-Hobson, 1993). All four spleens harboured HIV-specific CTL which were derived from total SMC, i.e. both the red and white pulp. As could be seen for patient I, the 190bp Vβ5 peak in both bulk CTL lines was also the major peak in 22/25 white pulps (Fig. 4). The presence of such a clone within the anti-HIV bulk CTL cultures as well as cell sorted CD8+ cells, 98.3% of which show the killer cell specific marker TIA-1, argues in favour of HIV-specific CTL infiltration of splenic white pulps. Thus white pulps may not only represent sites of antigen driven HIV production, but also CD4+ T cell destruction via the recruitment of HIV-specific CTL in response to processed HIV antigen presentation by the class I molecules on the surface of infected CD4+ cells. The above data parallel those of Devergne et al. who showed CTL specific markers, such as serine esterase B, within HIV infected lymph node GC (Devergne et al., 1991; Laman et al., 1992).

T cell activation is invariably in response to pathogens or antigens and is obviously beneficial to the host in terms of resolving the infection. In the case of the HIV-infected individual there is a price to pay for T cell activation: HIV replication. Thus the very helper cells destined to combat the pathogen in question will find themselves identified as targets for the host's anti-HIV specific immunity. After repeated or constant exposure to the same microbe, there must come a point where pathogen specific helper/memory T cell responses are sufficiently compromised such that symptoms prevail. It is perhaps not surprising that Pneumocystis carinii or Mycobacterium tuberculosis, both powerful stimulators of cell mediated immunity, are among the catalogue of opportunistic infections which makes up AIDS.

It would seem that prophylaxis aimed at treating concurrent infections should have a direct effect on curtailing HIV replication. The extreme situation, blocking T cell activation via drugs such as cyclosporin, might be envisioned, although this would necessitate handling the opportunistic infections. Vaccination against common pathogens might have to be viewed in terms of risk assessment with the merits of vaccination being weighed against activation and spread of HIV (Ho, 1992). With the onset of symptomatic HIV infection, there is an increased T cell anergy (Miedema et al., 1990). Among the many immunological abnormalities, cytokine imbalances also characterize late stage disease some of which, e.g. tumour necrosis factor α, may activate HIV expression from resting T cells (Fauci, 1993). Thus the iterative and deleterious process of antigenic stimulation, HIV activation and CD4 cell destruction may be more appropriate to the long clinically asymptomatic period characterized by efficient cellular immunity to pathogens and HIV, rather than to late stage disease when other factors might help drive HIV replication. As long as cell mediated immune responses remain, antigen driven T cell activation may prove to be among the most important sources of HIV production. HIV infected CD4 T cell destruction may be seen as an inevitable corollary of anti-HIV immunity.

ACKNOWLEDGMENTS

This work was supported by grants from Institut Pasteur, l'Agence Nationale de Recherches sur le SIDA (ANRS), and le Ministère de la Recherche et de l'Enseignement.

REFERENCES

Armstrong, J. A. and Horne, R. (1984). Follicular dendritic cells and virus-like particles in AIDS-related lymphadenopathy. Lancet ii:370-372.

Biberfeld, P., Chayt, K. J., Marselle, L. M., Biberfeld, G., Gallo, R. C. and Harper, M. E. (1986). HTLV-III expression in infected lymph nodes and relevance to pathogenesis of lymphadenopathy. Am. J. Pathol. 133:516-524.

Brinchmann, J. E., Gaudernack, G., Thorsby, E. and Vartdal, F. (1992). Staphylococcal exotoxin superantigens induce human immunodeficiency virus type 1 expression in naturally infected CD4+ T cells. J. Virol. 66:5924-5928.

Butcher, E. C., Rouse, R. V., Coffman, R. L., Nottenburg, C. N., Hardy, R. R. and Weissman, I. L. (1982). Surface phenotype of Peyer's patch germinal center cells: implications for the role of germinal centers in B cell differentiation. J. Immunol. 129:2698-2707.

Cochet, M., Pannetier, C., Regnault, A., Darche, S., Leclerc, C. and. Kourilsky, P. (1992). Molecular detection and in vivo analysis of the specific T cell response to a protein antigen. Eur. J. Immunol. 22:2639-2647.

Delassus, S., Cheynier, R. and Wain-Hobson, S. (1992). Inhomogeneous distribution of HIV proviruses in spleen. J. Virol. 66:5642-5645.

Devergne, O., Peuchmaur, M., Crevon, M. C., Trapani, J. A., Maillot, M. C., Galanaud, P. and Emilie, D. (1991). Activation of cytotoxic cells in hyperplastic lymph nodes from HIV-infectecd patients. AIDS 5:1071-1079.

Embretson, J., Zupancic, M., Ribas, J. L., Burke, A., Racz, P., Tenner-Racz, K. and Haase, A. T. (1993). Massive covert infection of helper T lymphocytes and macrophages by HIV during the incubation period of AIDS. Nature 362:359-362.

Epstein, L. G., Kuiken, C., Blumberg, B. M., Hartman, S., Sharer, L. R., Clement, M., and Goudsmit, J. (1991). HIV-1 V3 domain variation in brain and spleen of children with AIDS: Tissue-specific evolution within host-determined quasispecies. Virology 180:583-590.

Fauci, A. S. (1993). Multifactorial nature of human immunodeficiency virus disease: implications for therapy. Science 262:1011-1018.

Fuller, K. A., Kanagawa, O. and Nahm, M. H. (1993). T cells within germinal centers are specific for the immunizing antigen. J. Immunol. 151:4505-4512.

Hadida, F., Parrot, A., Kieny, M. P., Sadat-Sowdi, B., Mayaud, C., Debré, P. and Autran, B. (1992). Carboxy-terminal and central regions of human immunodeficiency virus-1 nef recognized by cytotoxic T lymphocytes from lymphoid organs. J. Clin. Invest. 89:53-60.

Ho, D. D. (1992). HIV-1 viremia and influenza. Lancet 339:1549.

Holland, J. J., de la Torre, J. C. and Steinhauer, D. A. (1992). RNA virus populations as quasispecies. Curr. Top. Microbiol. Immunol. 176:1-20.

Jacob, J., Kassir, R. and Kelsoe, G. (1991). In situ studies of the primary immune response to (4-hydroxy-3-nitrophenyl)acetyl. I. The architecture and dynamics of responding cell populations. J. Exp. Med. 173:1165-1175.

Janoff, E. N., O'Brien, J., Thompson, P., Ehret, J., Meiklejohn, G., Duvall, G. and Douglas, J. M. (1993). Streptococcus pneumoniae colonization, bacteremia, and immune response among persons with human immunodeficiency virus infection. J. Inf. Dis. 167:49-56.

Kimura, N., Toyonaga, B., Yoshikai, Y., Triebel, F., Debre, P., Minden, M. D. and Mak, T. W. (1986). Sequences and diversity of human T cell receptor β chain variable region genes. J. Exp. Med. 164:739-750.

Laman, J. D. and van der Eetwegh, A. J. M. (1992). Cytotoxic potential of CD8+ T cells in lymphoid follicles during HIV-1 infection. AIDS 6:333-334.

Le Tourneau, A., Audouin, J., Diebold, J., Marche, C., Tricottet, V. and Reynes, M. (1986). LAV-like particles in lymph node germinal centers in patients with the persistent lymphadenopathy syndrome and the acquired immunodeficiency syndrome-related complex. An ultrastructural study of 30 cases. Hum. Pathol. 17:1047-1053.

Liu, Y. L., Zhang, J., Lane, P. J. L., Chan, E. Y. T. and MacLennan, I. C. M. (1991). Sites of B cell activation in primary and secondary responses to T cell-dependent and T cell-independent antigens. Eur. J. Immunol. 21:2951-2962.

Lu, W. and Israèl-Biet, D. (1993). Virion concentration in bronchoalveolar lavage fluids of HIV infected patients. Lancet 342, 298.

Meyerhans, A., Cheynier, R., Albert, J., Seth, M., Kwok, S., Sninsky, J. J., Morfeldt-Manson, L., Åsjö, B. and Wain-Hobson, S. (1989). Temporal fluctuations in HIV quasispecies in vivo are not reflected by sequential HIV isolation. Cell 58:901-910.

Miedema, F., Tersmette, M. and van Lier, R. A. W. (1990) AIDS pathogenesis: a dynamic interaction between HIV and the immune system. Immunol. Today 11, 293-296.

Myers, G., Korber, B., Wain-Hobson, S., Smith, R. F. and Pavlakis, G. N. (1993). Human retroviruses and AIDS. Los Alamos National Laboratory, New Mexico.

Oksenhendler, E., Autran, B., Gorochov, G., D'Agay, M. F., Seligman, M. and Clauvel, J. P. (1992). CD8 lymphocytosis and pseudotumoral splenomegaly in HIV infection. Lancet 340:207-208.

Pannetier, C., Cochet, M., Darche, S., Casrouge, A., Zöller, M. and Kourilsky, P. (1993). The sizes of the CDR3 hypervariable regions of the murine T-cell receptor chains vary as a function of the recombined germ-line segments. Proc. Natl. Acad. Sci. USA. 90:4319-4323.

Pantaleo, G., Graziosi, C., Demareset, J. F., Butini, L., Montoroni, M., Fox, C. H., Orenstein, J. M., Kotler, D. P. and Fauci, A. S. (1993). HIV infection is active and progressive in lymphoid tissue during the clinically latent stage of disease. Nature 362:355-358.

Pedroza Martins, L., Chenciner, N. and Wain-Hobson, S. (1992). Complex intrapatient sequence variation in the V1 and V2 hypervariable regions of the HIV-1 gp120 envelope sequence. Virology 191:837-845.

Peluso, R., Haase, A., Stowring, L., Edwards, M. and Ventura, P. (1985). A trojan horse mechanism for the spread of visna virus in monocytes. Virology 147:231-236.

Racz, P., Tenner-Racz, K., Kahl, C., Feller, A. C., Kern, P. and Dietrich, M. (1986). The spectrum of morphologic changes of lymph nodes from patients with AIDS or AIDS-related complexes. Progr. Allergy 37:81-181.

Tenner-Racz, K., Racz, P., Dietrich, M. and Kern, P. (1985). Altered follicular dendritic cells and virus-like particles in AIDS and AIDS-related lymphadenopathy. Lancet i:105-106.

Tong-Starksen, S. E., Luciw, P. A. and Peterlin, B. M. (1987). Human immunodeficiency virus long terminal repeat responds to T cell activation signals. Proc. Natl. Acad. Sci. USA. 84:6845-6849.

Sala, M., Zambruno, G., Vartanian, J. P., Marconi, A., Bertazzoni U. and Wain-Hobson, S. (1994). Spatial discontinuities in human immunodeficiency virus type 1 quasispecies derived from epidermal Langerhans cells of an AIDS patient and evidence for double infection. Journal of Virology 68:5280-5283.

Sonigo, P., Alizon, M., Staskus, K., Klatzmann, D., Cole, S., Danos, O., Retzel, E., Tiollais, P., Haase, A. T. and Wain-Hobson, S. (1985). Nucleotide sequence of the visna lentivirus: relationship to the AIDS virus. Cell 42:369-382.

Steinman, R. M. (1991). The dendritic cell system and its role in immunogenicity. Ann. Rev. immunol. 9:271-296.

Van den Eertwegh, A. J. M., Laman, J. D., Schellekens, M. M., Boersma, W. J. A. and Claassen, E. (1992). Complement-mediated follicular localization of T-independent type-2 antigens: the role of marginal zone macrophages revisited. Eur. J. Immunol. 22:719-726.

Wain-Hobson, S. (1993). Viral burden and AIDS. Nature 366:22.

Wallis, R. S., Vjecha, M., Amir-Tahmasseb, M., Okewera, A., Byekwaso, F., Nyole, S., Kabengera, S., Mugerwa, R. D. and Ellner, J. J. (1993). Influence of tuberculosis on human immunodeficiency virus (HIV-1): enhanced cytokine expression and elevated b2-microglobulin in HIV-1 associated tuberculosis. J. Inf. Dis. 167:43-48.

Weinstein, P. D., Schweitzer, P. A., Cebra-Thomas, J. A. and Cebra, J. J. (1991). Molecular genetic features reflecting the preference for isotype switching to IgA expression by Peyer's patch germinal center B cells. Int. Immunol. 3:1253-1263.

Wolfs, T. F. W., Zwart, G., Bakker, M., Valk, M., Kuiken, C. and Goudsmit, J. (1991). Naturally occurring mutations within HIV-1 V3 genomic RNA lead to antigenic variation dependent on a single aminoacid substitution. Virology 185:195-205.

Zhu, T., Mo, H., Wang, N., Nam, D. S., Cao, Y., Koup, R. A. and Ho, D. D. (1993). Genotypic and phenotypic characterization of HIV-1 patients with primary infection. Science 261:1179-1181.

16

AUTOIMMUNITY, APOPTOSIS DEFECTS AND RETROVIRUSES

J. D. Mountz, J. Cheng, X. Su, J. Wu, and T. Zhou

The University of Alabama at Birmingham
Department of Medicine
Division of Clinical Immunology and Rheumatology and
Birmingham Veterans Administration Medical Center
Birmingham, Alabama 35294-0007

ABSTRACT: AUTOIMMUNITY, APOPTOSIS DEFECTS AND RETROVIRUSES

Autoimmune disease in both mice and humans is associated with increased expression of endogenous retroviruses in the thymus and T cells, and loss of self-tolerance by T cells. The basic genetic defect underlying autoimmune disease has been identified as a mutation of the Fas apoptosis antigen in MRL-*lpr/lpr* mice or a mutation of the Fas ligand in C3H-*gld/gld* mice. In MRL-*lpr/lpr* mice, the *lpr* mutation results from a 5.3 kb insertion of the *ETn* retrotransposon in the second intron of the Fas gene. In contrast to normal mice, which express a 2.2 kb normal size Fas cDNA, MRL-*lpr/lpr* mice express multiple Fas RNA transcripts ranging from 2-10.5 kb. In addition, a 5.7 kb full-length *ETn* transcript is highly expressed in the thymus of younger MRL-*lpr/lpr* mice. To determine if high *ETn* expression was dependent on abnormal Fas expression, CD2-*fas* transgenic mice were produced using the full-length murine Fas cDNA under the regulation of the CD2 promoter and enhancer. This resulted in normalization of Fas expression and also elimination of expression of the *ETn* retrotransposon. The *ETn* regulatory sequence contains potential DNA binding sites found in the enhancers of many genes activated during early T cell development in the thymus including enhancer regions for the TCR, CD3 and IL-2 genes. Therefore we propose that *ETn* expression is increased during early T cell development in the thymus, or after T cell activation, and that the integration of *ETn* in the Fas apoptosis gene leads to abnormal T cell apoptosis or development.

Human autoimmune disease has also been found to result from production of a soluble inhibitor of apoptosis. The full-length cDNA and genomic clones for human Fas were cloned and sequenced. Patients with SLE produced high levels of an alternatively spliced soluble Fas (sFas) RNA lacking the transmembrane (exon 6) resulting in high circulating levels of the Fas molecule. This human sFas molecule was able to inhibit apoptosis *in vitro* at levels found in serum of SLE patients (200 ng/ml). The same levels of mouse sFas were able to inhibit apoptosis *in vivo* in mice resulting in a 3-fold increase in spleen size, and altered thymocyte maturation consisting of increased production of CD4⁻ CD8⁻ T cells and decreased CD4⁺CD8⁺ T cells. Regulation of Fas signaling in human T cells also plays a role in abnormal apoptosis. Fas signaling is mediated by the hematopoietic stem cell phosphatase, (Hcph) and is inhibited in the Hcph deficient Molt-4 T cell, the phosphatase deficient motheaten (*me/me*) mice and by the tyrosine phosphatase inhibitor pervanadate. Multiple pathways of Fas apoptosis were also shown to exist, as Fas induced apoptosis is increased in the liver of *me/me* mice, and signaling likely also involves an sphingomylinase-ceramide activated kinase pathway as utilized by the TNF-R.

Fas ligand has been recently cloned in mice and humans, and is homologous to TNF-α. The Fas ligand defect in autoimmune C3H-*gld/gld* mice is due to a point mutation resulting in a single amino acid change in the hydrophobic region of the Fas ligand trimer. These results indicate that T cell apoptosis can be dramatically increased or decreased by cellular interactions which in turn regulate either the levels of production or signaling activity of the Fas and Fas ligand. Retroviruses and their products can influence apoptosis by altering expression of Fas or Fas-L, or altering apoptotic signaling after Fas/Fas-L interactions. Further insights into the regulation of apoptosis molecules will be important in normalizing this activity when it is decreased as in the case of autoimmune disease, or when it is in excess, as is the case with HIV disease.

1. IMMUNE FUNCTION MODIFICATION BY RETROVIRUSES

Increased expression of endogenous retroviral sequences (ERS) in the thymus of autoimmune strains has been proposed to be related to development of autoimmune disease (1-3). Inhibition of translation of retroviral transcripts by antisense RNA has been reported to result in increased proliferation of lymphocytes from NZB mice. It was proposed that full-length retroviral transcripts and protein products are a compensatory mechanism capable of decreasing lymphocyte proliferation in autoimmune mice. ERS can modify immune function and effect autoimmune disease through at least three mechanisms as summarized in Table 1.

First, retroviruses or retroviral proteins can have a direct immunologic effect which includes inhibition of protein kinase C (PK-C) and *trans*activation genes (4-20). Immuno-suppression linked to retroviral infection has been related to the envelope protein p15E and can be mimicked by a synthetic peptide CKS-17 linked to BSA (8-12). The immune effects of p15E and CKS-17-BSA include inhibition of interleukin (IL)-2 secretion, natural killer (NK) cell function and γ-interferon production. CKS-17-BSA also inhibits PK-C activity. Several other direct effects of immune modulation by retroviruses include immunosuppression by HIV-1 gp41 (13,14), increased expression of IL-2 or IL2R (15-17), or effects on MHC class I or class II gene expression (18-20).

Second, several retroviruses can effect the immune system indirectly via host immune responses to retroviral proteins. Mechanisms include idiotype and molecular mimicry leading to antibodies to viral components that bind to cell surface molecules might serve as antigens for anti-idiotypic antibodies (21), or the presence of amino acid homology between retroviral proteins and host proteins (22-27). Molecular mimicry of an 8-10 amino acid site of myelin based protein by hepatitis B virus polymerase can generate an autoimmune encephalitis (27). Endogenous retroviral envelope proteins (for example gp70) are present in the serum and surface of mouse cells (and cells of many other species) and loss of tolerance to these proteins could lead to a serum sickness syndrome (28). Reactivity against the endogenous type A particle on the pancreas of diabetic mice is caused by tolerance loss for the retroviral product (29,30).

Table 1. Immune Function Modification By Retroviruses

1. Direct Immunologic Effects of Retroviruses or Retroviral Proteins.

Name	Component	Effect/Reference
p15E	Transmembrane envelope protein	inhibition of protein kinase-C (4-12)
HIV-1 gp41	Transmembrane envelope protein	immunosuppressive (13,14)
HTLV-1 tax protein	transactivating protein	increases expression of IL-2, IL-2R (15-17)
Rad LV	radiation leukemia virus	increases class I antigen (18,19)
Mo-MuLV	Moloney murine leukemia virus	trans effect in MHC expression in fibroblast (20)

2. Indirect Effect on Host Immune Response

Name	Component	Effect/Reference
his-t-RNA	histidine - t-RNA	anti-Id myositis (21)
HIV-1 gp41	5AA homology with class II antigen	molecular mimicry (24,25)
p30gag	topoisomerase I	systemic sclerosis (26)
endogenous Type A particle	Type A endogenous retroviral	diabetes (29,30)
Mls	MMTV (Mouse Mammary Tumor Virus)	superantigen (31)
Mls	Mo-MuLV (Moloney Murine Leukemia Virus)	superantigen (32)

3. Disruption of Structure or Regulation of Host Gene

Name	Component	Effect/Reference
Mtv-8	Vκ upstream integration	Vκ expression (38)
Sine, R-C2	third intron human C2	regulating C2 expression (39)
ETn	integration in muscle chloride channel gene	myotonia (40)
ETn	present in cDNA	altered thymic gene expression (41)
ETn	upstream Vλ2	plasmacytoma (42)
ETn	switch region VH	plasmacytoma (43)
ETn	integration in Q6, Q8 mouse MHC	homology to ETn (44)
ETn	second intron in fas gene	fas expression, apoptosis defect (48)

The identity of minor lymphocyte stimulating (Mls) antigens, which are endogenous superantigens that can activate or induce the deletion of large portions of the T cell repertoire, has recently been revealed: they are encoded by mouse mammary tumor viruses (MMTV) that have integrated into the germ line as DNA proviruses. Hence, T cells bearing TCR Vβ-specific for the superantigen Mls-1a (encoded in the open reading frame of the 3' long terminal repeat of endogenous MMTV) can lead to deletion of T cells expressing Mls reactive Vβ regions (31). However, it has been proposed that Mls-mediated modulation may be only the tip of the retrovirus iceberg; already murine leukemia virus (MuLV) with similar superantigen properties have been discovered. A rapid activation and proliferation of CD4[+] T cells is associated with the development of an immunodeficiency syndrome of mice caused by a replication-defective MuLV (32). The responses of normal spleen cells to B cell-lines that express the defective virus indicate that these lines express a cell surface determinant that shares "superantigenic" properties with some microbial antigens and Mls-like self antigens. This antigen-elicited a potent proliferative response that was dependent on the presence of CD4[+] T cells and was associated with selective expansion of cells bearing Vβ5.

This response was markedly inhibited by a mAb-specific for the MuLV *gag*-encoded p30 antigen.

Infectious retroviruses are now suspect as potential autoimmunologic agents. Numerous autoimmune, arthritic, and dermatologic manifestations as well as a diffuse lympho-proliferative disorder can occur as a consequence of human immunodeficiency virus (HIV) infection (33). Some patients with systemic lupus erythematosus (SLE), Sjogren's Syndrome (SS) and scleroderma make antibodies which are reactive with the p24 *gag*-protein of HIV-1 (34-36). The antigenic genotype is rich in proline as is Sm which is also reactive (37). In SLE, this response is linked to a conserved immunodominant idiotype. If the immunogen is a proline-rich epitope expressed from an autoimmune retrovirus or ERS, this antibody would be another example of molecular mimicry. There is a unique 8.4-kb RNA transcript derived from a mink cell focus-forming (MCF) MuLV expressed in all autoimmune but not in normal mice as early as one day of age. A new human endogenous retroviral DNA related to HTLV-1 and HTLV-2 has been isolated from T cells obtained from a patient with mixed cryoglobu-linemia (33).

A third mechanism by which retroviruses can alter immune function is by integration and disruption of either the structure or regulation of the host gene. Retrotransposons are retroviral sequences that are especially capable of this type of immune disfunction. Mtv retroviral sequences can also effect transcription of adjacent genes. Mtv-8 is an endogenous retrovirus located 4.6-kb upstream of a Vκ region gene (called Vκ9M) within the κ-Ig locus. The proximity of these two genes results in reciprocal transcriptional activation (38). Mtv-8 transcription can be detected after juxtaposition of the κ-enhancers to the normal silent provirus. Reciprocally, the frequency of Vκ9M rearrangement is 5- to 10-fold higher in spleens from Mtv-8-positive mice compared to spleens from mice that lacked the Mtv-8 provirus. A variable number of tandem repeats (VNTR) locus has been identified within the third intron at the human complement C2 gene where it is associated with a short interspersed sequence retroposon (SINE.R-C2). SINE.R-C2 is a part of a larger retrotransposon family derived from a human ERS (HERV) which is homologous to MMTV (40).

The *ETn* retrotransposon has been identified in several autosomal recessive disease states in mice and man. The *ETn* transposon has inserted into the major mammalian-skele-tal-chloride-channel (CIC-1) in myotonia mice, destroying its coding potential for several membrane-spanning domains (40). Genes induced by glucocorticoids in murine thymocytes and in the WEHI-7TG cell line contain sequences for the remnants of a mouse *ETn* (41). *ETn* integration has occurred upstream of Vλ2 in the P3X63Ag8 cell line (42). The transposon is strongly expressed not only in embryonic cells but also in plasmacytomas, B lymphomas and T cell lines. Similarly, the *ETn* sequence has been inserted into separate Ig heavy-chain switch regions in plasmacytoma P3.26Bu4 (43). A unique 2.2-kb mRNA is transcribed from Q6 and Q8 genes of the mouse MHC. The 3' portion of Q8 contains extensive homology with the *ETn* transposon (44).

2. ET*n* RETROTRANSPOSON EXPRESSION IN MRL-*lpr/lpr* AUTOIMMUNE MICE

The possible role of retroviruses in autoimmune diseases, such as lupus and RA, has been of interest for several years. Both endogenous and exogenous retrovirus have been thought to play a role, but direct evidence has been lacking. The homozygous expression of the *lpr/lpr* gene leads to autoimmunity and lymphadenopathy in different strains of mice including MRL, C57BL/6, C3H, AKR, and BALB/c mice (45). The *lpr* gene has been identified as a point mutation in the intracellular region of the *fas* gene in CBA/J-lpr^cg mice

a

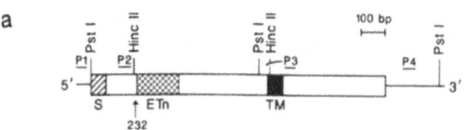

b

PCR Product of *lpr/lpr* and Normal Fas

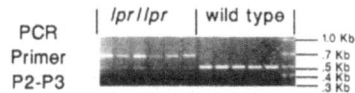

c

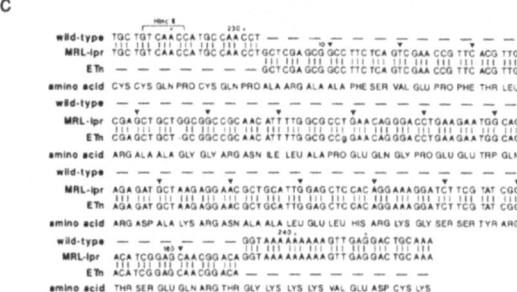

Figure 1. MRL-*lpr/lpr* mice express an abnormal *fas* RNA containing *ETn*. **1a)** The position of the *ETn* sequence inserted within the *fas* gene was determined by sequence analysis of cDNA prepared from the thymus of MRL-*lpr/lpr* and MRL-+/+ mice. The PCR primers used and their relative locations within the *fas* gene are indicated as P1, P2, P3 and P4. Also shown is the location of the 170 bp 5' probe which is the PstI-HincII fragment, and the 345 bp extracellular domain probe which is the HincII fragment derived from the normal *fas* cDNA clone. **1b)** The PCR products using primers P2-P3 were subjected to agarose gel electrophoresis and visualized by ultraviolet illumination in the presence of ethidium bromide. A unique larger PCR product was observed using thymic RNA from six different MRL-*lpr/lpr* mice. **1c)** The wild-type sequence of the *fas* gene is numbered as previously described (11). The *ETn* sequence found within the otherwise normal extracellular coding region of *fas* cDNA from MRL-*lpr/lpr* mice is 98% homologous to a portion of an *ETn* previously found to be integrated into the Ig locus of mice (12,14,15). The 168 bp *ETn* insert in the *fas* gene of MRL-*lpr/lpr* mice results in an in-frame amino acid sequence shown below the cDNA sequence. Reproduced from the *Journal of Experimetnal Medicine*, 1993, Vol. 178:461–468, by copyright permission from the Rockefeller University Press.

(2). The *fas* gene also has been found to be abnormal in MRL-*lpr/lpr* mice in which Southern blot analysis indicated altered restriction enzyme digestion (46,47) and *fas* RNA expression was not detectable in the thymus (46). These results led to the conclusion that the *fas* mutation in MRL-*lpr/lpr* mice was different from the mutation in CBA/J-lpr^{cg} mice, and that in MRL-*lpr/lpr* mice the mutation leads to disruption of normal transcription of the *fas* gene (48).

To determine if the *lpr/lpr* mutation in the extracellular domain of the *fas* gene results in abnormal *fas* RNA, cDNA corresponding to the extracellular domain was derived from thymus RNA from several MRL-*lpr/lpr* and MRL-+/+ mice using the polymerase chain reaction and primers P2-P3 (Fig. 1*a*). All RNA samples from the thymus of different MRL-*lpr/lpr* mice yielded a unique polymerase chain reaction product that was 168 bp larger than that of wild-type MRL-+/+ mice (Fig. 1*b*). The mutation of the *fas* gene in MRL-*lpr/lpr* mice was confirmed to be in the extracellular domain by sequencing, using full length

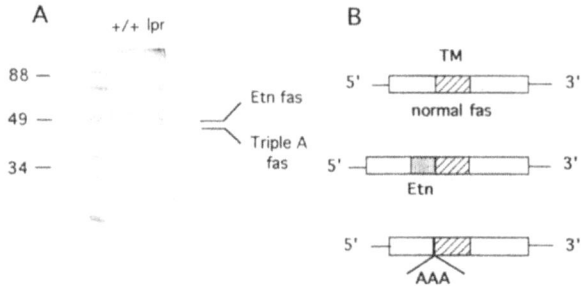

Figure 2. Characterization of the mutant Fas protein in MRL-*lpr/lpr* T cells. a) Western blot analysis of anti-Fas immunoprecipitated protein; A Fas protein of molecular weight 46 kD was precipitated from thymocytes from MRL-+/+ mice, whereas, two Fas proteins of 46 kD and 50 kD were precipitated from thymocytes from MRL-*lpr/lpr* mice. 2b) the structure of the cDNA of corresponding mutations. Sequence analysis indicated that the two sizes of the Fas proteins represented different mutations, one resulting from the *ETn* insertion and one resulting from a triple "A" insertion in the extracellular domain of Fas cDNA.

primers P1-P4 (Figure 1*a*) and using the extracellular *fas* cDNA clones from MRL-*lpr/lpr* and MRL-+/+ mice. The sequence of the transmembrane and cytoplasmic domains were identical in MRL-*lpr/lpr* and MRL-+/+ mice. Complete sequence analysis of cDNA corresponding to the extracellular domain of the *fas* gene was carried out using two different MRL-*lpr/lpr* mice and indicated that there was a 168 bp insert into the *fas* cDNA sequence at position 232 of an otherwise normally encoded extracellular domain (5) (Fig. 1*c*). The 268 bp *ETn* sequence found within the *fas* gene was 99% homologous to sequence Mus *ETn* Xi (42) (bp 1120-1285) and Mus *ETn* IgM (43) (bp 270-435) as determined by searching the GenBank.

To determine if the RNA containing the *ETn* retrotransposon sequence could lead to a protein product, MRL-*lpr/lpr* and MRL-+/+ mice were analyzed by Western blot analysis using an anti-murine Fas antibody. There was a 66 kD glycoprotein corresponding to the full-length Fas in both mice, and a unique 76 kD protein product in MRL-*lpr/lpr* mice, but not MRL-+/+ mice (Fig. 2). Thymocytes from MRL-+/+ and MRL-*lpr/lpr* mice were surface labeled with biotin followed by lysis of the cells. Biotin labeled Fas protein was immunoprecipitated using anti-Fas mAb and protein A sepharose, analyzed by SDS-PAGE, and western blotted and probed with alkaline phosphatase conjugated avidin. The mutant *fas* cDNA of interest were sequenced by standard methods. A Fas protein with an approximate molecular weight of 46 kD was precipitated from MRL-+/+ thymocytes, whereas two proteins with an approximate molecular weight of 46 kD and 50 kD were precipitated from MRL-*lpr/lpr* T cells (Fig. 2a). Sequence analysis indicated that the two sizes of the Fas proteins represented different mutations, one resulting from the *ETn* insertion and one resulting from a triple "A" insertion in the extracellular domain of Fas cDNA (Fig. 2b). These results support our previously study that indicated that the mutation of the *fas* gene in MRL-*lpr/lpr* mice is not due to the termination of Fas transcription, and that integration of *ETn* into the *fas* gene leads to abnormally spliced Fas mRNA which decreases Fas expression and results in non-functional Fas. Significantly, MRL-*lpr/lpr* T cells bearing the non-functional Fas antigen can be recognized by this antibody and their induction and developmental pathways traced.

A full length *fas* cDNA was used to probe northern blots of poly-A RNA prepared from the thymus of MRL-+/+, MRL-*lpr/lpr*, MRL-*lpr*/+, BXSB male and NZB mice and from the BW5147 cell line (Fig. 3). In MRL-+/+ mice there was a 2.2 kb normal sized *fas* cDNA. In contrast, in 1 mo old MRL-*lpr/lpr* mice there were multiple bands ranging from

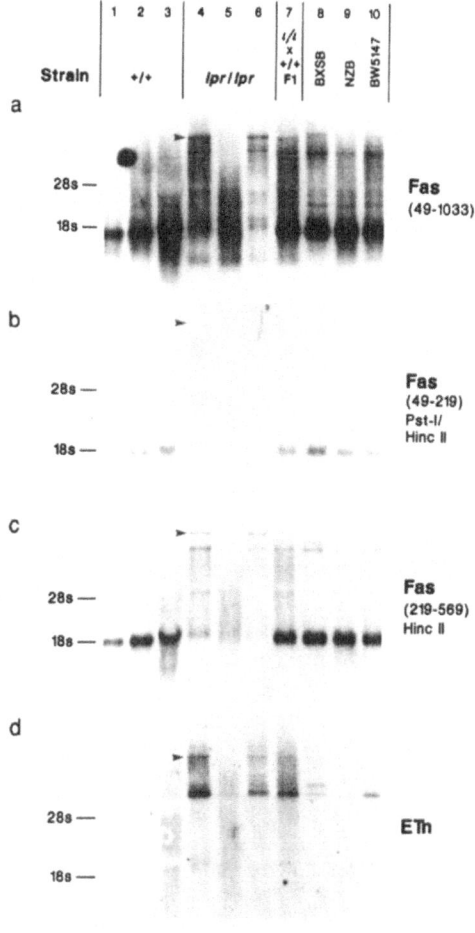

Figure 3. Northern blot analysis of *fas* RNAs from the thymus of wild-type MRL-+/+ and MRL-*lpr/lpr* mice. Thymus poly-A⁺ RNA from the indicated mouse strains were analyzed by probing four identical blots with (a) a full length *fas* cDNA probe, (b) a 5' Pst-I/HincII *fas* cDNA probe corresponding to position 49-219, (c) a *fas* cDNA probe corresponding to the 345 bp HincII fragment of extracellular domain, and (d) a 168 bp *ETn* probe derived from *ETn* sequences within the abnormal sized *fas* transcript obtained by PCR amplification of the extracellular domain of *fas* cDNA from *lpr/lpr* mice. MRL-+/+, BXSB male and NZB female mice were 2 mo of age. MRL-*lpr/lpr* mice were 1 mo old (lanes 4,6) and 3 mo old (lane 5). The upper arrows in panels a,b and c indicate the abnormal *fas* transcripts in MRL-*lpr/lpr* mice which correspond in size to a unique transcript which also hybridizes to the *ETn* probe used in panel d. Reproduced from the *Journal of Experimental Medicine*, 1993, Vol. 178:461–468, by copyright permission of the Rockefeller University Press.

2 kb to 10.5 kb. Fas expression was highest in the thymus of 1 mo old MRL-*lpr/lpr* mice, and decreased in 3 mo old mice. When identical blots were hybridized with a 170 bp PstI/HincII *fas* cDNA fragment corresponding to the first and second exons, *fas* expression in MRL-*lpr/lpr* mice was very low compared to *fas* expression in MRL-+/+ mice. A faint abnormal high molecular weight species of 10.5 kb was present using this 5' probe. When blots were probed with a 345 bp HincII *fas* cDNA fragment corresponding to the extracellular domain of *fas*, the primary species of RNA expressed in the thymus of young MRL-*lpr/lpr* mice was a high molecular weight 10.5 kb and 9.5 kb transcript. These results indicate that the *fas* mutation leads to production of abnormal high molecular weight *fas* transcripts in the thymus. There was high expression of the 2.2 kb *fas* transcript in (MRL-*lpr/lpr* x MRL-+/+)F₁ mice, and also in BXSB male and NZB autoimmune mice. Expression of normal levels of *Fas* RNA in BXSB and NZB mice indicates that autoimmune disease in these mice is not related to defective expression of *fas* RNA.

The 168 bp *ETn* probe, derived from within the *fas* cDNA prepared from thymus RNA of MRL-*lpr/lpr* mice, strongly hybridized to a 5.7 kb full-length *ETn* transcript which was expressed in the thymus of younger MRL-*lpr/lpr* mice, but not strongly expressed in the thymus of older MRL-*lpr/lpr* mice or in the thymus of MRL-+/+ mice (Fig. 3*d*, lanes

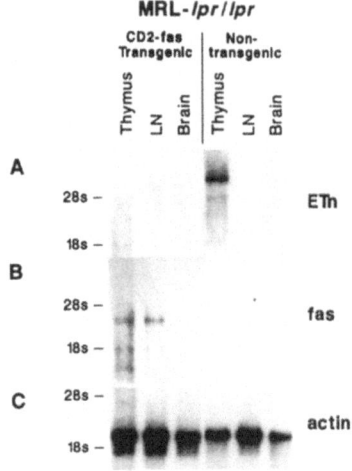

Figure 4. Decreased *ETn* expression in CD2-*fas* transgenic MRL-*lpr/lpr* mice. Poly-A RNA from thymus, lymph node (LN) and brain of 4 wk old CD2-*fas* transgenic and non-transgenic MRL-*lpr/lpr* mice was blotted and probed. **4A)** *ETn* expression is decreased in the thymus of 4 wk old CD2-*fas* transgenic MRL-lpr/lpr mice but not in age-matched non-transgenic littermate control mice. **4B)** CD2-fas transgenic MRL-*lpr/lpr* mice have high levels of fas RNA in the thymus and LN but not in non-T cell sites including the brain. Non-transgenic litter mate control mice do not express Fas. **4C)** The blot was stripped and hybridized with a β-actin probe to ensure that nearly equivalent amounts of RNA were present in all samples. Reproduced from the *Journal of Experimental Medicine*, 1993, Vol. 178:461–468, by copyright permission from the Rockefeller University Press.

1-3). RNA corresponding to the full-length 5.7 kb *ETn* transcripts was also abundant in the thymus of MRL-*lpr/+* and BXSB mice, and also in the BW5147 cell line. The largest *fas* transcript corresponds in size to an abnormal 10.5 kb *ETn* transcript in MRL-*lpr/lpr* mice suggesting the presence of the *ETn* sequence within one of the abnormal sized high molecular weight *fas* transcripts of MRL-*lpr/lpr* mice. A higher approximately 10.5 kb molecular weight *fas* transcript was also present in the thymus of MRL-*lpr/+* and BXSB mice, but not NZB mice or the BW5147 cell line.

To determine if high *ETn* expression was dependent on abnormal *fas* expression, CD2-*fas* transgenic mice were produced that utilized a full-length murine *fas* cDNA under the regulation of the CD2 promoter and enhancer (49) to correct defective *fas* expression in T cells of MRL-*lpr/lpr* mice. The presence of the *fas* transgene resulted in reduction of expression of *ETn* in the thymus, suggesting that high *ETn* expression is related to abnormal *fas* expression (Fig. 4a) (50). Northern blot analysis indicated that there was high expression of the *fas* transgene in the thymus and lymph node, but not in the brain of 4 wk old CD2-*fas* transgenic MRL-*lpr/lpr* mice (Fig. 4b).

These results suggest that increased retroviral expression may be related to defective *fas* expression in MRL-*lpr/lpr* mice.

We have also observed that *ETn* expression is decreased and *fas* expression is partially normalized in TCRβ transgenic mice (Wu, J., *et. al.*, manuscript in preparation). We have previously demonstrated that in TCRβ transgenic mice, there is nearly total elimination of the CD4⁻CD8⁻B220⁺ subpopulation of T cells and lymphoproliferation, but not elimination of autoimmunity (51,52). We have recently demonstrated that there is decreased apoptosis of thymocytes of MRL-*lpr/lpr* mice and an increase of a large, proliferating CD4⁺CD8⁺ subpopulation of thymocytes (52). The TCRβ transgene was found to reduce these large, proliferating CD4⁺CD8⁺ thymocytes and there was no difference between this population in TCRβ transgenic MRL-*lpr/lpr* mice the same population in MRL-+/+ mice. These results suggested that the presence of the TCRβ transgene corrected the defect in early T cell development related to lymphoproliferation despite the presence of a germline mutation of the *fas* apoptosis gene. Rearrangement of the TCRβ chain gene has been proposed to play a critical role in early T cell development in the thymus (53,54). The TCRβ transgene suppresses rearrangement of the endogenous TCRβ gene (55). Suppression of rearrangement of the endogenous TCRβ gene might accelerate T cell maturation resulting in decreased levels of retroviral LTR and eukaryotic gene enhancer binding proteins associated with T cell development (56). The *ETn* sequence contains potential DNA binding sites for the *Ets* oncogene (Wu, unpublished observation). These same DNA binding sequences are found in the enhancers of many genes that are activated during early T cell development in the thymus, including the enhancer region for TCRα, TCRβ, TCRγ, CD3γ, CD3ζ, CD2, IL-2 and GM-CSF (57). Potential Ets binding sites are also found in the LTR of MSV, HTLV-1, and HIV-2 (58,59). We propose that *ETn* expression is increased during early T cell development in the thymus due to the presence of common DNA binding protein motifs which are found in both the *ETn* LTR and the enhancers of several genes which undergo activation during early T cell development in the thymus. Prevention of aberrant transcription initiation at the site of the *ETn* integration within the second intron of the murine *fas* gene could result in normal transcription initiation from the 5' end of the *fas* gene. This would lead to the observed increased levels of *fas* expression in the thymus of the TCRβ transgenic MRL-*lpr/lpr* mice. This interpretation is consistent with the concept that *ETn* expression and abnormal *fas* expression are functionally related in *lpr* mice.

3. SOLUBLE Fas ANTIGEN AS AN INHIBITOR OF APOPTOSIS

Surface expression of the human Fas molecule has been described in various cell types, including activated T- and B-lymphocytes (60). However, a soluble form of Fas antigen has not been described. Soluble forms of various receptors including cytokine receptors and hormone receptors, and of other membrane molecules including major histocompatibility complex (MHC) class I and CD60 molecules, have been characterized previously (61). They are thought to be produced through either proteolytic cleavage of membrane-bound receptors as is the case for the interleukin (IL)-2 receptor (62) and human tumor necrosis factor (TNF) receptor (63), or as translation products of alternatively spliced mRNA as is the case for murine IL-4 receptor (64) and murine and human IL-7 receptor (65). The secreted receptors represent truncated forms of the membrane-bound receptors. They lack the transmembrane domains but retain the ability to bind ligand with a similar affinity to that of their membrane-bound counterparts. As a result, they are effective inhibitors and play an important role in the regulation of receptor activity.

The human Fas cDNA encodes a Fas molecule of 335 amino acids, with a calculated molecular weight of 37,729. It consists of a signal peptide of 16 amino acid residues at its amino terminus, an extracellular domain of 157 amino acid residues, a hydrophobic transmembrane domain of 17 amino acid residues and a cytoplasmic tail of 146 amino acids at its carboxyl terminus. The extracellular domain can be divided into three cysteine-rich subdomains. The cytoplasmic region contains the domain that is required for initiation of the apoptotic response (66). Structural homology places Fas in the superfamily including TNF receptors, NGF receptor and CD40 (60).

To investigate the possible presence of abnormal Fas transcripts in human subjects with autoimmune disease, we isolated cellular RNA from the PBMC of two systemic lupus erythematosus (SLE), two angioimmunoblastic lymphadenopathy (AILD) patients, and two normal controls (67). The Fas mRNA transcripts were then analyzed after amplification using oligonucleotide primers derived from the 5'-untranslated region (UTR) starting at nucleotide (nt) 170 and 3'-UTR and ending at nt 1336 (46). The amplified product was expected to be 1167-bp in size, and to encompass the entire translation region, as well as portions of the 5'- and 3'-UTR of the Fas mRNA. However, in addition to the anticipated full-length Fas cDNA fragment, a distinct smaller 1104 bp DNA fragment was also observed. In some patients, the relative intensity of this smaller Fas mRNA fragment was increased over that of the full-length Fas mRNA.

The structure and significance of the smaller PCR product was determined by cloning, DNA sequence analysis and comparison of the deduced amino acid sequence with that of the

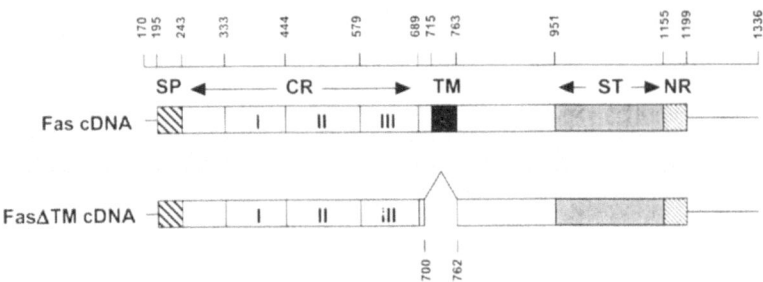

Figure 5. Human FasΔTM structure. A schematic representation of alternatively spliced Fas mRNA variants. The translated and UTR regions are indicated by boxes and thick solid lines, respectively. Regions lacking in the FasΔTM variant are indicated by broken lines and nt positions. SP, CR, TM, ST, and NR represent signal peptide, cysteine-rich subdomains, transmembrane domain, signal transduction domain, and negative regulation domain, respectively. Nt regions encoding each domain are shown above. For genomic PCR, primers were designed to flank each of the putative introns. Reproduced from *Science*, J. Cheng et al., "Protection from Fas-mediated apoptosis by a soluble from of the Fas molecule," Vol. 263:1759–1762, 3/25/94, and ©AAAS.

previously reported human Fas antigen (60). A schematic representation of the alternately spliced Fas mRNA is shown in Fig. 5. The DNA sequence analysis confirmed that the longer insert represented the anticipated 1167-bp Fas cDNA fragment, and contained the intact open reading frame. The smaller 1104 bp clone, designated FasΔTM, had a 63bp deletion starting at nt sequence 700-GATCC AGA and ending at nt sequence GTT TGG G-762. This deletion does not affect the open reading frame, but results in a Fas protein product lacking the 21 amino acid residues corresponding to the last 5 amino acid residues of the Fas extracellular domain and 16 of the 17 amino acid residues of the Fas hydrophobic transmembrane (TM) domain. Thus, this product is likely to be expressed as a soluble, secreted form of Fas.

To confirm the existence of the soluble Fas product, the Fas cDNA and FasΔTM coding region were inserted into a mammalian expression vector (pcDNA-1) and transfected into COS cells. Flow cytometry and immunohistochemical analysis were performed by staining the transfected COS cells with anti-human Fas Ab (67). RT-PCR analysis indicated that the transfected cells expressed the corresponding Fas transcript. Immunofluorescence and flow cytometry analysis revealed that the antibody stained the surface of the cells that were transfected with the full-length Fas cDNA, but not those cells transfected with the FasΔTM-expression plasmid. It also revealed that there were no apparent differences in the degree of cytoplasmic staining between those cells transfected with the full-length Fas cDNA and those cells transfected with the FasΔTM variant. Taken together, these data confirmed that the FasΔTM transcript produced the expected Fas protein product as did the Fas cDNA, and in addition, suggested that FasΔTM protein was not retained in the membrane of the cell, but was present in the cytoplasm as a soluble form.

Confirmation of the presence of a secreted FasΔTM protein was sought by using a inhibition assay for apoptosis induced by the anti-Fas Ab (Fig. 6). Phytohemagglutinin (PHA-P)-stimulated PBMC from normal subjects were used for this experiment as it has been shown that stimulated cells undergo apoptosis after culture with the anti-Fas Ab (66). The PHA-P-stimulated PBMC were cultured with anti-Fas Ab in the presence of supernatant derived from COS cells transiently expressing FasΔTM antigen from the FasΔTM-expression recombinant. As a control, the same PBMC cells were similarly treated with the anti-human Fas Ab except that the added supernatant was derived from COS cells transiently expressing Fas antigen from the full-length Fas cDNA-expression recombinant. The percentage of cells undergoing apoptosis was determined 12 h later by the TdT method. There was a dose-dependent increase in cell survival rate in the medium supplemented with the

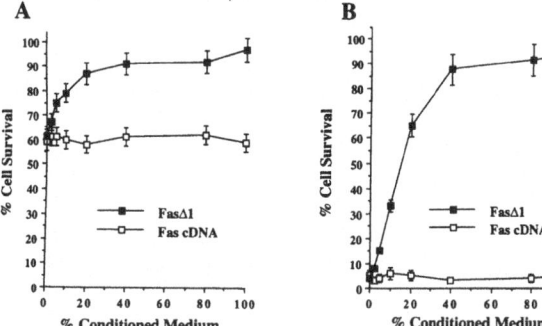

Figure 6. Inhibition assay for apoptosis induced by anti-Fas Ab. Normal human PBMC were stimulated with PHA-P and then incubated in RPMI 1640 with 200 ug/ml murine anti-human Fas mAb in the presence of various concentrations of supernatant harvested from COS cells transfected with either full length Fas cDNA or FasΔTM. Cells undergoing apoptosis were determined by the TdT method. A total of 200 cells including apoptotic cells and live cells were counted in 10 randomly selected microscopic fields. The percentage of viable cells not undergoing apoptosis is indicated. Fas cDNA, open squares; FasΔTM, filled squares. Reproduced from *Science*, J. Cheng et al., "Protection from Fas-mediated apoptosis by a soluble from of the Fas molecule," Vol. 263:1759–1762, 3/25/94, and ©AAAS.

supernatant from COS cells transfected with the FasΔTM-expression plasmid but not in the medium supplemented with the supernatant from COS cells transfected with the full-length Fas cDNA-expression plasmid. This higher survival rate observed in cells treated with the FasΔTM supernatant can be explained by the secretion of the soluble FasΔTM antigen into the supernatant, resulting in interaction of the soluble FasΔTM antigen with anti-human Fas Ab, neutralization of the Ab and consequently, inhibition of the Ab-mediated apoptosis.

The finding that the Fas apoptosis molecule can exist in a secreted form may be of physiological significance since a secreted molecule that is capable of ligand binding could compete with the surface expressed Fas molecule for interaction with the Fas ligand. This would inhibit Fas antigen-mediated apoptosis. In this regard, increased production of soluble forms of Fas antigen may contribute to the etiology and development of human autoimmune diseases including SLE and AILD. A soluble form of Fas was present at increased concentration in approximately 60% of patients with SLE (Fig. 7). In normal controls and patients with rheumatoid arthritis, serum levels of soluble Fas were less than 100 ng/ml. Although soluble Fas is only

Figure 7. Increased serum levels of soluble Fas in SLE. Sera from 10 normal individuals, 10 RA patients, or 10 SLE patients assayed for the presence of soluble Fas (sFas) by enzyme-linked immunosorbent assay. The concentrations were determined by the inclusion of dilutions of purified recombinant soluble Fas to create a standard curve. Reproduced from *Science*, J. Cheng et al., "Protection from Fas-mediated apoptosis by a soluble from of the Fas molecule," Vol. 263:1759–1762, 3/25/94, and ©AAAS.

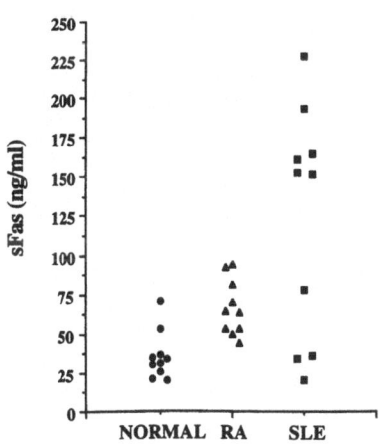

increased approximately twofold in 60% of SLE patients, much higher physiological concentrations may be present at limited site where there is high expression of Fas and Fas ligand. Also, in light of the fact that Fas-mediated apoptosis has been implicated in lymphocyte apoptosis in HIV infection (68), it will be of great importance to investigate a role for FasΔTM in immunodeficiencies, and whether or not blockade of Fas-mediated apoptosis *in vivo,* using recombinant FasΔTM molecules will be of clinical utility in such disease conditions.

4. A SINGLE POINT MUTATION IN A CONSERVED 3' REGION OF THE CODING REGION THE Fas LIGAND IN C3H/HeJ-*gld/gld* MICE

The rat and mouse Fas ligands has been cloned and found to be a member of the tumor necrosis factor (TNF) family (69-71). As this family exhibits highly conserved regions of sequence corresponding to antiparallel β strands in the extracellular carboxyl terminal domain, we exploited this homology to clone the murine Fas ligand from C3H/HeJ-*gld/gld* and +/+ mice. The greatest homology between rat Fas ligand, TNF-α and TNF-β was in a region containing the third major β strand corresponding to bp 626-652 and region C (Fig. 8). Therefore, PCR cDNA cloning was carried out using RNA

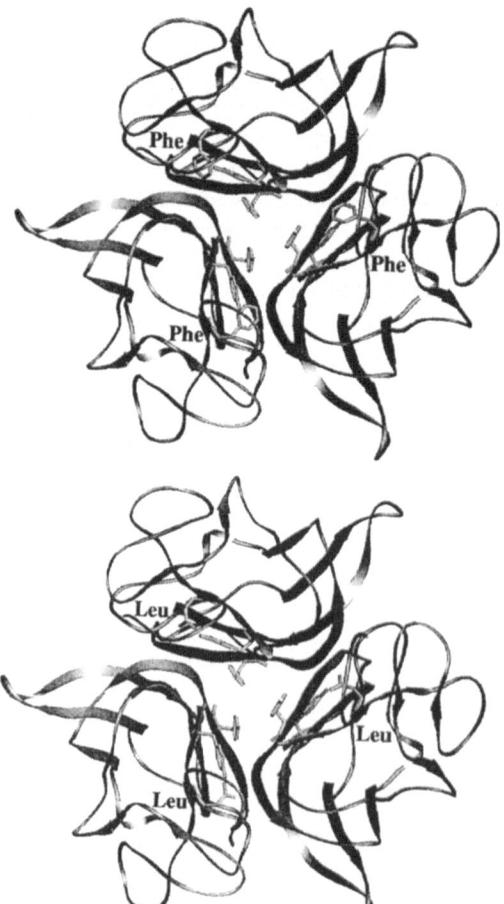

Figure 8. Alignment of amino acid sequence of the conserved region of Fas ligand in wild type and, *gld* mice and rat. Amino acid substitution at position 272 in *gld* mice. Phe to Leu amino acid substitution in conserved region H in *gld* mice.

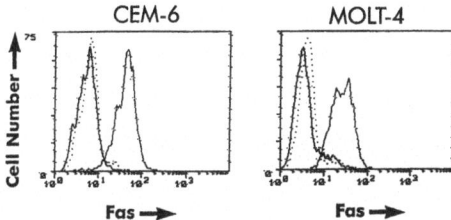

Figure 9. Flow Cytometry Analysis of Fas Expression on CEM-6 and MOLT-4 Cell Lines. 10^6 of cells were stained with anti-human Fas antibody followed by anti-mouse IgM FITC conjugated second antibody. 5000 cells were then analyzed by FACScan. The histograms of FITC fluorescence density are presented. Dotted lines represent the second antibody control showing no non-specific binding by the second antibody as compared to the unstained cells (lower intensity solid line). The higher intensity solid line represents staining with the Fas monoclonal antibody with a separated positive peak.

from PMA stimulated spleen cells of C3H/HeJ-+/+ and C3H/HeJ-*gld/gld* mice, oligonucleotide primers homologous to this region of the rat Fas ligand, and oligo dT. This yielded a 985 bp clone from both C3H/HeJ-+/+ and -*gld/gld* mice. Using the 5' RACE technique, full length cDNA clones were obtained and sequenced. There was complete sequence identity between cDNA clones from C3H/HeJ-+/+ and -*gld/gld* mice except for bp 889. This is predicted to result in a phenylalanine to leucine substitution in the last β strand of Fas ligand in the *gld* mice.

5. REGULATION OF Fas SIGNALING AND APOPTOSIS

Mouse anti-human Fas antibody induces apoptosis-like cytolytic activity against certain cells expressing the Fas antigen, such as U937 and HL-60 (72-74), but not the others. This suggests that anti-Fas apoptosis is not only regulated by Fas-Fas ligand interaction, but also by a permissive Fas signaling pathway. Deletion analysis of the human Fas antigen from the C terminus indicated that the region homologous to TNF type I receptor is essential for the Fas antigen to transduce the signal for cell death into cells (66). This C terminus region of the Fas antigen does not contain domains for kinases or phosphatases, suggesting that this region might interact with cytoplasmic proteins involved in the signal transduction. However, the mechanisms by which the intracellular death signal transduced by Fas antigen remain unclear.

Ten human cell lines were screened for expression of Fas and susceptibility to anti-Fas induced apoptosis. The cell lines were first incubated with mouse anti-human Fas monoclonal antibody and then stained with a FITC-conjugated anti-mouse IgM. Two of the ten cell lines, CEM-6 and MOLT-4, expressed nearly equivalent levels of cell surface Fas antigen (Fig. 9).

These two cell lines were further characterized for their ability to undergo Fas-induced apoptosis. The capability of Fas molecule to transduce apoptotic signal was demonstrated by analysis of Fas-induced internucleosomal DNA cleavage in these two cell lines. Total DNA was extracted after 4 hr-culture with anti-Fas followed by electrophoresis. A DNA ladder indicating extensive internucleosomal DNA cleavage was observed in the CEM-6 cell line after incubation with anti-Fas whereas no DNA breakdown was observed in the MOLT-4 cell line incubated under the same conditions. These data suggest that despite equal Fas expression, there was a defect in the Fas signaling pathway in the MOLT-4 cell line after

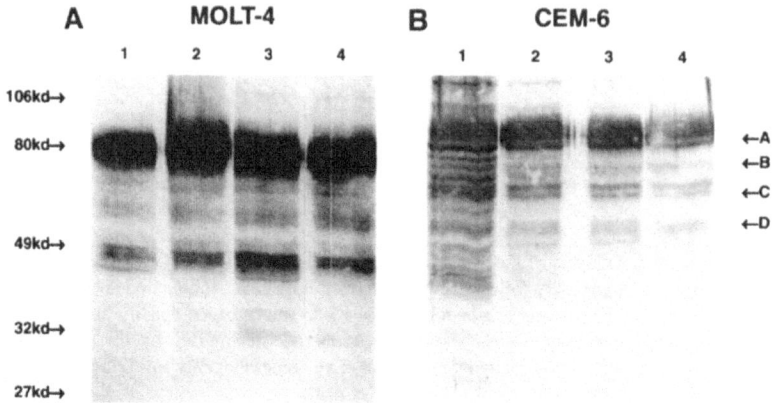

Figure 10. Anti-Fas induced protein tyrosine dephosphorylation. The CEM-6 (A) and MOLT-4 (B) cell lines were treated with anti-Fas mAb for various amounts of time. Lane 1 was untreated cells. Lane 2-4 were cells treated with anti-Fas mAb for 15, 30 or 60 min, respectively. The cells were lysed in lysis buffer and the cell lysates (20mg/ml) were electrophoresed by 10% SDS-PAGE gel, transferred to nitrocellulose membrane and analyzed by anti-phosphotyrosine mAb. The sizes of the standard markers are indicated to the left of the figure.

anti-Fas crosslinking, which led to defective apoptosis. Thus, the CEM-6 and MOLT-4 cell lines were used as a system to study Fas-induced apoptosis signaling.

Protein phosphorylation and dephosphorylation have been shown to exert opposing function in apoptosis in many systems, but little is known concerning their role in Fas-mediated apoptosis. Preincubation for 12 hr with the protein kinase inhibitor genistein had no effect on Fas-induced apoptosis. In contrast, there was a dramatic dose-dependent decrease in the percent of cells undergoing apoptosis after a 12 hr incubation with different concentrations of the protein tyrosine phosphatase inhibitor pervanadate (74). These results suggest that Fas signaling might be mediated by activation of a phosphatase, followed by dephosphorylation of a substrate protein. This was investigated by preincubation of the CEM-6 and MOLT-4 cell line with ^{32}P for 1 hr, followed by addition of anti-Fas antibody. The cells were incubated for different time periods followed by protein extraction and electrophoresis on a 10% SDS PAGE gel and autoradiography (Fig. 10). There were prominent phosphorylated substrates in the CEM-6 cell line (Lane 1).

Following Fas signaling in the CEM-6 cell line, there was a rapid dephosphorylation of these substrates which was evident within 30 minutes. In contrast, no phosphorylation was observed in the MOLT-4 cell line. These results indicate that MOLT-4 has a defect in a phosphatase related to Fas signaling.

Although there has been no intrinsic kinase or phosphatase activity in its cytoplasmic region, a domain has been identified in the cytoplasmic region of Fas that is required to transduce the signal for cell death (66). Whether this apoptotic signal-transducing domain, which is significantly conserved in type I TNF receptor, exerts its function through the interaction with a phosphatase remains to be clarified. In addition, a sphingomyelinase-ceramide signaling mechanism for phosphatase activation by the TNF-R has been described, and may be operative for Fas signaling (75-80). These results provides promising intervention points for apoptosis signaling (Fig. 11). The apoptosis defect observed in MOLT-4 cells could conceivably be overcome by supplying a phosphatase activity or inhibiting a phosphorylation activity. Further understanding of the interplay between phosphorylation and dephosphorylation events mediated by protein tyrosine kinase and phosphatase will be critical pharmacologic targets for modulation of apoptosis.

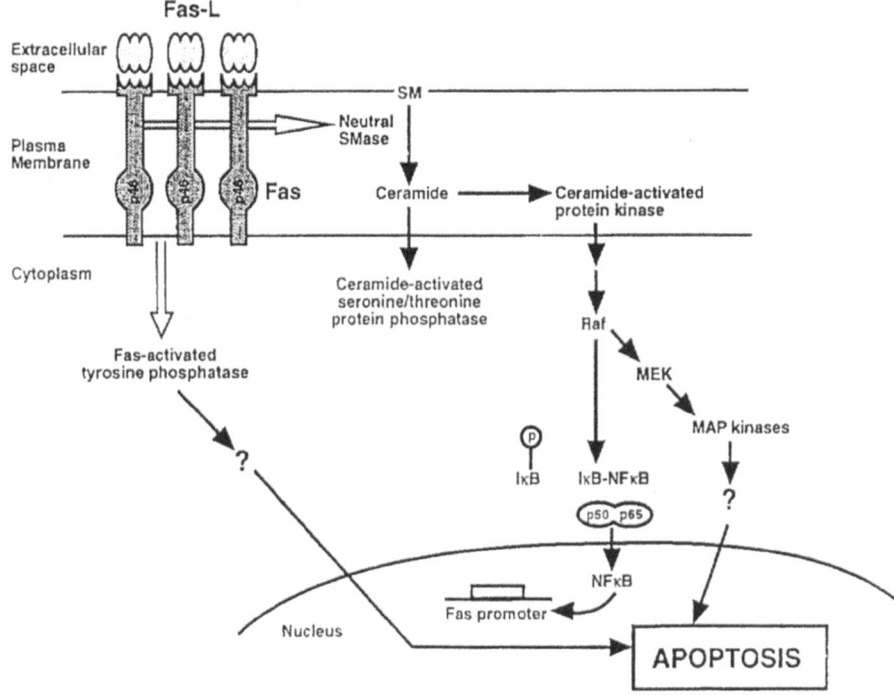

Figure 11. Proposed Fas signaling pathways. Fas-L forms a trimer which crosslinks the cell surface Fas molecule. This leads to intracellular signaling utilizing a phosphatase signaling pathway and a sphingomyelinase signaling pathway.

SUMMARY

Autoimmunity and AIDS both share the common feature of increased expression of retroviral protein products and abnormal apoptosis of immune cells (81). This leads to a more global immunomodulatory defect (82-84). The challenge in the future will be to devise compounds that can either regulate the effect of the retroviral products on apoptosis, or that can inhibit apoptosis pathways in order to restore normal immune system function.

ACKNOWLEDGEMENTS

We thank Dr. M. Luo for performing 3D structure analysis of mouse Fas Ligand, Dr. W.J. Koopman, Dr. S. Gay, and Dr. N. Talal for helpful discussions and B.K. Bunn for expert secretarial assistance in typing the manuscript. This work was supported in part by a VA Merit Review Award, a VA Career Development Award, P60 AR20614, P50 AI23694, P01 AR03555, R01 AI30744 from the National Institutes of Health.

REFERENCES

1. Krieg, A. M., Gause, W. C., Gourley, M. F. and Steinberg, A. D. 1989. A role for endogenous retroviral sequences in the regulation of lymphocyte activation. *J. Immunol.* 143:2448-2451.

2. Kreig, A. M., Gourley, M. F. and Steinberg, A. D. 1991. Association of murine lupus and thymic full-length endogenous retroviral expression maps to a bone marrow stem cell. *J. Immunol.* 146:3002-3006.

3. Gourley, M. F., Kisch, W. J., Mojcik, C. F., King, L. B., Krieg, A. M. and Steinberg, A. D. 1992. Molecular aspects of system lupus erythematosus: murine endogenous retroviral expression. *Cell Biol.* 11:253-264.

4. Hebebrand, L. C., Olsen, R. G., Mathes, L. E. and Nichols, W. S. 1979. Inhibition of human lymphocyte mitogen and antigen response by a 15,000 dalton protein from feline leukemia virus. *Cancer Res.* 39:443-447.

5. Orosz, C. G., Zinn, N. E., Olsen, R. G. and Mathes, L. E. 1985. Retrovirus-mediated immunosuppression II. FeLV-UV alters *in vitro* murine T lymphocyte behavior by reversibly impairing lymphokine secretion. *J. Immunol.* 135:583-590.

6. Cianciolo, G. J., Matthews, T. J., Bologneis, D. P. and Snyderman, R. 1980. Macrophage accumulation in mice is inhibited low molecular weight products from murine leukemia viruses. *J. Immunol.* 124:2900-2905.

7. Schmidt, D. M., Sidhu, N. K., Cianciolo, G. J. and Snyderman, R. 1987. Recombinant hydrophilic region of murine retroviral protein p15E inhibits stimulated T-lymphocyte proliferation. *Proc. Natl. Acad. Sci, USA.* 84:7290-7294.

8. Ruegg, C. L., Monell, C. R. and Strand, M. 1989. Identification, using synthetic peptides, of the minimum amino acid sequence from the retroviral transmembrane protein p15E required for inhibition of lympho-proliferation and its similarity to gp21 of human T-lymphotrophic virus types I and II. *J. Virol.* 63:3250-3256.

9. Cianciolo, G. J., Copeland, T. D., Oroszlan, S. and Snyderman, R. 1985. Inhibition of lymphocyte proliferation by a synthetic peptide homologous to retroviral envelope proteins. *Science* 230:453-455.

10. Harris, D. T., Cianciolo, G. J., Snyderman, R., Argov, S. and Koren,H. S. 1987. Inhibition of human natural killer cell activity by a synthetic peptide homologous to a conserved region in the retroviral protein, p15E. *J. Immunol.* 138:889-894.

11. Gottlieb, R. A., Lennarz, W. J., Knowles, R. D., Cianciolo, G. J., Dinarello, C. A., Lachman, L. B. and Kleinerman, E. S. 1989. Synthetic peptide corresponding to a conserved domain of the retroviral protein p15E blocks IL-1-mediated signal transduction. *J. Immunol.* 142:4321-4328.

12. Cianciolo, G. J., Bogerd, H. and Snyderman, R. 1988. Human retrovirus-related synthetic peptides inhibit T lymphocyte proliferation. *Immunol. Letters* 19:7-14.

13. Ruegg, C. L., Monell, C. R. and Strand, M. 1989. Inhibition of Lymphoproliferation by a synthetic peptide with sequence identity to gp41 of human immunodeficiency virus type I. *J. Virol.* 63:3257-3260.

14. Chattopadhyay, S. K., Morse, III, H. C., Makino, M., Ruscetti, S. K. and Hartley, J. W. 1989. Defective virus is associated with induction of murine retrovirus-induced immunodeficiency syndrome. *Proc. Natl. Acad. Sci. USA* 86:3862-3866.

15. Siekevitz, M., Feinberg, M. B., Holbrook, N., Wong-Staal, F. and Greene, W. C. 1987. Activation of interleukin 2 and interleukin 2 receptor (Tac) promoter expression by the trans-activator (tat) gene product of human T-cell leukemia virus type I. *Proc. Natl. Acad. Sci., USA* 84:5389-5393.

16. Leung, K. and Nabel, G. J. 1988. HTLV-I transactivator induces interleukin-2 receptor expression through an NF-κB-like factor. *Nature* 333: 776-778.

17. Green, J. E., Hinrichs, S. H., Vogel, J. and Jay, G. 1989. Exocrinopathy resembling Sjogren's syndrome in HTLV-I *tax* transgenic mice. *Nature* 341:72-74.

18. Wilson, L. D., Flyer, D. C. and Faller, D. V. 1987. Murine retroviruses control class I major histocom-patibility antigen gene expression via a *trans* effect at the transcriptional level. *Mol. Cell Biol.* 7:2406-2415.

19. Merulo, D., Nimelstein, S. H., Jones, P. P., Lieberman, M. and McDevitt, H. O. 1978. Increased synthesis and expression of H-2 antigens on thymocytes as a result of radiation leukemia virus infection: a possible mechanism for H-2 linked control of virus-induced neoplasia. *J. Exp. Med.* 147:470-487.

20. Wettstein, P. J., Colombo, M. P. and Jaenisch, R. 1988. Non-H-2 histocompatibility antigens encoded by Moloney-murine leukemia virus in MOV mouse strains are detectable by skin grafting and cytolytic T lymphocytes. *J. Immunol.* 140:4337-4341.

21. Plotz, P. H. 1983. Autoantibodies are anti-idiotype antibodies to antiviral antibodies. *Lancet* ii:824-826.

22. Gaulton, G. N. and Greene, M. I. 1989. Inhibition of cellular DNA synthesis by retrovirus occurs through a receptor-linked signaling pathway that is mimicked by anti-idiotypic, antireceptor antibody. *J. Exp. Med.* 169:197-211.

23. Query, C. C. and Keene J. D. 1987. A human autoimmune protein associated with U1 RNA contains a region of homology that is cross-reactive with retroviral p30 *gag* antigen. *Cell* 51:211-220.

24. Golding, H., Robey, F. A., Gates, III, F. T., Linder, W., Beining, P. R., Hoffman, T. and Golding, B. 1988. Identification of homologous regions in human immunodeficiency virus I gp41 and human MHC class

II β1 domain. I. Monoclonal antibodies against the gp41-derived peptide and patients' sera react with native HLA class II antigens, suggesting a role for autoimmunity in the pathogenesis of acquired immune deficiency syndrome. *J. Exp. Med.* 167:914-923.

25. Golding, H., Shearer, G. M., Hillman, K., Luca, P., Manischewitz, J. R., Zajac, A., Clerici, M. M., Gress, R. E., Boswell, R. N. and Golding,B. 1989. Common epitope in human immunodeficiency virus (HIV) I-gp41 and HLA class II elicits immunosuppressive autoantibodies capable of contributing to immune dysfunction in HIV-infected individuals. *J. Clin. Invest.* 83:1430-1435.

26. Maul, G. G., Jimenez, S. A., Riggs, E. and Ziemnicka-Kotula, D. 1989. Determination of an epitope of the diffuse systemic sclerosis marker antigen DNA topoisomerase I-sequence similarity with retroviral p30*gag* protein suggests a possible cause for autoimmunity in systemic sclerosis. *Proc. Natl. Acad. Sci., USA* 86:8492-8496.

27. Fujinami, R. S. and Oldstone, M. B. A. 1985. Amino acid homology between the encephalitogenic site of myelin basic protein and virus: mechanism for autoimmunity. *Science* 230:1043-1045.

28. Siliciano, R. F., Lawton, T., Knall, C., Karr, R. W., Berman, P., Gregory, T. and Reinherz E. L. 1988. Analysis of host-virus interactions in AIDS with anti-gp120 T-cell clones: effect of HIV sequence variation and mechanism for CD4+ cell depletion. *Cell* 54:561-575.

29. Adams, T. E., Alpert, S. and Hanahan, D. 1987. Non-tolerance and autoantibodies to a transgenic self antigen expressed in pancreatic-β cells. *Nature* 325:223-228.

30. Leiter, E. H., Fewell, J. W. and Kuff, E. L. 1986. Glucose induces intracisternal type A retroviral gene transcription and translation in pancreatic β cells. *J. Exp. Med.* 163:87-100.

31. Acha-Orbea, H. and Palmer, E. 1991. Mls-a retrovirus exploits the immune system. *Immunol. Today* 12:356-361.

32. Ambros/Hugin, W. H., Vacchio, M. S. and Morse, H. C., III. 1991. A virus-encoded "superantigen" in a retrovirus-induced immunodeficiency syndrome of mice. *Science* 252:424-431.

33. Talal, N., Flescher, E. and Dang, H. 1992. Evidence of possible retroviral involvement in autoimmune disease. *Ann. Allergy* 69:1-4.

34. Talal, N., Garry, R. F., Schur, P. H., Alexander, S., Dauphinee, M. J., Livas, I. H., Ballester, A., Takei, M. and Dang, H. 1990. A conserved idiotype and antibodies to retroviral proteins in systemic lupus erythematosus. *J. Clin. Invest.* 85:1866-1871.

35. H. Dang., Dauphinee, M. J., Talal, N., Garry, R. F. and Alexander, S. 1991. Serum antibodies to retroviral *gag* in systemic sclerosis. *Arth. Rheum.* 34:1336-1343.

36. Talal, N., Dauphinee, M. J., Dang, H., Alexander, S., Hart, D. J. and Garry, R.F. 1990. Detection of serum antibodies to retroviral proteins in patients with primary Sjogrens syndrome (autocrine exocrinopathy). *Arth. Rheum.* 33:774-781.

37. DeKeyser, F. S., Hoch, O., Takei, M., Dang, H., DeKeyser, H., Rokeach, C. O. and Talal, N. 1992. Cross-reactivity of B/B' subunit of the Sm ribonucleoprotein autoantigen with proline-rich polypeptides. *Clin. Immunol. Immunopathol.* 62:285-290.

38. Yang, J. -N. and Dudley, J. 1992. Endogenous Mtv-8 or a closely linked sequence stimulates rearrangement of the downstream Vκ9 gene. *J. Immunol.* 149:1242-1251.

39. Zhu, Z. B., Hsieh, S. L., Bentley, D. R., Campbell, R. D. and Volanakis, J. E. 1992. A variable number of tandem repeats locus within the human complement C2 gene is associated with a retrotransposon derived from a human endogenous retrovirus. *J. Exp. Med.* 175:1783-1787.

40. Stelmmeyei, K., Klocke, R., Ortland, C., Gronemeier, M., Jockusch, H., Grunder, S. and Jentsch, T. J. 1991. Inactivation of muscle chloride channel by transposon insertion in myotonic mice. *Nature* 354:304-308.

41. Baughman, G., Harrigan, M. T., Campbell, N. F., Nurrish, S. J. and Bourgeois, S. 1991. Genes newly identified as regulated by glucocorticoids in murine thymocytes. *Mol. Endocrinol.* 5:637-644.

42. Weiss, S. and Johansson, B. 1989. Integration of the transposon-like element *ETn* upstream of Vλ 2 in the cell line P3X63Ag8. *J. Immunol.* 143:2384-2391.

43. Shell, B., Szurek, P. and Dunnick, W. 1987. Interruption of two immunoglobulin heavy-chain switch regions in murine plasmacytoma P3.26Bu4 by insertion of retrovirus-like element ETn. *Mol. Cell. Biol.* 7:1364-1370.

44. Elliott, E., Rathbun, D., Ramsingh, A., Garberi, J. and Flaherty, L. 1989. Genetics and expression of the Q6 and Q8 genes. An LTR-like sequence in the 3' untranslated region. *Immunogenet.* 29:371-379.

45. Cohen, P. L. and Eisenberg R. A. 1991. *Lpr* and *gld*: single gene models of systemic autoimmunity and lymphoproliferation. *Ann. Rev. Immunol.* 9:243-269.

46. Watanabe-Fukunaga, R., Brannan C. I., Copeland, N. G., Jenkins, N. A. and Nagata S. 1992. Lymphoproliferation disorder in mice explained by defects in Fas antigen that mediates apoptosis. *Nature* 356:314-318.

47. Watson, M. L., Rao, J. K., Gilkeson, G. S., Ruiz, P., Eicher, E. M., Pisetsky, D. S., Matsuzawa, A., Rochelle, J. M. and Seldin, M. F. 1992. Genetic analysis of MRL-*lpr* mice: relationship of the Fas apoptosis gene to disease manifestations and renal disease-modifying loci. *J. Exp. Med.* 176:145-150.

48. Wu, J., Zhou, T., He, J. and Mountz, J. D. 1993. Autoimmune disease in mice due to integration of an endogenous retrovirus in an apoptosis gene. *J. Exp. Med.* 178:461-468.

49. Greaves, D. R., Wilson, F. D., Lang, G. and Kioussis, D. 1989. Human CD2 3′-flanking sequences confer high-level, T cell-specific, position-independent gene expression in transgenic mice. *Cell* 56:979-986.

50. Wu, J., Zhou, T., Zhang, J., He, J., Gause, W. C. and Mountz, J. D. 1994. Correction of accelerated autoimmune disease by early replacement of the mutated *lpr* gene with the normal *fas* apoptosis gene in the T cells of transgenic MRL-*lpr/lpr* mice. *Proc. Natl. Acad. Sci., USA* 91:2344-2348.

51. Mountz, J. D., Zhou, T., Eldridge, J., Berry, K. and Blüthmann, H. 1990. Transgenic rearranged T-cell receptor gene inhibits lymphadenopathy and accumulation of CD4⁻CD8⁻CD8⁻B220⁺ T cells in MRL-*lpr/lpr* mice. *J. Exp. Med.* 172:1805-1817.

52. Zhou, T., Blüthmann, H., Eldridge, J., Berry, K. and Mountz, J. D. 1993. Origin of CD4⁻CD8⁻B220⁺ T cells in MRL-*lpr/lpr* mice: clues from a TCR β mouse. *J. Immunol.* 150:3651-3667.

53. Huesmann, M., Scott, B., Kisielow, P. and von Boehmer, H. 1991. Kinetics and efficacy of positive selection in the thymus of normal and T cell receptor transgenic mice. *Cell* 66:533-539.

54. Teh, H. S., Kishi, H., Scott, B., Borgulya, P., von Boehmer, H. and Kisielow, P. 1992. Early deletion and late positive selection of T cells expressing a male-specific receptor in T-cell receptor transgenic mice. *Dev. Immunol.* 1:1-22.

55. Uematsu, Y., Ryser, S., Dembic, Z., Borgulya, P., Krimpenfort, P., Berns, A., von Boehmer, H. and Steinmetz, H. 1988. In transgenic mice the introduced functional T cell receptor beta gene prevents expression of endogenous beta genes. *Cell* 52:831-837.

56. Thompson, C. B., Wang, C. Y., Ho, I. C., Bohjanen, P. R., Petryniak, B., June, C. H., Miesfeldt, S., Zhang, L., Nabel, G. J. and Karpinski, B. 1992. *cis*-acting sequences required for inducible interleukin-2 enhancer function bind a novel Ets-related protein, Elf-1. *Mol. Cell. Biol.* 12:1043-1056.

57. Wang, C. Y., Petryniak, B., Ho, I. C., Thompson, C. B. and Deiden, J. M. 1992. Evolutionarily conserved Ets family members display distinct DNA binding specificities. *J. Exp. Med.* 175:1391-1398.

58. Leiden, J. M, Wang, C. Y, Petryniak, B., Markovitz, D. M., Nabel, G. J. and Thompson, C. B. 1992. A novel Cts-related transcription factor, Elf-1, binds to human immunodeficiency virus type 2 regulatory elements that are required for inducible transactivation in T cells. *J Virol* 66:5890-5994.

59. Bosselut, R., Duvall, J. F., Gegonne, A., Bailly, M., Hemar, A., Brady, J. and Ghysdael, J. 1990. The product of the c-ets-1 proto-oncogene and the related Ets2 protein act as transcriptional activators of the long terminal repeat of human T cell leukemia virus HTLV-1. *EMBO J* 9:3137-3149.

60. Itoh, N., Yonehara, S., Ishii, A., Yonehara, M., Mizushima, S.I., Sameshima, M., Hase, A., Seto, Y. and Nagata,S. 1991. The polypeptide encoded by the cDNA for human cell surface antigen Fas can mediate apoptosis. *Cell* 66:233-243.

61. Fernandez-Botran, R. 1991. Soluble cytokine receptors: their role in immunoregulation. *FASEB J.* 5:2567-2574.

62. Josimovic-Alasevic, O., Herrmann, T. and Diamantstein, T. 1988. Demonstrations of two distinct forms of released low-affinity type interleukin 2 receptors. *Eur. J. Immunol.* 18:1855-1857.

63. Schall, T. J., Lewis, M., Koller, K. J., Lee, A., Rice, G. C., Wong, G. W. H., Gatanaga, T., Granger, G. A., Lentz, R., Raab, H., Kohr, W. J. and Goeddel, D. V. 1990. Molecular cloning and expression of a receptor for human tumor necrosis factor. *Cell* 61:361-370.

64. Mosley, B., Beckmann, M. P., March, C. J., Idzerda, R. L., Gimpel, S. D., VandenBos, T., Friend, D., Alper, A., Anderson, D., Jackson, J., Wignall, J. M., Smith, C., Gallis, B., Sims, J. E., Urdal, D., Widmer, M. B. and Park, L. S. 1989. The murine interleukin-4 receptor: molecular cloning and characterization of secreted and membrane bound forms. *Cell* 59:335-348.

65. Goodwin, R. G., Friend, D., Ziegler, S. F., Jerzy, R., Falk, B. A., Gompel, S., Cosman, D., Dower, S. K., March, C. J., Namen, A. E. and Park, L. S. 1990. Cloning of the human and murine interleukin-7 receptors: demonstration of a soluble form and homology to a new receptor superfamily. *Cell* 60:941-951.

66. Itoh, N. and Nagata, S. 1993. A novel protein domain required for apoptosis. Mutational analysis of human Fas antigen. *J. Biol. Chem.* 268:10932-10937.

67. Cheng, J., Zhou, T., Liu, C., Shapiro, J. P., Brauer, M. J., Kiefer, M. C., Barr, P. J. and Mountz, J. D. 1994. Protection from Fas-mediated apoptosis by a soluble form of the Fas molecule. *Science* 263:1759-1762.

68. Krowka, J. F., Cuevas, B., Ascher, M. S. and Sheppard, H. W. 1994. Increased soluble Fas in AIDS. *J. Immunol.*, submitted for publication.

69. Suda, T., Takahashi, T., Golstein, P. and Nagata, S. 1993. Molecular cloning and expression of the Fas ligand, a novel member of the tumor necrosis factor family. *Cell* 75:1169-1178.

70. Takahashi, T., Tanaka, M., Brannan, C. I., Jenkins, N. A., Copeland, N. G., Suda, T. and Nagata, S. 1994. Generalized lymphoproliferative disease in mice, caused by a point mutation in the Fas ligand. *Cell* 76:969-976.

71. Suda, T. and Nagata, S. 1994. Purification and characterization of the Fas-ligand that induces apoptosis. *J. Exp. Med.* 179:873-879.

72. Trauth, B. C., Klas, C., Peters, A. M. J., Matzuku, S., Moller, P., Falk, W., Debatin, K. -M. and Krammer, P. H. 1989. Monoclonal antibody-mediated tumor regression by induction of apoptosis. *Science* (Wash. DC). 245:301-312.

73. Yonehara, S., Ishii, A. and Yonehara, M. 1989. A cell-killing monoclonal antibody (anti-Fas) to a cell surface antigen co-downregulated with the receptor of tumor necrosis factor. *J. Exp. Med.* 169:1747-1753.

74. Su, X., Zhou, T., Wu, J., Jope, R. and Mountz, J. D. 1994. Dephosphorylation of a 65 Kd protein associated with a signal for Fas mediated apoptosis. *J. Immunol.* 152:A3004.

75. Pumiglia, K. M., Lau, L., Huang, C., Burroughs, S. and Feinstein, M. B. 1992. Activation of signal transduction in platelets by the tyrosine phosphatase inhibitor pervanadate (vanadyl hydroperoxide). *Biochem. J.* 286:441-450.

76. Oehm, A., Behrmann, I., Falk, W., Pawlita, M., Maier, G., Klas, C., Li-Weber, M., Richards, S., Dhein, J., Trauth, B. C., Ponstingl, H. and Krammer, P. H. 1989. Purification and molecular cloning of the APO-1 cell surface antigen, a member of the tumor necrosis factor/nerve growth factor receptor family. *J. Biol. Chem.* 267:10709-10714.

77. Kolesnick, R. and Golde, D. W. 1994. The sphingomyelin pathway in tumor necrosis factor and interleukin-1 signaling. *Cell* 77:325-327.

78. Mathias, S., Dressler, K. A. and Kolesnick, R. N. 1991. Characterization of a ceramide-activated protein kinase: stimulation by tumor necrosis factor a. *Proc. Natl. Acad. Sci. USA.* 88:10009-10014.

79. Ballou, L. R. 1992. Spingolipids and cell function. *Immunol. Today* 13:339-342.

80. Alderson, M. R., Armitage, R. J., Maraskovsky, E., Tough, T. W., Roux, E., Schooley, K., Ramsdell, F. and Lynch, D.H. 1993. Fas transduces activation signals in normal human T lymphocytes. *J. Exp. Med.* 178:2231-2238.

81. Gougeon, M. L., Laurent-Crawford, A. G., Hovanessian, A. G. and Montagnier, L. 1993. Direct and indirect mechanisms mediating apoptosis during HIV infection: contribution to *in vivo* CD4 T cell depletion. *Seminars in Immunol.* 5:187-194.

82. Walker, C. M. 1993. Non-cytolytic control of HIV replication by CD8+ T cells. *Seminars in Immunol.* 5:195-201.

83. Poli, G. and Fauci, A. S. 1993. Cytokine modulation of HIV expression. *Seminars in Immunol.* 5:165-173.

84. Clark, S. J. and Shaw, G. M. 1993. The acute retroviral syndrome and the pathogenesis of HIV-1 infection. *Seminars in Immunol.* 5:149-155.

17

AIDS AS IMMUNE SYSTEM ACTIVATION
Key questions that remain

Michael S. Ascher, Haynes W. Sheppard, John F. Krowka, and
Hans J. Bremermann

Viral and Rickettsial Disease Laboratory
California Department of Health Services
Berkeley, California 94704

INTRODUCTION

Since 1987, when we first formulated the hypothesis that AIDS and HIV disease are
the result of inappropriate immune system activation triggered by viral gp120 signalling at
CD4 [1-3], the concept has been supported by several developments. First is a better
understanding of the natural history of HIV disease. Second is the elucidation of the role of
CD4 in T cell activation. Third is the appreciation of the prominent role of programmed cell
death or apoptosis in the normal dynamic equilibrium of the immune system. Last is the
failure of antiviral strategies to affect the clinical course of disease in infected individuals.

We present herein our current view of the following critical questions that remain in
fully understanding AIDS as an activation disease: What is the source of the signal? What
is the role of CD4 in the immune system? What is the natural history for which we are trying
to develop models? Does HIV kill T cells in vivo? What is the regenerative capacity of the
immune system? Is the apoptosis seen in HIV infection special? What is the role of
superantigens in the HIV disease process? What are the implications for treatment?

Answers to these questions should allow us to shift the paradigm from the view that
AIDS is a conventional cytopathic viral disease to the view that the CD4 component of the
immune system can be completely destroyed by false physiological signalling, and lead to
the practical goal of a safe, effective and rational therapy for this inexorably fatal infection.

WHAT IS THE SOURCE OF THE SIGNAL?

The first question to be addressed is the source of the activation of the immune
system. Since our initial reviews, a large number of further examples of activation phenomena in HIV disease have appeared [4-8]. Several different potential sources have been
identified, recalling in some cases Sonnabend's original hypothesis that multiple concurrent
infectious diseases present in the affected individuals might effectively burn out the immune
system through overstimulation [9]. This idea was generally ignored after the discovery of

HIV but the discoverer of the virus has actually reemphasized it in the form of a role for mycoplasma in HIV disease progression [10]. It is unclear whether a mycoplasma cofactor has any role in controlled studies [11,12]. Another view of the source of the activation is that autoimmunity is triggered by molecular mimicry [13-16], and that reverberating circuits of response and response to response may be occurring [17]. A variant of this idea invokes an analogy with graft-versus-host disease, with the virus being either a modified host or serving as the graft [18]. More recently, the identification of the prototypical superantigen (Mls) as a retroviral product has led to the suggestion that HIV may encode a superantigen and act through a similar mechanism [19]. From our earliest publications, we have considered it most likely that HIV itself, through its glycoprotein gp120, with high affinity binding to the cellular CD4, provides a costimulatory signal contributing to T cell activation by lowering the threshold of the receptor complex [20]. This proposal predated a better appreciation of the functional role of CD4, which is now well established, as follows.

WHAT IS THE ROLE OF CD4?

A key feature of our early papers is the idea that the CD4 molecule has a central role in T cell activation. It had previously been identified as the phenotypic marker of a critical T cell population but was felt to be simply an adhesion molecule that facilitated cell to cell contact. It is now recognized as a major coreceptor contributing to the T cell receptor complex signalling mechanism by providing a critical regulatory threshold for T cell activation [21,22]. Ironically, the studies of the CD4 receptor which defined its functional activity, in the form of calcium mobilization effects, actually employed gp120 as the binding element [23]. Others have disputed these effects and been unable to reproduce these results under different conditions [24]. A recent study utilizing a mouse transgenic for human CD4 has shown the sort of CD4 depletion that is predicted by our model [25].

WHAT IS THE NATURAL HISTORY OF HIV DISEASE WE ARE TRYING TO MODEL?

The next critical question that one must answer in attempting to understand HIV pathogenesis is what is the natural history we are trying to model. A sequence of papers illustrates the evolution of the thinking in this area [26-31]. In the first analyses of data from HIV-infected subjects, cross-sectional data indicated that sick individuals had larger amounts of virus and more healthy individuals had less virus. The idea was then advanced that the natural history therefore included a virologic latency preceding an explosive emergence of virus, with destruction of the immune system [32]. This was the main rationale for the use of AZT. Based on continuing analysis of cross-sectional data, the burden obsession contin- ues, in that investigators are continually trying to show higher and higher viral burdens in the course of progression [33-41]. In our own studies, viral burden was an important factor in defining progression [42]. In the composite, a high mean burden early in disease is a bad prognosticator and a low mean burden a good prognosticator but large overlap is present and there is little change over time. It is the change over time and its translation into the underlying mechanism that we have questioned [43,44].

Later in our understanding of HIV natural history we began to adopt the view that the immune system undergoes a gradual but steady erosion throughout the entire "clinical latent period", with a variable course determined at the onset by immune response and degree of immune activation [45,46]. One unanswered questions from this model is whether the early loss of about 400 cells on the average is indeed an absolute loss of T cells or simply a tissue redistribution in response to persistent viral signalling.

DOES HIV KILL T CELLS IN VIVO?

The next question to answer in a full understanding of the HIV process is whether virus kills T cells at all *in vivo*. *In vitro* experiments which put virus together with cells in rather unphysiological conditions such as crowding and mitogen activation will produce killing. One very intriguing experiment using a single virus and cell preparation showed that T cells could either be killed or expanded clonally depending on the conditions [47]. *In vitro* studies can't answer the question definitively, but the variability of cell killing by HIV under physiologic conditions suggests that direct virus-mediated cytopathology is of little importance in HIV pathogenesis. The model we have proposed does not require it and suggests that most of the cells that are lost in the course of infection are actually uninfected. This is reflected in studies in which 10 times more apoptotic cells are present in HIV-infected individuals compared to infected cells [48]. Our view of normal T cell dynamics indicates that many more T cells die during everyday immune responses than are ever infected. A different way to look at this problem, in light of the relative stability of burden in the face of overall loss of T cell numbers, is that the infected T cell population might be stable in number, immortal and antigenic-specific [1]. This might explain the V-beta preference in the growth of virus in cells [49]. This idea has dramatic implications for the control of the infection, leading to the possibility that a clonal deletion could eliminate a home for the virus and be the ultimate sort of immunity. One interesting feature of recent experiments in SCID-hu mice is the finding that virus strains with the most prominent *in vitro* cytopathic effects are the mildest in this system and vice versa [50].

WHAT IS THE REGENERATIVE CAPACITY OF THE IMMUNE SYSTEM?

If the dynamic equilibrium of the immune system is the central process that is destabilized in HIV infection, the key question in this system is what is the regenerative capacity of the immune system [51-53]. Many studies say it is very large, in that it is possible to remove approximately 1% of the T cell population every day, and get very little short term effect on T cell numbers and rapid recovery when the removal is stopped [54]. It is therefore hard to understand how a very low infectious virus burden can kill such a resilient system. We have suggested that the critical feature in the dynamic stability of a T cell population, revealed by experiments of T cell cloning, is the recovery of memory cells from previous responses. Thymic replacement of specificities from potential stem cells is not the primary source of new T cells in the adult periphery. Thus HIV, by interfering with the recovery of memory cells, causes the loss of the total system. This proposed feature of immunologic memory is not established, but clearly it is an important issue that must be addressed in the course of our understanding AIDS.

WHAT IS THE RELATIONSHIP TO APOPTOSIS OR PROGRAMMED CELL DEATH?

The next question that arises is based on the observation that programmed cell death or apoptosis is increased in HIV disease [48,55-60]. The questions that result from this finding are whether the apoptosis seen with HIV infection is special and why is the frequency of lymphocyte death in HIV-infected individuals orders of magnitude greater than the frequency of HIV-infected cells?. In our view, as above, it is the normal dominant phenomenon of the immune system for T cell progeny to die. This prevents the development of lymphoma from everyday responses [61,62]. An increased rate of apoptosis just reflects a heightened activation/heightened destruction as in the case of CD8's, and should not be associated with the death of the population [53,63,64]. It is not how many new cells are made and then killed but the survival of precursors for the next response that matters. It is not the cells that die that are important but the cells that survive. Recent studies have indicated that CD4 signalling has the ability to delete memory cells but the mechanism has not been defined [65].

WHAT IS THE RELATIONSHIP TO SUPERANTIGENS?

The identification of retroviral components as the superantigen responsible for the Mls phenomenon in mice emphasizes that viral products can have major effects on the immune system, including clonal deletion. This system is the basis for a number of models including immunologic tolerance [66-70]. There are clearly some major differences from HIV in that the target cells of an individual superantigen have V-beta specificity [71]. The preliminary findings of V-beta restriction for HIV loss have not been substantiated by further studies [72-74]. In our view, HIV gp120 is analogous to a superantigen, but instead of effecting a specific subpopulation of T cells, it signals the coreceptor of all the CD4 cells [75]. One useful feature of thinking of HIV from the superantigen perspective is that the signal intensity can be variable, ranging from a virus like PBJ14 which is rapidly pathogenic for primates, to HIV in chimpanzees which appears not to cause discernible disease in the face of chronic infection. Our model would predict that HIV and SIV strains with higher affinity for CD4 would be more virulent than weaker ones. In conclusion, we consider it unlikely that a separate superantigen is present in HIV, and we can account for all of the phenomena simply by the gp120 signalling at CD4 [76].

WHAT ARE IMPLICATIONS FOR TREATMENT?

The last question that derives from the model we have outlined is what are the implications for treatment. A strategy aimed at blocking excess activation is implicit. This approach is similar to providing antipyretics to someone with fever. It is not the goal to lower the body temperature below normal but simply to restore the normal state. Thus, suppression, or particularly, immunosuppression, is not the goal. One such approach has used an anticytokine, pentoxiphylline [77-79]. Cyclosporin (CsA) has been used extensively for this purpose with mixed results. After an initial trial showed promise in relatively early infection [80], a later uncontrolled trial in AIDS cases claimed adverse effects and cooled the enthusiasm from the earlier studies [81]. Further followup of CsA recipients continues to show promise [82] and further *in vitro* work with related drugs shows positive effects [83]. A rather remarkable study of transplant recipients has shown little or no adverse effects of using CsA in HIV-infected transplants, and perhaps a slight benefit [84]. Thus, the issue is not settled and is clearly worthy of further study.

In the course of such studies, it is critical to select patients who have signs and laboratory markers of activation and make sure that the trial design is stratified on these levels. This was not done in previous trials of CsA and may partially explain the absence of consistent effects in various trials. It is also critical to measure activation markers serially and correlate them with things like levels of programmed cell death. This has only been done on a limited scale [85]. Next, the dose needed to reduce HIV-inducted activation may be very different from that required to produce transplant survival and drugs deemed weak in their activity towards protecting a transplant may have sufficient activity in reducing the HIV signal. It is also possible that an intermittent dosing schedule could minimize from toxic side-effects. In the course of all of our thinking toward treatment it is critical to remember and avoid the *in vivo/in vitro* paradox, in which an individual may appear to have a deficient response *in vitro* because of a maximal response *in vivo*. For example, T cells are deficient in their production of IL-2 when removed from the HIV-infected subjects and it was a natural thought to prescribe IL-2. If, on the other hand, the system is overstimulated *in vivo* and has too much IL-2 contributing to the immunopathogenesis, giving more would certainly not be a good idea. One must be careful in both the design and evaluation of treatments to understand the relationship between *in vivo* and *in vitro* events. If one were to approach apoptosis directly as a target for therapy [86-88], it is possible that release of CD8 cells from the dominant and protective cell death may result in immunopathologic consequences [89]

SUMMARY

Immune system activation is gaining attention as a central part of HIV pathogenesis. Although there is no consensus yet as to the source of the signal or the result of the signalling, this line of thinking represents a significant shift in the paradigm away from considering HIV disease like any other cytopathic viral infection. Hopefully, completion of studies focussed on this approach will lead to more complete understanding of AIDS and more effective therapies, and will at least bring to the fore some of the central unanswered questions in modern cellular immunology.

REFERENCES

1. Ascher MS, Sheppard HW. AIDS as immune system activation: a model for pathogenesis. Clin Exp Immunol 1988;73:165-167.
2. Ascher MS, Sheppard HW. AIDS as immune system activation II: the panergic imnesia hypothesis. JAIDS 1990;3:177-191.
3. Sheppard HW, Ascher MS. The natural history and pathogenesis of HIV infection. Ann Rev Micro 1992;46:533-564.
4. Godfried MH, van der Poll T, Weverling GJ, Mulder JW, Jansen J, van Deventer SJH, Sauerwein HP. Soluble receptors for tumor necrosis factor as predictors of progression to AIDS in asymptomatic human immunodeficiency virus type 1 infection. J Inf Dis 1994;169:739-745.
5. Plaeger-Marshall S, Isacescu V, O'Rourke S, Bertoli J, Bryson YJ, Stiehm ER. T cell activation in pediatric AIDS pathogenesis: three-color immunophenotyping. Clin Immunol Immunopathol 1994;71:19-26.
6. Dondorp AM, Veenstra J, van der Poll T, Mulder JW, Reiss P. Activation of the cytokine network in a patient with AIDS and the recalcitrant erythematous desquamating disorder. Clin Inf Dis 1994;18:942-945.
7. Kestens L, Vanham G, Vereecken C, Vandenbruaene M, Vercauteren G, Colebunders RL, Gigase PL. Selective increase of activation antigens HLA-DR and CD38 on CD4+CD45RO+ T lymphocytes during HIV-1 infection. Clin Exp Immunol 1994;95:436-441.
8. Aukrust P, Liabakk NB, Muller F, Lien E, Espevik T, FrolandSS. Serum levels of tumor necrosis factor-alpha(TNF-alpha) and soluble TNF receptors in human immunodeficiency virus type 1 infection-correlations to clinical, immunologic, and virologic parameters. J Inf Dis 1994;169:420-424.
9. Sonnabend J, Witkin SS, Purtillo DT. Acquired immunodeficiency syndrome, opportunistic infections, and malignancies in male homosexuals. JAMA 1983;249:2370-2374.

10. Montagnier L, Blanchard A. Mycoplasma as cofactors in infection due to the human immunodeficiency virus. Clin Inf Dis 1993;17(Suppl 1):S309-S315.

11. Lo SC, Hayes MM, Wang RYH, Pierce PF, Kotani H, Shih JWK. Newly discovered mycoplasma isolated from patients infected with HIV. Lancet 1991;338:1415-1418.

12. Katseni VL, Gilroy CB, Ryait BK, Ariyoshi K, Bieniasz PD, Weber JN, Taylor-Robinson D. Mycoplasma fermentans in individuals seropositive and seronegative for HIV-1. Lancet 1993;341:271-273.

13. Andrieu JM, Even P, Vener A. AIDS and related syndromes as a viral-induced autoimmune disease of the immune system: an anti-MHC II disorder. AIDS Res 1986;2:163-174.

14. Even P, Venet A, Israel-Biet D, Tourani JM, Lowenstein W, Andrieu JM. Autoimmunity and immunopathy in viral diseases: an overview. In Autoimmune Aspects of HIV Infection, ed. J-M. Andrieu, J-F. Bach and P. Even, 1988, pp. 7-22. Pub. by Royal Soc. Med. Serv. Ltd.

15. Even P, Andrieu JM, Venet A, Beldjord K, Tourani JM, Israel-Biet D. The human immune deficiency virus disease (HIVD) as a virus-induced immunopathic and autoimmune disorder. In Autoimmune Aspects of HIV Infection, ed. J-M. Andrieu, J-F. Bach and P. Even, 1988, pp. 79-107. Pub. by Royal Soc. Med. Serv. Ltd.

16. Ziegler JL, Stites DP. Hypothesis: AIDS is an autoimmune disease directed at the immune system and triggered by a lymphotropic virus. Clin Immunol Immunopathol 1986;41:305-313.

17. Hoffmann GW, Kion TA, Grant MD. An idiotypic network model of AIDS immunopathogenesis. Proc Natl Acad Sci USA 1991;88:3060-3064.

18. Habeshaw JA. HLA mimicry by HIV-1 gp120 in the pathogenesis of AIDS. Immunol Today 1994;15:39-40.

19. Janeway C. Mls: makes a little sense. Nature 1991;349:459-461.

20. Ameglio F, Capobianchi MR, Castilletti C, Fei PC, Fais S, Trento E, Dianzani F. Recombinant gp120 induces IL-10 in resting peripheral blood mononuclear cells; correlation with the induction of other cytokines. Clin Exp Immunol 1994;95:455-458.

21. Janeway CA. The co-receptor function of CD4. Sem in Immunol 1991;3:153-160.

22. Janeway CA. The T cell receptor as a multicomponent signalling machine: CD4/CD8 coreceptors and CD45 in T cell activation. Ann Rev Imm 1992;10:645-674.

23. Neudorf SML, Jones MM, McCarthy BM, Harmony JAK, Choi EM. The CD4 molecule transmits biochemical information important in the regulation of T lymphocyte activity. Cell Immunol 1990;125:301-314.

24. Kaufmann R, Laroche D, Buchner K, et al. The HIV-1 surface protein gp120 has no effect on transmembrane signal transduction in T cells. JAIDS 1992;5:760-770.

25. Wang ZQ, Orlikowsky T, Dudhane A, et al. Deletion of T lymphocytes in human CD4 transgenic mice induced by HIV-gp120 and gp120-specific antibodies from AIDS patients. Eur J Immunol 1994;24:1553-1557.

26. Francis DP, Jaffe HW, Fultz PN, Getchell JP, McDougal JS, Feorino PM. The natural history of infection with the lymphadenopathy-associated virus human T-lymphotropic virus type III. Ann Intern Med 1985;103:719-722.

27. Fauci AS, Masur H, Gelmann EP, Markham PD, Hahn BH, Lane HC. The acquired immunodeficiency syndrome: an update. Ann Intern Med 1985;102:800-803.

28. Fauci AS. The human immunodeficiency virus: Infectivity and mechanisms of pathogenesis. Science 1988;239:617-622.

29. Fauci AS, Schnittman SM, Poli G, Koenig S, Pantaleo G. Immunopathogenic mechanisms in human immunodeficiency virus (HIV) infection. Ann Intern Med 1991;114:678-693.

30. Fauci AS. Immunopathogenesis of HIV infection. JAIDS 1993;6:655-662.

31. Fauci AS. Multifactorial nature of human immunodeficiency virus disease: implications for therapy. Science 1993;262:1011-1018.

32. Nowak MA, Anderson RM, McLean AR, Wolfs TFW, Goudsmit J, May RM. Antigenic diversity thresholds and the development of AIDS. Science 1991;254:963-969.

33. Piatak M, Saag MS, Yang LC, Clark SJ, et al. High levels of HIV-1 in plasma during all stages of infection determined by competitive PCR. Science 1993;259:1749-1754.

34. Maddox J. Where the AIDS virus hides away. Nature 1993;362:287.

35. Pantaleo G, Graziosi C, Demarest JF, et al. HIV infection is active and progressive in lymphoid tissue during the clinically latent stage of disease. Nature 1993;362:355-358.

36. Embretson J, Zupancic M, Ribas JL, Burke A, Racz P, Tenner-Racz K, Haase AT. Massive covert infection of helper T lymphocytes and macrophages by HIV during the incubation period of AIDS. Nature 1993;362:359-362.

37. Rosenberg YJ, Zack PM, Leon EC, et al. Immunological and virological changes associated with decline in CD4/CD8 ratios in lymphoid organs of SIV-infected macaques. AIDS Res Hum Retrovir 1994;10:863-

38. Chevret S, Kirstetter M, Mariotti M, Lefrere MF, Frottier J, Lefrere JJ. Provirus copy number to predict disease progression in asymptomatic human immunodeficiency virus type 1 infection. J Inf Dis 1994;169:882-885.

39. Schnittman SM, Greenhouse JJ, Psallidopoulos MC, et al. Increasing viral burden in CD4+ T cells from patients with human immunodeficiency virus (HIV) infection reflects rapidly progressive immunosuppression and clinical disease. Ann Intern Med 1990;113:438-443.

40. Lu W, Shih WK, Tourani JM, Eme D, Alter HJ, Andrieu JM. Lack of isolate-specific neutralizing activity is correlated with an increased viral burden in rapidly progressing HIV-1-infected patients. AIDS 1993;(suppl 2):S91-S99.

41. Nuovo GJ, Becker J, Burk MW, Margiotta M, Fuhrer J, Steigbigel RT. In situ detection of PCR-amplified HIV-1 nucleic acids in lymph nodes and peripheral blood in patients with asymptomatic HIV-1 infection and advanced stage AIDS. JAIDS 1994;7:916-923.

42. Lee TH, Sheppard HW, Reis M, Dondero D, Osmond D, Busch MP. Circulating HIV 1-infected cell burden from seroconversion to AIDS: importance of postseroconversion viral load on disease course. JAIDS 1994;7:381-388.

43. Ascher MS, Sheppard HW, Arnon JM, Lang W. Viral burden in HIV disease. JAIDS 1991;4:824-830.

44. Sheppard HW, Ascher MS, Krowka JF. Viral burden and HIV disease. Nature 1993;364:291.

45. Sheppard HW, Ascher MS, McRae B, Anderson RE, Lang W, Allain JP. The initial immune response to HIV and immune system activation determine the outcome of HIV disease. JAIDS 1991;4:704-712.

46. Simmonds P, Lainson FA, Cuthbert R, Steel CM, Peutherer JF, Ludlam CA. HIV antigen and antibody detection: variable responses to infection in the Edinburgh haemophiliac cohort. Br Med J 1988;296:593-598.

47. Langhoff E, McElrath J, Bos HJ, Pruett J, Granelli-Piperno A, Cohn ZA, Steinman RM. Most CD4+ T cells from human immunodeficiency virus-1 infected patients can undergo prolonged clonal expansion. J Clin Invest 1989;84:1637-1643.

48. Gougeon ML, Olivier R, Garcia S, Guetard D, Dragie T, Dauguet C, Montagnier L. Evidence for an engagement process towards apoptosis in lymphocytes of HIV-infected patients. Comptes Rendu 1991;312:529-537.

49. Laurence J, Hodtsev AS, Posnett DN. Superantigen implicated in dependence of HIV-1 replication in T cells on TCR V-beta expression. Nature 1992;358:255-259.

50. Mosier DE, Gulizia RJ, MacIsaac PD, Torbett BE, Levy JA. Rapid loss of CD4+ T cells in human-PBL-SCID mice by noncytopathic HIV isolates. Science 1993;260:689-692.

51. Michie CA, McLean A. Lymphocyte lifespan, immunological memory and retroviral infections. Immunol Today 1993;14:235.

52. Michie CA, McLean A, Alcock C, Beverley PCL. Lifespan of human lymphocyte subsets defined by CD45 isoforms. Nature 1992;360:264-265.

53. McLean A, Michie C. Viral burden in AIDS. Nature 1993;365:301.

54. Tough DF, Sprent J. Turnover of naive- and memory-phenotype T cells. J Exp Med 1994;179:1127-1135.

55. Ameisen JC, Capron A. Cell dysfunction and depletion in AIDS: the programmed cell death hypothesis. Immunol Today 1991;12:102-105.

56. Ameisen JC. Programmed cell death and AIDS: from hypothesis to experiment. Imm Today 1992;13:388-391.

57. Groux H, Monte D, Bourrez JM, Capron A, Ameisen JC. A mechanism for CD4+ T-cell dysfunction and depletion in AIDS: activation-induced programmed cell death by apoptosis. Immunology 1991;312:599-606.

58. Gougeon ML, Montagnier L. Apoptosis in AIDS. Science 1993;260:1269-1270.

59. Re MC, Zauli G, Gibellini et al. Uninfected haematopoietic progenitor (CD34+) cells purified from the bone marrow of AIDS patients are committed to apoptotic cell death in culture. AIDS 1993;7:1049-1055.

60. Banda NK, Bernier J, Kurahara DK, Kurrle R, Haigwood N, Sekaly RP, Finkel TH. Crosslinking CD4 by human immunodeficiency virus gp120 primes T cells for activation-induced apoptosis. J Exp Med 1992;176:1099-1106.

61. Kerr JFR, Wyllie AH, Currie AR. Apoptosis: a basic biological phenomena with wide-ranging implications in tissue kinetics. Br J Cancer 1972;26:239-257.

62. Iseki R, Mukai M, Iwata M. Regulation of T lymphocyte apoptosis. J Immunol 1991;147:4286-4292.

63. Sheppard HW, Ascher MS. AIDS and programmed cell death. Immunol Today 1999;12:423.

64. Lewis DE, Tang DSN, Adu-Oppong A, Schober W, Rodgers JR. Anergy and apoptosis in CD8+ T cells from HIV-infected persons. J Immunol 1994;153:412-420.

65. Howie SEM, Sommerfield AJ, Gray E, Harrison DJ. Peripheral T lymphocyte depletion by apoptosis after CD4 ligation in vivo: selective loss of CD44- and "activating" memory T cells. Clin Exp Imm 1994;95:195-200.

66. Palmer E. Infectious origins of superantigens: one of the mysteries of the Mls antigens of mice has been solved by the discovery that they are encoded by endogenous retroviruses. Curr Biol 1991;1:74-76.

67. Hugin AW, Vacchio MS, Morse HC. A virus-encoded "superantigen" in a retrovirus-induced immunodeficiency syndrome of mice. Science 1991;252:424-427.

68. Coffin JM. Superantigens and endogenous retroviruses: a confluence of puzzles. Science 1992;255:411-413.

69. McCormack JE, Callahan JE, Kappler J, Marrack PC. Profound deletion of mature T cells in vivo by chronic exposure to exogenous superantigen. J Immunol 1993;150:3785-3792.

70. Held W, Acha-Orbea H, MacDonald HR, Waanders GA. Superantigens and retroviral infection: insights from mouse mammary tumor virus. Immunol Today 1994;15:184-190.

71. Dadaglio G, Garcia S, Montagnier L, Gougeon ML. Selective anergy of VB8+ T cells in human immunodeficiency virus-infected individuals. J Exp Med 1994;179:413-424.

72. Imberti L, Sottini A, Bettinardi A, Puoti M, Primi D. Selective depletion in HIV infection of T cells that bear specific T cell receptor V-beta sequences. Science 1991;254:860-862.

73. Gougeon ML, Dadaglio G, Garcia S, Muller-Alouf H, Roue R, Montagnier L. Is a dominant superantigen involved in AID pathogenesis. Lancet 1993;342:50-51.

74. Weber GF, Cantor H. HIV glycoprotein as a superantigen. A mechanism of autoimmunity and implications for a vaccination strategy. Med Hypotheses 1993;41:247-250.

75. Sheppard HW, Ascher MS. Superantigens, alloreactivity, immunologic tolerance and AIDS: A unified hypothesis. In: Perelson A, Weissbuch G, Couthino A, eds. Theoretical and Experimental Insights into Immunology. New York, Springer-Verlag. 1992 (in press).

76. Theodore AC, Kornfeld H, Wallace RP, Cruikshank WW. CD4 modulation of noninfected human T lymphocytes by HIV-1 envelope glycoprotein gp120: contributions to the immunosuppression seen in HIV-1 infection by induction of CD4 and CD3 unresponsiveness. JAIDS 1994;7:899-907.

77. Landman D, Sarai A, Sathe SS. Use of pentoxifylline therapy for patients with AIDS-related wasting: pilot study. Clin Inf Dis 1994;18:97-99.

78. Dezube BJ. Pentoxifylline for the treatment of infection with human immunodeficiency virus. Clin Inf Dis 1994;18:285-287.

79. Mole L, Margolis D, Ghotbi L, Holodniy M. The use of pentoxifylline alone in HIV-infected patients. JAIDS 1994;7:519-521.

80. Andrieu J-M, Even P, Venet A, et al. Effects of cyclosporin on T-cell subsets in human immunodeficiency virus disease. Cl Im Impth 1988;46:181-198.

81. Phillips A, Wainberg M, Coates R, et al. Cyclosporine-induced deterioration in patients with AIDS. Can Med Assoc J 1989;140:1456-1460.

82. Andrieu JM, Even P, Tourani JM, Beldjord K, Audroin C. Results of a 2-year exploratory study with cyclosporin a in human immunodeficiency virus infection. In Autoimmune Aspects of HIV Infection, ed. J.-M. Andrieu, J.-F. Bach and P. Even, 1988, pp. 191-194.. Pub. by Royal Soc. Med. Serv. Ltd.

83. Karpas A, Lowdell M, Jacobson SK, Hill F. Inhibition of human immunodeficiency virus and growth of infected T cells by the immunosuppressive drugs cyclosporin A and FK 506. Proc Natl Acad Sci USA 1992;89:8351-8355.

84. Schwarz A, Offerman G, Keller F, Bennhold I, L'Age-Stehr J, Krause PH, Mihatsch MJ. The effect of cyclosporine on the progression of human immunodeficiency virus type 1 infection transmitted by transplantation-data on four cases and review of the literature. Transplantation 1993;55:95-103.

85. Bass HZ, Hardy D, Mitsuyasu RT, et al. The effect of zidovudine treatment on serum neopterin and beta2-microglobulin levels in mildly symptomatic, HIV type 1 seropositive individuals. JAIDS 1992;5:215-221.

86. Sarin A, ClericiM, Blatt SP, Hendrix CW, Shearer GM, Henkart PA. Inhibition of activation-induced programmed cell death and restoration of defective immune responses of HIV+ donors by cysteine protease inhibitors. J Immunol 1994;153:862-872.

87. Cheng J, Zhou T, Liu C, et al. Protection from fas-mediated apoptosis by a soluble form of the fas molecule. Science 1994;263:1759-1762.

88. Kroemer G, Martinez-A C. Pharmacological inhibition of programmed lymphocyte death. Immunol Today 1994;15:235-242.

89. Zinkernagel RM, Hengartner H. T-cell-mediated immunopathology versus direct cytolysis by virus: implications for HIV and AIDS. Immunol Today 1994;15:262-268.

18

INHIBITION OF T LYMPHOCYTE ACTIVATION AND APOPTOTIC CELL DEATH BY CYCLOSPORIN A AND TACROLIMUS (FK506)

Its Relevance to Therapy of HIV Infection

Angus W. Thomson[1]* and C. Andrew Bonham[2]

[1] Pittsburgh Transplantation Institute and
Department of Molecular Genetics and Biochemistry
University of Pittsburgh Medical Center
Pittsburgh, Pennsylvania 15213
[2] Pittsburgh Transplantation Institute and
Department of Surgery and
University of Pittsburgh Medical Center
Pittsburgh, Pennsylvania 15213

SUMMARY

Theoretically, drugs that inhibit programmed cell death could be used to inhibit the increased apoptotic decay of lymphocyte populations in human immunodeficiency virus (HIV) infection. The concept that immunopathologic processes cause immune suppression provides a further rationale for the use of agents such as cyclosporin A (CsA) or tacrolimus (formerly known as FK506) early in HIV infection to reduce cytotoxic CD8$^+$ T cell-mediated destruction of HIV-infected target cells.

MECHANISMS OF CELL DEATH IN HIV INFECTION

Modulation of HIV infection with immunosuppressants is not a new idea, but the molecular basis for such therapy is only now being elucidated. The pathogenetic mechanisms leading to acquired immune deficiency syndrome AIDS which may be altered by immuno-

---

* Correspondence to: Dr. A. W. Thomson, Pittsburgh Transplantation Institute, Department of Surgery, W1544 Biomedical Science Tower, University of Pittsburgh Medical Center, 200 Lothrop St., Pittsburgh, PA 15213. Tel. (412) 624-6392; Fax. (412) 624-1172.

modulation include 1) viral infection and replication, 2) HIV-induced dysregulation of cytokines, 3) apoptosis, 4) HIV-induced autoimmunity and cytotoxic T-lymphocyte mediated immunopathology.[1]

VIRAL INFECTION AND REPLICATION

HIV causes cytolysis and/or fusion of infected cells *in vitro*, but evidence for a direct cytopathic effect *in vivo* is lacking.[1-5] Viral infection occurs in cells expressing the CD4 cell surface molecule. The state of activation of host lymphocytes influences reverse transcription and viral expression. In quiescent lymphocytes, reverse transcription of viral RNA does not go to completion unless a mitogenic signal is applied shortly after infection. In contrast, non-dividing macrophages permit HIV virion production.[6] Antigen presenting cells (APC) infected by HIV may be unable to provide CD4$^+$ T helper (Th) cells with cytokines essential for activation.[1]

HIV AND APOPTOSIS

Programmed cell death, or the morphological changes of apoptosis in the immune system, is manifested by internucleosomal DNA fragmentation by endogenous endonucleases. This process is felt to be important in the regulation of lymphocyte growth and renewal.[7-11] The complexity of the process regulating programmed cell death is emphasized by the finding that the same stimulus can either promote or prevent apoptosis, depending on the presence of costimulators and the functional state of the cell. Thus CsA and protein kinase inhibitors prevent DNA fragmentation induced in T-cell hybridomas by anti-CD3, but not that by dexamethasone. Similarly, cAMP analogues can inhibit anti-CD3 but not glucocorticoid programmed cell death of T-cell hybridomas.[12,13] The stimuli which can induce apoptosis include binding of T and B cell antigen receptors, cytokines, ionizing irradiation, and drugs.[13] The molecular mechanisms that induce or prevent apoptosis are multiple. Hyper-crosslinking of surface IgM or IgD receptors on mature B-cells induces programmed cell death that is reversed by costimulation with IL-4 and anti-CD40.[14] B-cell hybridomas undergo apoptosis upon withdrawal of IL-6[15] or exposure to a calcium ionophore.[16] Interferon-γ and TNF-α upregulate Fas antigen expression - a cell molecule that mediates apoptosis.[13,17,18] HIV induces apoptosis in CD4 T cells.[19] CD4 crosslinking may cause apoptosis.[17] HIV gp120 inhibits the T cell receptor(TCR)/CD3 phospholipase C transduction pathway and primes cells for apoptosis upon activation.[20] The rate of T cell depletion in AIDS depends on the rate of cellular activation.[21-23] Alterations of the APC by HIV may result in T cells programmed for apoptosis.[24] HIV induces downregulation of *bcl-2* expression and death by apoptosis in EBV-immortalized B cells.[25] Conceivably, pharmacological agents which inhibit programmed cell death could be used to counteract the increased apoptotic decay of lymphocyte populations. Theoretically, such treatment might inhibit deletion of lymphocytes stimulated by modified self antigens or viral antigens. On the other hand, autoimmune responses could be initiated or aggravated.

HIV AND IMMUNOPATHOLOGY

Although in-situ hybridization analysis has revealed the percentage of HIV-infected mononuclear cells in peripheral blood to be less than 0.01%,[26] the number of circulating Th cells is often less than 10% of normal, and their function is suppressed. HIV induces a potent cytotoxic T cell response. There is an inverse relationship between HIV titers and HIV-specific CD8[+] T cells.[1] Infected CD4[+] T cells are destroyed, as are infected APC. Loss of these APC deprives CD4[+] T cells of relevant stimuli and essential cytokines.[27-29] The decline in APC and Th cells results in immunosuppression and inability to control otherwise trivial intracellular infections that are characteristic of AIDS. This concept of immunopathology causing immunosuppression provides a rationale for the use of immunosuppressants early in HIV infection to reduce or inhibit anti-HIV CD8[+] T cells.

PHARMACOLOGICAL MODULATION OF T CELL ACTIVATION

There have been several excellent reviews of the molecular actions of CsA and tacrolimus (formerly known as FK506), and the modes of action of these potent immunosuppressants will be addressed only briefly. CsA and tacrolimus are clinically important immunophilin-binding "pro-drugs" which inhibit TCR-mediated transcription of the IL-2 gene. The major target of the CsA-cyclophilin A and FK506-FK binding protein (FKBP) drug-immunophilin complexes is the heterodimeric, Ca^{2+}/calmodulin-regulated phosphatase calcineurin, a key enzyme in T cell signal transduction following ligation of the TCR. Calcineurin activity may result in dephosphorylation of the nuclear factor of activated T cells (NF-AT), inducing its translocation into the nucleus where it acts as a transcription factor for IL-2. Activation of the genes for IL-2 and its receptor determines progression from the G0 to the G1 phase of the T cell cycle.[30]

INHIBITION OF T CELL ACTIVATION AND HIV INFECTION

CsA and tacrolimus inhibit activation of HIV-infected T cells by blocking transition through G1 - thereby preventing the completion of reverse transcription of resident virus.[31,32] Quiescent cells that harbor the viral genome may be prevented from releasing infectious progeny.[33] CsA disrupts the interaction of HIV GAG polyprotein Pr55[gag] with host cell cyclophilins A and B, possibly interfering with protein folding and virion assembly.[34] The HIV long terminal repeat (LTR) contains binding sites for NF-AT. Inhibition of NF-AT activation can reduce viral expression.[35] CsA pretreatment renders T cells resistant to HIV infection.[36,37] This does not appear to be secondary to decreased CD4 expression, as this does not occur except in treated microglial cells.[38] Both CsA and tacrolimus reduce the yield of infectious HIV from infected cells by approximately 100-fold, as well as selectively inhibiting the growth of infected cells.[35] Obviously, the effects of CsA and tacrolimus extend to HIV-specific CD8[+] T cells, which if titrated sufficiently, could abrogate immunopathology due to these cells.

INHIBITION OF APOPTOSIS

Although the mechanisms whereby a cell undergoes apoptosis are myriad, several steps have been identified which are easily altered. The level of calcineurin activity correlates closely with the ability of T cells to undergo apoptosis.[39] Tissue transglutaminase (tTG) is a Ca^{2+}-dependent enzyme not active at Ca^{2+} levels normally detected in viable cells, and is involved in the effector phase of programmed cell death. CsA, by preventing increases in intracellular calcium, inhibits activation of tTG. Gp-120-dependent induction of apoptosis is blocked in a similar fashion.[20] CsA and tacrolimus prevent induction of apoptosis by anti-CD2 mAb.[40] Activation induced programmed cell death of CD4[+] T cells is prevented

Table 1. Inhibitory effects of CsA and FK 506 on apoptosis *in vitro* and *in vivo*

In vitro:T-cell lines	
Apoptosis is blocked by CsA or FK 506	Shi *etal Nature* **339**, 625, 1989
A CsA/FK506-sensitive protective mechanism exists	Cairns *etal Thymus* 21, 177, 1993
in a subpopulation of murine thymocytes	McCarthy *etal Transplantation* 54, 543, 1992
Apoptotic activity correlates with calcineurin activity	Fruman *etal Eur J Immunol* **22**, 2513, 1992
Inhibitory effect of FK506 is reversible by rapamycin	Staruch *etal Int J Immunopharmacol* **13**, 677, 1991
or by IFN-γ	Groux *etal Eur J Immunol* **23**, 1623, 1993
In vivo:Thymocytes	
Apoptosis is inhibited by CsA or FK 506	Jenkins *etal Science* **241**, 1655, 1988;
	Gao *etal Nature* **336,** 176, 1988

by CsA, cycloheximide, and mAb anti-CD28.[41] CsA and tacrolimus protect B-cell lymphoma cells from apoptosis induced by ionomycin or ligation of surface IgM.[42] Such treatment might have the advantage of inhibiting deletion of lymphocytes stimulated by modified self or viral antigens, but could also aggravate immunopathology.

CLINICAL EXPERIENCE

Studies with CsA in HIV-infected subjects to date have been inconclusive, and the role of immunosuppressants as therapeutic agents has remained controversial.[43-46] CsA in HIV patients has been shown to expand the CD4[+] T cell population and to inhibit the expansion of the CD8[+] T cell population.[45] On the other hand, CsA induced rapid deterioration in patients with AIDS.[46] The possibility that suppression of T-cell responses early in the disease might be beneficial was suggested from analysis of CsA-treated HIV[+] organ transplant recipients infected during or shortly after transplantation. Those patients receiving immunosuppression with CsA progressed less rapidly towards development of AIDS than those receiving immunosuppression without CsA (five year cumulative risk of AIDS - 31% vs. 90%).[44] However, no data were provided regarding the steroid dosages received by the patients in the two groups. Higher steroid dosages in the non-CsA treated group could have impacted on lymphocyte survival and progression to AIDS. The best results in HIV patients have been achieved when CsA was administered early after infection,[45] but the drug cannot totally prevent progression to AIDS. Tacrolimus and CsA may slow progression to AIDS by preventing virus binding to T cells, decreasing the number of activated T cells, preventing apoptosis, or eliminating autoreactive CD8[+] T cells and subsequent immunopathology. Further attention to tacrolimus and CsA is needed to determine if there is a place for them in the modulation of HIV infection.

REFERENCES

1. Zinkernagel RM, Hengartner H. T-cell-mediated immunopathology versus direct cytolysis by virus: implications for HIV and AIDS. *Immunol Today* 1994;15:262-68.
2. Rosenberg ZF, Fauci AS. Immunopathologic mechanisms of HIV infection. *Adv Immunol* 1989;47:377-431.
3. Levy JA. Mysteries of HIV: challenges for therapy and prevention. *Nature* 1988;333:519-22.
4. Mosier DE, Gulizia RJ, MacIsaac PD, et al. Rapid loss of CD4[+] T cells in human-PBL-SCID mice by noncytopathic HIV isolates. *Science* 1993;260:689-92.

5. Lo SC, Tsai S, Benish JR, et al. Enhancement of HIV-1 cytocidal effects in CD4$^+$ lymphocytes by the AIDS-associated mycoplasma. *Science* 1991;251:1074-6.

6. Stevenson M, Brichacok B, Hoinzingor N, et al. Molecular basis of cell-cycle dependent HIV-1 replication. *First International Symposium on Cellular Approaches to the Control of HIV Disease, Paris,* 1994;abstract.

7. Cohen JJ. Apoptosis. *Immunol Today* 1993;14:126-30.

8. Cohen JJ. Programmed cell death and apoptosis in lymphocyte development and function. *Chest* 1993;103(2 Suppl):99S-101S.

9. Williams GT. Apoptosis in the immune system. *J Pathol* 1994;173:1-4.

10. Cairns JS, Mainwaring MS, Cacchione RN, et al. Regulation of apoptosis in thymocytes. *Thymus* 1993;21:177-93.

11. McCarthy SA, Cacchione RN, Mainwaring MS, et al. The effects of immunosuppressive drugs on the regulation of activation-induced apoptotic cell death in thymocytes. *Transplantation* 1992;54:543-7.

12. Lee MR, Liou ML, Liou ML, et al. cAMP analogs prevent activation-induced apoptosis of T cell hybridomas. *J Immunol* 1993;151:5208-17.

13. Kroemer G, Martinez-AC. Pharmacological inhibition of programmed lymphocyte death. *Immunol Today* 1994;15:235-42.

14. Parry SL, Hasbold J, Holman M, et al. Hypercross-linking surface IgM or IgD receptors on mature B-cells induces apoptosis that is reversed by costimulation with IL-4 and anti-CD40. *J Immunol* 1994;152:2821-9.

15. Liu J, Li H, de Tribolet N, et al. IL-6 stimulates growth and inhibits constitutive, protein synthesis-independent apoptosis of murine B-cell hybridoma 7TD1. *Cellular Immunol* 1994;155:428-35.

16. Bonnefoy-Berard N, Genestier L, Flacher M, et al. The phosphoprotein phosphatase calcineurin controls calcium-dependent apoptosis in B cell lines. *Eur J Immunol* 1994;24:325-9.

17. Oyaizu N, McCloskey TW, Than SS, et al. Mechanisms of apoptosis in peripheral blood mononuclear cells of HIV-infected patients. *First International Symposium on Cellular Approaches to the Control of HIV Disease, Paris,* 1994;abstract.

18. Stalder T, Hahn S, Erb P. Fas antigen is the major target molecule for CD4$^+$ T cell-mediated cytotoxicity. *J Immunol* 1994;152:1127-33.

19. Corbeil J, Howell MI, Tremblay M, et al. HIV-induced apoptosis of CD4$^+$ T cells: viral infection and subsequent cell surface signalling are required. *First International Symposium on Cellular Approaches to the Control of HIV Disease, Paris,* 1994;abstract.

20. Amendola A, Lombardi G, Oliverio S, et al. HIV-1 gp-120-dependent induction of apoptosis in antigen-specific human T cell clones is characterized by 'tissue' transglutaminase expression and prevented by cyclosporine A. *FEBS Letters* 1994;339(3):258-64.

21. Ameisen JC, Capron A. Cell dysfunction and depletion in AIDS: the programmed cell death hypothesis. *Immunol Today* 1991;12:102-5.

22. Ameisen JC. Programmed cell death and AIDS: from hypothesis to experiment. *Immunol Today* 1992;13:388-91.

23. Ameisen JC, Estaquier J, Idziorek T, et al. Programmed cell death (PCD) (Apoptosis) and AIDS pathogenesis: significance, and potential mechanism. *First International Symposium on Cellular Approaches to the Control of HIV Disease, Paris,* 1994;abstract.

24. Meyaard L, Schuitemaker H, Miedema F. T-cell dysfunction in HIV infection: anergy due to defective antigen-presenting cell function? *Immunol Today* 1993;14:161-4

25. De Rossi A, Ometto L, Roncella S, et al. HIV-1 induces down-regulation of bcl-2 expression and death by apoptosis of EBV-immortalized B cells: a model for a persistent "self-limiting" HIV-1 infection. *Virology* 1994;198:234-44.

26. Harper ME, Marselle LM, Gallo RC, et al. Detection of lymphocytes expressing human T-lymphotropic virus type III in lymph nodes and peripheral blood from infected individuals by in situ hybridization. *PNAS USA* 1986;83:772-6.

27. Zinkernagel R. Immunopathogenesis of virus-induced immunodeficiency. *First International Symposium on Cellular Approaches to the Control of HIV Disease, Paris,* 1994;abstract.

28. Lafferty KJ, Cunningham AJ. A new analysis of allogeneic interactions. *Aust J Exp Biol & Med Science* 1975;53:27-42.

29. Schwartz RH. A cell culture model for T lymphocyte clonal anergy. *Science* 1990;248:1349-56.

30. Liu J. FK506 and cyclosporin, molecular probes for studying intracellular signal transduction. *Immunol Today* 1993;14:290-5.

31. Zack JA. The role of T-cell activation in HIV-1 infection. *First International Symposium on Cellular Approaches to the Control of HIV Disease, Paris,* 1994;abstract.

32. Lu W, Salerno-Goncalvez R, Yuan J, et al. Effects of immunoregulatory molecules on activation-induced and HIV-triggered apoptosis. *First International Symposium on Cellular Approaches to the Control of HIV Disease, Paris,* 1994;abstract.

33. Bell KD, Ramilo O, Vitetta ES. Combined use of an immunotoxin and cyclosporine to prevent both activated and quiescent peripheral blood T cells from producing type 1 human immunodeficiency virus. *PNAS USA* 1993;90:1411-5.

34. Luban J. Cyclophilin A and HIV-1 replication. *First International Symposium on Cellular Approaches to the Control of HIV Disease, Paris,* 1994;abstract.

35. Karpas A, Lowdell M, Jacobson S, et al. Inhibition of human immunodeficiency virus and growth of infected T cells by the immunosuppressive drugs cyclosporine A and FK 506. *PNAS USA* 1992;89:8351-5.

36. Wainberg MA, Dascal A, Blain N, et al. The effect of cyclosporine A on infection of susceptible cells by human immunodeficiency virus type 1. *Blood* 1988;72:1904-10.

37. Klatzmann D, Laporte JP, Achour A, et al. Functional inhibition by cyclosporin A of the lymphocyte receptor for the AIDS virus (HIV). *Comptes Rendus de l Academie des Sciences - Serie Iii, Sciences de la Vie* 1986;303:343-8.

38. Sawada M, Suzumura A, Marunouchi T. Down regulation of CD4 expression in cultured microglia by immunosuppressants and lipopolysaccharide. *Biochem & Biophys Res Comm* 1992;189:869-76.

39. Fruman DA, Mather PE, Burakoff SJ, et al. Correlation of calcineurin phosphatase activity and programmed cell death in murine T cell hybridomas. *Eur J Immunol* 1992;22:2513-7.

40. Wesselborg S, Prufer U, Wild M, et al. Triggering via the alternative CD2 pathway induces apoptosis in activated human T lymphocytes. *Eur J Immunol* 1993;23:2707-10.

41. Groux H, Torpier G, Monte D, et al. Activation-induced death by apoptosis in $CD4^+$ T cells from human immunodeficiency virus-infected asymptomatic individuals. *JEM* 1992;175:331-40.

42. Genestier L, Dearden-Badet MT, Bonnefoy-Berard N, et al. Cyclosporin A and FK506 inhibit activation-induced cell death in the murine WEHI-231 B cell line. *Cellular Immunol* 1994;155:283-91.

43. Tzakis AG, Cooper MH, Dummer JS, et al. Transplantation in HIV+ patients. *Transplantation* 1990;49:354-8.

44. Schwarz A, Offerman G, Keller F, et al. The effect of cyclosporine on the progression of human immunodeficiency virus type 1 infection transmitted by transplantation—data on four cases and review of the literature. *Transplantation* 1993;55:95-103.

45. Andrieu JM, Even P, Venet A, et al. Effects of cyclosporin on T-cell subsets in human immunodeficiency virus disease. *Clinical Immunol & Immunopathol* 1988;47:181-98.

46. Philips A, Wainberg MA, Coates R, et al. Cyclosporin-induced deterioration in patients with AIDS. *Can Med Assoc J* 1989;15:1456.

19

CYCLOPHILIN AND GAG IN HIV-1 REPLICATION AND PATHOGENESIS

Ettaly Kara Franke and Jeremy Luban

Department of Medicine
Columbia University
College of Physicians and Surgeons
701 West 168th Street
New York, New York 10032

INTRODUCTION

The *gag* gene products perform many functions in the retroviral life cycle. Recent work suggests that specific binding of HIV-1 Gag to the cellular proteins known as the cyclophilins is necessary for viral infectivity and perhaps of importance to the immunopathology associated with HIV infection. Cyclophilins are ubiquitous prolyl isomerases thought to function as chaperones. Members of this family of proteins are required for the immunosuppression induced by cyclosporin A and are suspected regulators of cellular activation pathways. Here we review the functions of the *gag* proteins, what is known about the Gag-cyclophilin interaction, and the possible relevence of this interaction for HIV-1 replication and pathogenesis.

THE GAG GENE PRODUCTS SERVE MANY FUNCTIONS FOR THE VIRUS

The *gag* gene of HIV-1 and related retroviruses is translated as a precursor polyprotein which contains information sufficient for assembly of virion particles (20, 36, 88, 99, 100). During this process the Gag polyprotein specifically incorporates several viral elements into the virion, including the viral genomic RNA (for review see (65)) and the Gag-Pol precursor (84, 103). In the case of the primate immunodeficiency viruses, the viral proteins Vpr and/or Vpx are also incorporated into virions in a process that requires the Gag polyprotein (52, 63, 68, 85, 121). Efficient virion release from some cell lines requires a viral protein called Vpu (37, 56, 109), though the mechanism underlying this effect is unknown.

At the time of virion release the Gag polyprotein is cleaved by the *pol*-encoded Protease to produce several proteins, including the matrix protein (MA), which lines the virion membrane envelope; the capsid protein (CA), which forms the core of the virion; and the nucleocapsid protein (NC), which coats the genomic RNA. Activation of the viral Protease is necessary for the formation of infectious virions (38, 59, 86) and Protease activation itself may be regulated by sequences within *gag* (72).

Gag polyprotein cleavage products serve important functions upon entry of the virus into a new host cell. Evidence for this was perhaps first provided by *FV-1*, a dominant genetic marker which limits the efficiency of integration of certain murine retroviral strains (64). Viral sensitivity to this restriction is determined by sequences coding for CA (21, 46). More recently, engineered mutations in *gag* have been identified which have no observable effect upon virion assembly but which disrupt the infectivity of virion particles early in the infectious cycle (47, 74, 108, 117). During these early steps of infection, the unintegrated viral genome is contained within a nucleoprotein complex comprised partly of *gag* gene products. Direct analysis of the complexes from cells acutely infected with Moloney murine leukemia virus has demonstrated that the unintegrated DNA is intimately associated with CA protein (12). HIV-1 differs in that MA, not CA, is detected as part of the pre-integration complex (15, 24). Thus, Gag protein not only plays an important role in virion assembly, but also in early events after infection.

DISCOVERY OF THE GAG-CYCLOPHILIN INTERACTION

Little is known about host proteins necessary for Gag polyprotein folding or transport to the cell membrane, although targeting to the cell surface generally requires cotranslational modification of the Gag polyprotein by the host N-myristoyl transferase (14, 38, 81, 90, 91, 94). Similarly, nothing is known about interactions between *gag*-encoded proteins and host proteins that occur during uncoating of the virion or transport of the pre-integration complex to the nucleus. At any of these stages in the retroviral life cycle Gag-host protein interactions could be required for viral replication.

To identify protein-protein interactions necessary for HIV-1 replication, we used the yeast two-hybrid system (25) to screen a cDNA library for encoded proteins which interact with the HIV-1 Gag polyprotein (70). Other labs have used the two-hybrid system to study interactions involving a range of proteins including cyclin-dependent kinase Cdk2 (44), p53 (49), proteins which interact with Max (122), H-Ras (114), and the retinoblastoma tumor suppresser protein (22). Previously, we had used the two-hybrid system to study Gag polyprotein multimerization (69). To screen a cDNA library with the two-hybrid system a strain of *Saccharomyces cerevisiae* with an integrated copy of a GAL1-*lacZ* fusion gene under the control of GAL4 upstream activation sequences is co-transformed with two GAL4-fusion protein expression plasmids. The first plasmid expresses the GAL4 DNA-binding domain fused to a given protein of interest. The second plasmid expresses the GAL4 activation domain fused to proteins encoded by a cDNA expression library. If a protein encoded by the library interacts with the protein of interest, the two domains of GAL4 co-localize to the upstream activation sequences and activate transcription from GAL4-responsive indicator genes. We transformed the indicator yeast strain with a plasmid encoding a GAL4 DNA binding domain-HIV-1 Gag Polyprotein fusion protein and a pool of plasmids expressing the GAL4 activation domain-fused to cDNA-encoded proteins. One million transformants were screened for β-gal activity, and six clones with binding activity were identified. All clones were either cyclophilin A or cyclophilin B.

In the two-hybrid system transcriptional activation is used as an indirect indication of protein-protein interactions. To directly demonstrate binding of the HIV-1 Gag polyprotein to the cyclophilins, we expressed the cyclophilin proteins as fusions with Glutathione S-transferase (GST). GST-fusion proteins may be purified from bacterial lysates in a single-step using glutathione-agarose beads (104) and this system is now commonly used

Table 1. Cloned mammalian cyclophilins

Name	Molecular weight (kD)	Localization
Cyclosporin A	18	Cytoplasm
Cyclosporin B	20	ER
Cyclosporin C	23	ER
Cyclosporin D	18	Mitochondria
Cyclosporin 40	40	Cytoplasm
NK-TR	150	Cell surface

to demonstrate protein-protein interactions *in vitro* (51). As a source of HIV-1 Gag polyprotein we used a lysate from bacteria transformed with an HIV-1 *gag* expression plasmid, pT7HG(pro-) (71). When Gag protein was incubated with the GST-cyclophilin fusion protein bound to glutathione-agarose beads, Gag was quantitatively recovered in a specific fashion indicating that Gag binds directly to cyclophilin proteins (70).

THE CYCLOPHILIN FAMILY OF PROTEINS

The cyclophilins are a family of ubiquitous proteins expressed in all organisms from primates to bacteria (31, 106, 116). All members share a conserved core of about 109 amino acids. They are differentiated from one another by unique extensions which function in organelle and membrane transport. Several mammalian cyclophilins have been cloned (Table 1). Cyclophilin A (40, 42, 43) is an abundant, cytosolic protein found in all tissues. Cyclophilins B and C are targeted to the endoplasmic reticulum (13, 30, 45, 87), while cyclophilin D is targeted to the mitochondria (9). Cyclophilins are present at the cell surface (16), and include a 150 kD molecule on NK cells which is thought to be component of the tumor-recognition complex (4). Recently, a cyclophilin was cloned which appears to be a component of the steroid receptor complex (55).

In light of the cyclophilin literature, our discovery that these proteins bind specifically to an HIV-1 protein had obvious implications for viral replication and for viral pathogenesis. First, cyclophilins are believed to function as chaperones (26, 35) and therefore might be important for folding or cellular trafficking of *gag*-encoded proteins. Cyclophilins catalyze the isomerization of peptidyl-prolyl bonds (27, 57), which is a rate-limiting step in protein folding (26). Drugs which block cyclophilin isomerase activity, disrupt collagen triple helix assembly in fibroblasts (107), and prevent formation of the correct disulfide bonded form of transferrin in HepG2 cells (67). Transit from the endoplasmic reticulum of specific isoforms of rhodopsin is blocked in *Drosophila* bearing mutations in a cyclophilin gene (19). A role for cyclophilins in protein folding is also suggested by a sub-cellular distribution reminiscent of the heat shock chaperone proteins. In addition, transcription of cyclophilin mRNA is stimulated by heat shock and disruption of cyclophilin genes in yeast leads to decreased survival following heat shock (110). Thus, binding to cyclophilins might be important for the proper folding or targeting of *gag*-encoded protein.

The discovery of the Gag-cyclophilin interaction was not only intriguing because of its possible relevence for viral replication. Cyclophilins are thought to play a role in T-cell activation (76, 93) and this suggested that the Gag-cyclophilin interaction might play a role in the immunopathology associated with HIV infection. Though there is precedent for pathogenic effects of *gag* gene products from other retroviruses (120) we had not expected that this would be the case for HIV-1 *gag* protein. The Cyclophilins were originally identified as cellular binding proteins for the immunosuppressive drug cyclosporin A (42). It has since been determined that the drug-Cyclophilin complex binds and inhibits the activity of the phosphatase calcineurin (31, 93). The substrates of calcineurin are important for several processes including activation of IL-2 gene transcription (18, 80), apoptosis in murine T-cell hybridomas (32), antigen-mediated degranulation of a murine cytotoxic T-cell clone (23), and perhaps thymic selection (10). NF-ATp is the first calcineurin substrate to be identified (50). As a complex with c-Fos and c-Jun this protein activates transcription from the IL-2 promoter (75). By blocking the activity of calcineurin the Cyclophilin-cyclosporin A complex blocks the transport to the nucleus of NF-ATp. Though there is no direct evidence that cyclophilins regulate these processes in the absence of cyclosporin A it has been postulated that the cyclophilins most likely regulate the activity of cellular ligands important for cell activation pathways (76, 93). The same prediction has been made for the cellular targets of the immunosuppressive drug FK506. Structurally unrelated to cyclosporin A, FK506 coincidently binds to a different family of cellular prolyl isomerases, the FKBPs. Of seemingly extraordinary coincidence, the FK506-FKBP complex also inhibits calcineurin. Recently, it was discovered that FKBP-12 binds specifically to the type I receptor for transforming growth factor-β in the absence of FK506 (118). Thus, the native function of some prolyl isomerases appears to involve the mediation of signalling events. These findings raise the possibility that *gag*-encoded proteins might disrupt the normal interactions between cyclophilins and their substrates and thus perturb the immune function of HIV-1 infected cells.

Many theories have been proposed to explain the qualitative immune deficits, as well as the frank CD4$^+$ T cell depletion which are observed with HIV-1 infection (82). These include direct toxicity due to the interaction between CD4 and viral gp120 (58, 105, 119); depletion of thymic T cells due to the downregulation of CD4 expression induced by the viral Nef protein (33, 54, 73, 102); and depletion due to HIV-1-encoded superantigens (48, 89). One of the leading theories is that a viral product alters T-cells so that activation initiates a program for cell death (apoptosis) rather than proliferation (3). This model is consistant with the specific deficit in recall function that has been observed with HIV-1 infected cells *in vitro* (39, 61, 97) and several groups have demonstrated the association of apoptosis with HIV-1 infection (1, 11, 39, 62, 77, 111). Apoptosis might be caused by inappropriate signals delivered to the cell as a result of CD4-gp120 binding (7, 95) or secondary to the high levels of Class II antigen carried on the surface of virions (6), and may be enhanced by interactions with specific antigen-presenting cells (17). Interestingly, apoptosis in HIV-1 infected cells (39), in thymocytes (98), or in T-cell hybridomas (98), is blocked by cyclosporin A. Our observation that Gag binds to cyclophilins, the cellular targets of cyclosporin A, raises the possibility that *gag* gene products might play a role in the apoptosis associated with HIV-1.

To date we have no evidence that Gag plays a role in the immunopathology associated with HIV-1 infection. Gag binds to cyclophilin but the Gag-cyclophilin complex is not capable of binding calcineurin (70). Thus, Gag cannot directly mimic cyclosporin A. It remains a possibility that Gag binding to cyclophilin perturbs aspects of cyclophilin function that have not yet been elucidated such as binding to as yet unidentified ligands (76, 93).

MINIMAL GAG SEQUENCE REQUIREMENTS FOR CYCLOPHILIN BINDING

To localize the portion of Gag that mediates binding to the cyclophilins, we have examined the effect of engineered mutations in *gag* on binding to cyclophilin (29, 70). To date we have identified a 350 nucleotide sequence within CA coding sequence which is sufficient for binding to cyclophilin. This region does not overlap with sequences required for Gag polyprotein multimerization (28). Thus, one could imagine a Gag polyprotein monomer binding simultaneously to cyclophilin and another Gag molecule during virion assembly. Also, the fact that sequences within CA are sufficient for binding indicates that the biologically relevant partner in the Gag-cyclophilin interaction could be either the Gag polyprotein at the time of virion assembly, or CA early after viral infection. Thus, the Gag-cyclophilin interaction might be of functional importance for virion assembly or for early events such as virion uncoating, reverse transcription, and transport to the nucleus of the pre-integration complex.

CYCLOPHILIN-BINDING IS NOT A SHARED PROPERTY OF ALL RETROVIRAL GAGS

The Gag polyproteins of retroviruses distantly related to HIV-1, such as Moloney murine leukemia virus (MLV) and Mason-Pfizer monkey virus, do not bind to cyclophilin (70). This indicates that the Gag-cyclophilin interaction must not be required for the replication of all retroviruses. Interestingly, the Gag polyproteins of other primate immunodeficiency viruses, such as SIV_{MAC239}, bind Cyclophilin B, but not Cyclophilin A (Table 2). Unlike the cytoplasmic protein Cyclophilin A, Cyclophilin B is targeted to the endoplasmic reticulum (45). Since Gag proteins are primarily cytoplasmic we cannot easily envision a role for Cyclophilin B in Gag function. Therefore current binding data would suggest that among primate immunodeficiency viruses, only HIV-1 replication might require the cyclophilin interaction.

We expect that the Gag-cyclophilin interaction will be restricted to a sub-group of primate immunodeficiency retroviruses. Sequence alignments between HIV/SIV isolates have led to the identification of five viral lineages (2, 41, 78): SIV_{CPZ} from chimpanzees and the closely related HIV-1; SIV_{SM} from sootey mangabeys, captive macaques and the closely related HIV-2; SIV_{SYK} from Sykes' monkey; SIV_{MND} from mandrill; and SIV_{AGM} from African Green Monkeys. One of the distinguishing features of primate lentiviruses is the presence of the *vpr/vpx* genes (78). Different SIVs and HIVs possess either one or the other gene, or both, and it has been suggested that *vpx* arose by duplication of *vpr* (113). Interestingly, both gene products seem to be incorporated into virion particles via interactions with *gag* proteins (52, 68, 85). SIV_{MAC239}, a virus with both a *vpr* and a *vpx* gene, does not bind to Cyclophilin A (70). Since HIV-1 possesses only the *vpr* gene, it might be that cyclophilin A substitutes for *vpx* in those viruses which do not possess it. On the other hand,

Table 2. Interactions between primate immunodeficiency virus Gag polyproteins and cyclophilin proteins

| Clone Name | In Vitro Binding to | | CyP A Incorporation into Virions |
	CyP A	CyP B	
HIV1$_{HXB2}$	+	+	+
HIV1$_{NL43}$	+	+	+
HIV2$_{ROD}$	–	+	–
SIV$_{MAC239}$	–	+	–
SIV$_{BK28}$	–	+	–
SIV$_{SMMPBJ}$	–	+	–
SIV$_{SAB384}$	–	+	–

if the Gag-Cyclophilin interaction is restricted to the HIV-1/SIV$_{CPZ}$ group of viruses then perhaps the Gag-cyclophilin interaction is related to the function of Vpu, an accessory protein which is only found in this subgroup of viruses.

CYCLOSPORIN A INHIBITS THE GAG-CYCLOPHILIN INTERACTION AND HIV-1 REPLICATION

The cyclophilins are the intracellular target of the immunosuppressive drug cyclosporin A. Cyclosporin A disrupts binding of the HIV-1 Gag polyprotein or CA to cyclophilin *in vitro* (70). If the Gag-cyclophilin interaction were necessary for HIV-1 infectivity one would predict that cyclosporin A would block viral replication. A review of the clinical literature is not inconsistent with this proposal (5, 96). Experiments in tissue culture have shown that cyclosporin A blocks HIV-1 replication (8, 53, 115). However, one still cannot conclude from these studies that the anti-HIV effects of cyclosporin A are due to a block of the Gag-cyclophilin interaction, especially since the HIV-1 promoter responds to transcription factors which are blocked by cyclosporin A (34, 79).

Evidence that cyclosporin A blocks HIV-1 via mechanisms independent of transcriptional effects has been provided by experiments in which cyclosporin A was shown to inhibit HIV-1 replication in the presence of IL-2, a lymphokine which bypasses the T-cell activation block of cyclosporin A (83). More convincing data comes from studies with non-immunosuppressive derivatives of cyclosporin A. These compounds bind to cyclophilin as tightly as the parent compound (101), but the complex that these drugs form with cyclophilin binds calcineurin about one thousand-fold less efficiently than the complex formed by the parent compound (66). Thus, the non-immunosuppressive derivative compounds have insignificant effects on known T-cell signal transduction pathways. Non-immunosuppressive cyclosporin A analogues are as effective at blocking Gag binding to cyclophilin *in vitro* and HIV-1 replication in tissue culture as is the parent compound (92, 112) and (E.K. Franke and J. Luban, unpublished data). Inhibition curves with these compounds are identical to those obtained with cyclosporin A. Whichever drug is used, the effects require drug concentrations 10-100-fold greater than are necessary for immunosuppression, but equimolar to the concentration of Cyclophilin A in the cytoplasm (60). The structurally unrelated immunosuppressive drug FK506 has no effect on the Gag-cyclophilin interaction *in vitro* nor on HIV-1 replication in tissue culture. FK506 binds to a different family of cellular prolyl isomerases, the FKBPs, but like cyclosporin A it inhibits T-cell activation pathways through binding of the drug-receptor complex to calcineurin (93). These studies demonstrate that cyclosporin A disrupts HIV-1 replication via mechanisms that are distinct from the known effects of the drug on signal transduction pathways.

CYCLOPHILIN A IS SPECIFICALLY INCORPORATED INTO HIV-1 VIRIONS AND APPEARS TO BE NECESSARY FOR HIV-1 REPLICATION

HIV-1 virions contain an 18 kD protein which is recognized by anti-Cyclophilin A antibodies (29, 112). The fact that other cyclophilins, and the unrelated cytoplasmic immunophilin FKBP12, are not incorporated, suggests that Cyclophilin A is incorporated specifically and not simply as a result of it's abundance in the cytoplasm. The Gag polyprotein is all that is required for incorporation and mutations in *gag* which disrupt binding to cyclophilin *in vitro*, block incorporation of cyclophilin into virions. Cyclosporin A also blocks incorporation of Cyclophilin A into virions at the same concentrations that are required for disruption of HIV-1 infectivity. Primate immunodeficiency viruses other than HIV-1 do not encode Gag polyproteins capable of binding to Cyclophilin A *in vitro* and do not incorporate detectable amounts of Cyclophilin A into virions (Table 2). Cyclosporin A has no effect on the replication of these viruses (92, 112). Taken together these observations suggest that cyclosporin A blocks HIV-1 replication by competing directly with Gag for binding to Cyclophilin A, and that HIV-1 virion infectivity uniquely requires the formation of Gag-Cyclophilin A hetero-multimers. The Gag-cyclophilin interaction is not required for virion assembly, but for the formation of infectious virions.Thus, the Gag-cyclophilin interaction seems to play a vital role in the life cycle of HIV-1.

CONCLUSION

To date there is no evidence that the Gag-cyclophilin interaction is of any significance to the immunopathology associated with HIV-1 infection. In contrast, we believe that the interaction is required for the formation of infectious virions. Ultimate proof will perhaps require a combination of approaches including experiments with compounds or fragments of Gag or cyclophilin which disrupt the interaction, experiments with mutant viruses, and experiments with host cell lines in which the *cyclophilin A* gene has been disrupted by homologous recombination.

It remains to be determined what specific role the Gag-cyclophilin interaction plays in viral replication. It is not necessary for the formation of virions but perhaps it assists virion uncoating, or transport of the pre-integration complex to the nucleus. We do not know if cyclophilin prolyl-isomerase activity is necessary for viral infectivity or if cyclophilin merely binds to Gag and serves a structural role in the virion. Quantitative estimates with radiolabeled virion protein indicate that there is at least as much virion-associated Cyclophilin A as there are *pol*-encoded proteins (29, 112). This observation suggests that Cyclophilin A may serve a structural function. Hopefully disruption of the Gag-cyclophilin interaction will one day prove to be the basis for novel therapies which disrupt the replication of HIV-1 in infected individuals.

ACKNOWLEDGMENTS

This work was supported by grant AI 00988 from the NIAID and grant 91-49 from the James S. McDonnell Foundation.

REFERENCES

1. Aldrovandi, G. M., G. Feuer, L. Gao, B. Jamieson, M. Kristeva, I. S. Y. Chen and J. A. Zack. 1993. The SCID-hu mouse as a model for HIV-1 infection. Nature. 363:732-736.
2. Allan, J. S. 1992. Viral evolution and AIDS. J. NIH Res. 4:51-54.
3. Ameisen, J. C. and A. Capron. 1991. Cell dysfunction and depletion in AIDS: the programmed cell death hypothesis. Immunol. Today. 12:102-105.
4. Anderson, S. K., S. Gallinger, J. Roder, J. Frey, H. A. Young and J. R. Ortaldo. 1993. A cyclophilin-related protein involved in the function of natural killer cells. Proc. Natl. Acad. Sci. USA. 90:542-546.
5. Andrieu, J.-M., P. Even, A. Venet, J.-M. Tourani, M. Stern, W. Lowenstein, C. Audroin, D. Eme, D. Masson, H. Sors, D. Israel-Biet and K. Beldjord. 1988. Effects of cyclosporin on T-cell subsets in human immunodeficiency virus disease. Clin. Immunol. Immunopathol. 46:181-198.

6. Arthur, L. O., J. W. Bess, R. C. Sowder, R. E. Benveniste, D. L. Mann, J.-C. Chermann and L. E. Henderson. 1992. Cellular proteins bound to immunodeficiency viruses: Implications for pathogenesis and vaccines. Science. 258:1935-1938.

7. Banda, N. K., J. Bernier, D. K. Kurahara, R. Kurrle, N. Haigwood, R.-P. Sekaly and T. H. Finkel. 1992. Crosslinking CD4 by human immunodeficiency virus gp120 primes T cells for activation-induced apoptosis. J. Exp. Med. 176:1099-1106.

8. Bell, K. D., O. Ramilo and E. S. Vitetta. 1993. Combined use of an immunotoxin and cyclosporine to prevent both actvated and quiescent peripheral blood T cells from producing type 1 human immunodeficiency virus. Proc. Natl. Acad. Sci. USA. 90:1411-1415.

9. Bergsma, D. J., C. Eder, M. Gross, H. Kersten, D. Sylvester, E. Appelbaum, D. Cusimano, G. P. Livi, M. M. McLaughlin, K. Kasyan, W. P. Prichett, M. J. Bossard, M. Brandt and M. A. Levy. 1991. The cyclophilin multigene family of peptidyl-prolyl isomerases. J. Biol. Chem. 266:23204—23214.

10. Bierer, B. E., G. Hollander, D. A. Fruman and S. J. Burakoff. 1993. Cyclosporin A and FK506: molecular mechanisms of immunosuppression and probes for transplantation biology. Curr. Opin. Immunol. 5:763-773.

11. Bonyhadi, M. L., L. Rabin, S. Salimi, D. A. Brown, J. Kosek, J. M. McCune and H. Kaneshima. 1993. HIV induces thymus depletion in vivo. Nature. 363:728-732.

12. Bowerman, B., P. O. Brown, J. M. Bishop and H. E. Varmus. 1989. A nucleoprotein complex mediates the integration of retroviral DNA. Gene Dev. 3:469-478.

13. Bram, R. J., D. T. Hung, P. K. Martin, S. L. Schreiber and G. Crabtree. 1993. Identification of the immunophilins capable of mediating inhibition of signal transduction by cyclosporin A and FK506: Role of calcineurin-binding and cellular location. Mol. Cell. Biol. 13:4760-4769.

14. Bryant, M. and L. Ratner. 1990. Myristoylation-dependent replication and assembly of human immunodeficiency virus 1. Proc. Natl. Acad. Sci. USA. 87:523-527.

15. Bukrinsky, M. I., S. Haggerty, M. P. Dempsey, N. Sharova, A. Adzhubel, L. Spitz, P. Lewis, D. Goldfarb, M. Emerman and M. Stevenson. 1993. A nuclear localization signal within HIV-1 matrix protein that governs infection of non-dividing cells. Nature. 365:666-669.

16. Cacalano, N. A., B.-X. Chen, W. L. Cleveland and B. F. Erlanger. 1992. Evidence for a functional receptor for cyclosporin A on the surface of lymphocytes. Proc. Natl. Acad. Sci. USA. 89:4353-4357.

17. Cameron, P. U., M. Pope, S. Gezelter and R. M. Steinman. 1994. Infection and apoptotic cell death of CD4+ T cells during an immune response to HIV-1-pulsed dendritic cells. Aids Res. Hum. Retro. 10:61-71.

18. Clipstone, N. A. and G. R. Crabtree. 1992. Identification of calcineurin as a key signalling enzyme in T-lymphocyte activation. Nature. 357:695-697.

19. Colley, N., E. Baker, M. Stamnes and C. Zuker. 1991. The cyclophilin homolog ninaA is required in the secretory pathway. Cell. 67:255-263.

20. Delchambre, M., D. Gheysen, D. Thines, C. Thiriart, E. Jacobs, E. Verdin, M. Horth, A. Burny and F. Bex. 1989. The Gag precursor of simian immunodeficiency virus assembles into virus-like particles. EMBO J. 8:2653-2660.

21. DesGroseillers, L. and P. Jolicoeur. 1983. Physical mapping of the Fv-1 tropism host range determinant of BALB/c murine leukemia viruses. J.Virol. 48:685-696.

22. Durfee, T., K. Becherer, P.-L. Chen, S.-H. Yeh, Y. Yang, A. E. Kilburn, W.-H. Lee and S. J. Elledge. 1993. The retinoblastoma protein associates with the protein phosphatase type 1 catalytic subunit. Genes Dev. 7:555-569.

23. Dutz, J. P., D. A. Fruman, S. J. Burakoff and B. E. Bierer. 1993. A role for calcineurin in degranulation of murine cytotoxic lymphocytes. J. Immunol. 150:2591-2598.

24. Farnet, C. M. and W. A. Haseltine. 1991. Determination of viral proteins present in the human immunodeficiency virus type 1 preintegration complex. J. Virol. 65:1910-1915.

25. Fields, S. and O. Song. 1989. A novel genetic system to detect protein-protein interactions. Nature. 340:245-246.

26. Fischer, G. and F. X. Schmid. 1990. The mechanism of protein folding. Implications of in vitro refolding models for de novo protein folding and translocation in the cell. Biochemistry. 29:2205-2212.

27. Fischer, G., B. Wittmann-Liebold, K. Lang, T. Kiefhaber and F. X. Schmid. 1989. Cyclophilin and peptidyl-prolyl cis-trans isomerase are probably identical proteins. Nature. 337:476-478.

28. Franke, E. K., H. E.-H. Yuan, K. L. Bossolt, S. P. Goff and J. Luban. 1994. Specificity and sequence requirements for interactions between various retroviral Gag proteins. J. Virol. 68:5300-5305.

29. Franke, E. K., H. E.-H. Yuan and J. Luban. 1994. Specific incorporation of Cyclophilin A into HIV-1 virions. Submitted.

30. Friedman, J. and I. Weissman. 1991. Two cytoplasmic candidates for immunophilin action are revealed by affinity for a new cyclophilin: one in the presence and one in the absence of CsA. Cell. 66:799-806.

31. Fruman, D. A., S. J. Burakoff and B. E. Bierer. 1994. Immunophilins in protein folding and immunosuppression. FASEB J. 8:391-400.

32. Fruman, D. A., P. E. Mather, S. J. Burakoff and B. E. Bierer. 1992. Correlation of calcineurin phosphatase activity and programmed cell death in murine T cell hybridomas. Eur. J. Immunol. 22:2513-2517.

33. Garcia, V. and A. D. Miller. 1991. Serine phosphorylation-independent downregulation of cell-surface CD4 by nef. Nature. 350:508-511.

34. Gaynor, R. B., M. D. Kuwabara, F. K. Wu, J. A. Garcia, D. Harrich, M. Briskin, R. Wall and D. S. Sigman. 1988. Proc. Natl. Acad. Sci. USA. 85:9406-9410.

35. Gething, M.-J. and J. Sambrook. 1992. Protein folding in the cell. Nature. 355:33-45.

36. Gheysen, D., E. Jacobs, F. de Foresta, C. Thiriart, M. Francotte, D. Thines and M. DeWilde. 1989. Assembly and release of HIV-1 precursor Pr55gag virus-like particles from recombinant baculovirus-infected insect cells. Cell. 59:103-112.

37. Gottlinger, H. G., T. Dorfman, E. A. Cohen and W. A. Haseltine. 1993. Vpu protein of human immunodeficiency virus type 1 enhances the release of capsids produced by gag gene constructs of widely divergent retroviruses. Proc. Natl. Acad. Sci. USA. 90:7381-7385.

38. Gottlinger, H. G., J. G. Sodroski and W. A. Haseltine. 1989. Role of capsid precursor processing and myristoylation in morphogenesis and infectivity of human immunodeficiency virus type 1. Proc. Natl. Acad. Sci., USA. 86:5781-5785.

39. Groux, H., G. Torpier, D. Monte, Y. Mouton, A. Capron and J. Ameisen. 1992. Activation-induced death by apoptosis in CD4+ T cells from human immunodeficiency virus-infected asymptomatic individuals. J. Exp. Med. 175:331-340.

40. Haendler, B., R. Hofer-Warbinek and E. Hofer. 1987. Complementary DNA for human T-cell cyclophilin. EMBO J. 6:947-950.

41. Hahn, B. H. 1994. Viral genes and their products. 21-43. In Textbook of AIDS Medicine, ed. Broder, Merigan and Bolognesi. Williams and Wilkins., Baltimore.

42. Handschumacher, R., M. Harding, J. Rice and R. Drugge. 1984. Cyclophilin: A specific cytosolic binding protein for cyclosporin A. Science. 226:544-547.

43. Harding, M. W., R. E. Handschumacher and D. W. Speicher. 1986. Isolation and amino acid sequence of cyclophilin. J. Biol. Chem. 261:8547-8555.

44. Harper, J. W., G. R. Adami, N. Wei, K. Keyomarsi and S. J. Elledge. 1993. The p21 Cdk-interacting protein Cip1 is a potent inhibitor of G1 cyclin-dependent kinases. Cell. 75:805-816.

45. Hasel, K. W., J. R. Glass, M. Godbout and J. G. Sutcliffe. 1991. An endoplasmic reticulum-specific cyclophilin. Mol. Cell. Biol. 11:3484-3491.

46. Hopkins, N., J. Schindler and R. Hynes. 1977. Six NB-tropic murine leukemia viruses derived from a B-tropic virus of BALB/c have altered P30. J Virol. 21:309-318.

47. Hsu, H. W., P. Schwartzberg and S. P. Goff. 1985. Point mutations in the p30 domain of the gag gene of Moloney leukemia virus. Virology. 142:211-214.

48. Imberti, L., A. Sottini, A. Bettinardi, M. Puoti and D. Primi. 1991. Selective depletion in HIV infection of T cells that bear specific T cell receptor VB sequences. Science. 254:860-862.

49. Iwabuchi, K., B. Li, P. Bartel and S. Fields. 1993. Use of the two-hybrid system to identify the domain of p53 involved in oligomerization. Oncogene. 8:1693-1696.

50. Jain, J., P. G. McCaffrey, Z. Miner, T. K. Kerppola, J. N. Lamert, G. L. Verdine, T. Curran and A. Rao. 1993. The T-cell transcription factor NFATp is a substrate for calcineurin and interacts with Fos and Jun. Nature. 365:352-355.

51. Kaelin, W., D. Pallas, J. DeCaprio, F. Kaye and D. Livingston. 1991. Identification of cellular proteins that can interact specifically with the T/E1A-binding region of the retinoblastoma gene product. Cell. 64:521-532.

52. Kappes, J. C., J. S. Parkin, J. A. Conway, J. Kim, C. G. Brouillette, G. M. Shaw and B. H. Hahn. 1993. Intracellular transport and virion incorporation of vpx requires interaction with other virus type-specific components. Virology. 193:222-233.

53. Karpas, A., M. Lowdell, S. Jacobson and F. Hill. 1992. Inhibition of human immunodeficiency virus and growth of infected T cells by the immunosuppressive drugs cyclosporin A and FK506. Proc. Natl. Acad. Sci. USA. 89:8351-8355.

54. Kestler, J. W., D. J. Ringler, K. Mori, D. L. Panicali, P. K. Sehgal, M. D. Daniel and R. C. Desrosiers. 1991. Importance of the nef gene for maintenance of high virus loads and for development of AIDS. Cell. 65:651-663.

55. Kieffer, L. J., T. W. Seng, W. Li, D. G. Osterman, R. E. Handschumacher and R. M. Bayney. 1993. Cyclophilin-40, a protein with homology to the P59 component of the steroid receptor complex. J. Biol. Chem. 268:12303-12310.

56. Klimkait, T., K. Strebel, M. D. Hoggan, M. A. Martin and J. M. Orenstein. 1990. The human immunodeficiency virus type -specific protein Vpu is required for efficient virus maturation and release. J. Virol. 64:621-629.

57. Kofron, J. L., P. Kuzmic, V. Kishore, E. Colon-Bonilla and D. H. Rich. 1991. Determination of kinetic constants for peptidyl prolyl cis-trans isomerases by an improved spectrophotmetric assay. Biochemistry. 30:6127-6134.

58. Koga, Y., M. Sasaki, H. Yoshida, H. Wigzell, G. Kimura and K. Nomoto. 1990. Cytopathic effect determined by the amount of CD4 molecules in human cell lines expressing envelope glycoprotein of HIV. J. Immunol. 144:94-102.

59. Kohl, N. E., E. A. Emini, W. A. Schleif, L. J. Davis, J. C. Heimbach, R. A. Dixon, E. M. Scolnick and I. S. Sigal. 1988. Active human immunodeficiency virus protease is required for viral infectivity. Proc. Natl. Acad. Sci. USA. 85:4686-4690.

60. Koletsky, A. J., M. W. Harding and R. E. Handschumacher. 1986. Cyclophilin: distribution and variant properties in normal and neoplastic tissues. J. Immunol. 137:1054-1059.

61. Lane, H., J. Depper, W. Greene, G. Whalen, T. Waldmann and A. Fauci. 1985. Qualitative analysis of immune function in patients with the acquired immunodeficiency syndrome. N Eng J Med. 313:79-84.

62. Laurent-Crawford, A., B. Krust, S. Muller, Y. Riviere, M.-A. Rey-Cuille, J.-M. Bechet, L. Montagnier and A. Hovanessian. 1991. The cytopathic effect of HIV is associated with apoptosis. Virology. 185:829-839.

63. LaVallee, C., X. J. Yao, A. Ladha, H. Gottlinger, W. A. Haseltine and E. A. Cohen. 1994. Requirement of the Pr55gag precursor for incorporation of the Vpr product into human immunodeficiency virus type 1 viral particles. J. Virol. 68:1926-1934.

64. Lilly, F. and T. Pincus. 1973. Genetic control of murine viral leukemogenesis. Adv. Cancer Res. 17:231-277.

65. Linial, M. L. and A. D. Miller. 1990. Retroviral RNA packaging: sequence requirements and implications. Curr. Top. Microbiol. Immunol. 157:125-152.

66. Liu, J., M. Alber, T. Wandless, S. Luan, D. Alberg, P. Belshaw, P. Cohen, C. MacKintosh, C. Klee and S. Schreiber. 1992. Inhibition of T cell signaling by immunophilin-ligand complexes correlates with loss of calcineurin phosphatase activity. Biochem. 31:3896-3901.

67. Lodish, H. and N. Kong. 1991. Cyclosporin A inhibits an initial step in folding of transferrin within the endoplasmic reticulum. J. Biol. Chem. 266:14835-14838.

68. Lu, Y.-L., P. Spearman and L. Ratner. 1993. Human immunodeficiency virus type 1 viral protein R localization in infected cells and virions. J. Virol. 67:6542-6550.

69. Luban, J., K. B. Alin, K. L. Bossolt, T. Humaran and S. P. Goff. 1992. Genetic assay for multimerization of retroviral gag polyproteins. J. Virol. 66:5157-5160.

70. Luban, J., K. A. Bossolt, E. K. Franke, G. V. Kalpana and S. P. Goff. 1993. Human immunodeficiency virus type 1 gag protein binds to cyclophilins A and B. Cell. 73:1067-1078.

71. Luban, J. and S. Goff. 1991. Binding of human immunodeficiency virus type 1 (HIV-1) RNA to recombinant HIV-1 gag polyprotein. J. Virol. 65:3203-3212.

72. Luban, J., C. Lee and S. P. Goff. 1993. Effect of linker insertion mutations in the human immunodeficiency virus type 1 gag gene on activation of viral protease expressed in bacteria. J. Virol. 67:3630-3634.

73. Luria, S., I. Chambers and P. Berg. 1991. Expression of the type 1 human immunodeficiency virus Nef protein in T cells prevents antigen receptor-mediated induction of interleukin 2 mRNA. Proc. Natl. Acad. Sci. USA. 88:5326-5330.

74. Mammano, F., A. Ohagen, S. Hoglund and H. G. Gottlinger. 1994. Role of the major homology region of human immunodeficiency virus type 1 in virion morphogenesis. J. Virol. In press.:

75. McCaffrey, P. G., C. Luo, T. K. Kerppola, J. Jain, T. M. Badalian, A. M. Ho, E. Burgeon, W. S. Lane, J. N. Lambert, T. Curran, G. L. Verdine, A. Rao and P. G. Hogan. 1993. Isolation of the cyclosporin-sensitive T cell transcription factor NFATp. Science. 262:750-754.

76. McKeon, F. 1991. When worlds collide: immunosuppressants meet protein phosphatases. Cell. 66:823-826.

77. Meyaard, L., S. Otto, R. Jonker, M. Mijnster, R. Keet and F. Miedema. 1992. Programmed death of T cells in HIV-1 infection. Science. 257:217-219.

78. Myers, G., K. MacInnes and B. Korber. 1992. The emergences of simian/human immunodeficiency viruses. AIDS Res. Human Retrovir. 8:373.

79. Nabel, G. and D. Baltimore. 1987. An inducible transcription factor activates expression of human immunodeficiency virus in T cells. Nature. 326:711-713.

80. O'Keefe, S. J., J. Tamura, R. L. Kincaid, M. J. Tocci and E. A. O'Neill. 1992. FK-506- and CsA-sensitive activation of the interleukin-2 promoter by calcineurin. Nature. 357:692-694.

81. Pal, R., M. S. Reitz Jr., E. Tschachler, R. C. Gallo, M. G. Sarnagadharan and F. D. M. Veronese. 1990. Myristylation of gag proteins of HIV-1 plays an important role in virus assembly. AIDS Res. Hum. Retroviruses. 6:721-730.

82. Pantaleo, G., C. Graziosi and A. Fauci. 1993. The immunopathogenesis of human immunodeficiency virus infection. N. Engl. J. Med. 328:327-335.

83. Pantaleo, G., M. Vaccarezza, O. J. Cohen, R. H. Hohman and A. S. Fauci. Cyclosporin A suppresses HIV-1 infection in primary T lymphocytes acutely infected in vitro. IXth International Conference on AIDS. 246, 1993.

84. Park, J. and C. D. Morrow. 1992. The nonmyristylated Pr160gag-pol polyprotein of human immunodeficiency virus type 1 interacts with Pr55gag and is incorporated into viruslike particles. J. Virol. 66:6304-6313.

85. Paxton, W., R. I. Connor and N. R. Landau. 1993. Incorporation of Vpr into human immunodeficiency virus type 1 virions: requirement for p6 region of *gag* and mutational analysis. J. Virol. 67:7229-7237.

86. Peng, C., B. Ho, T. Chang and N. Chang. 1989. Role of human immunodeficiency virus type 1 specific protease in core maturation and viral infectivity. J. Virol. 63:2550-2556.

87. Price, E. R., L. D. Zydowsky, M. Jin, C. H. Baker, F. D. McKeon and C. T. Walsh. 1991. Human cyclophilin B: a second cyclophilin gene encodes a peptidyl-prolyl isomerase with a signal sequence. Proc. Natl. Acad. Sci. USA. 88:1903-1907.

88. Ramsay, G. and M. J. Hayman. 1980. Analysis of cells transformed by defective leukemia virus OK10: production of noninfectious particles and synthesis of Pr76gag and an additional 200,000-dalton protein. Virology. 106:71-81.

89. Rebai, N., G. Pantaleo, J. F. Demarest, C. Ciurli, H. Soudeyns, J. W. Adelsberger, M. Vaccarezza, R. E. Walker, R. P. Sekaly and A. S. Fauci. 1994. Analysis of the T-cell receptor beta-chain variable-region (V beta) repertoire in monozygotic twins discordant for human immunodeficiency virus: evidence for perturbation of specific V beta segments in CD4+ T cells of the virus-positive twins. Proc. Natl. Acad. Sci. USA. 91:1529-1533.

90. Rein, A., M. McClure, N. Rice, R. Luftig and A. Schultz. 1986. Myristylation site in Pr65gag is essential for virus particle formation by Moloney murine leukemia virus. Proc. Natl. Acad. Sci., USA. 83:7246-7250.

91. Rhee, S. S. and E. Hunter. 1987. Myristylation is required for intracellular transport but not for assembly of D-type retrovirus capsids. J. Virol. 61:1045-1053.

92. Rosenwirth, B., A. Billich, R. Datema, P. Donatsch, F. Hammerschmid, R. Harrison, P. Hiestand, H. Jaksche, P. Mayer, P. Peichl, V. Quesniaux, F. Schatz, H.-J. Schuurman, R. Traber, R. Wenger, B. Wolff, G. Zenke and M. Zurini. 1994. Inhibition of HIV-1 replication by SDC NIM 811, a non-immunosuppressive cyclosporin A analogue. Antimicro. Agents Chemother. 38:1763-1772.

93. Schreiber, S. L. and G. R. Crabtree. 1992. The mechanism of action of cyclosporin A and FK506. Immunology Today. 13:136-142.

94. Schultz, A. M. and A. Rein. 1989. Unmyristoylated Moloney murine leukemia virus Pr65gag is excluded from virus assembly and maturation events. J. Virol. 63:2370-2373

95. Schwartz, O., M. Alizon, J. M. Heard and O. Danos. 1994. Impairment of t cell receptor-dependent stimulation in CD4+ lymphocytes after contact with membrane-bound HIV-1 envelope glycoprotein. Virology. 198:360-365.

96. Schwarz, A., G. Offermann, F. Keller, I. Bennhold, J. L'Age-Stehr, P. H. Krause and M. J. Mihatsch. 1993. The effect of cyclosporine on the progression of human immunodeficiency virus type 1 infection transmitted by transplantation - Data on four cases and review of the literature. Transplantation. 55:95-103.

97. Shearer, G. and M. Clerici. 1991. Early T-helper cell defects in HIV infection. AIDS. 5:245-253.

98. Shi, Y., B. M. Sahai and D. R. Green. 1989. Cyclosporin A inhibits activation-induced cell death in T-cell hybridomas and thymocytes. Nature. 339:625-626.

99. Shields, A., O. N. Witte, E. Rothenberg and D. Baltimore. 1978. High frequency of aberrant expression of Moloney murine leukemia virus in clonal infections. Cell. 14:601-609.

100. Shioda, T. and H. Shibuta. 1992. Production of human immunodeficiency virus (HIV)-like particles from cells infected with recombinant vaccinia viruses carrying the *gag* gene of HIV. Virology. 175:139-148.

101. Sigal, N. H., F. Dumont, P. Durette, J. J. Siekierka, L. Peterson, D. H. Rich, B. E. Dunlap, M. J. Staruch, M. R. Melino, S. L. Koprak, D. Williams, B. Witzel and J. M. Pisano. 1991. Is cyclophilin involved in

the immunosuppressive and nephrotoxic mechanism of action of cyclosporin A? J. Exp. Med. 173:619-628.

102. Skowronski, J., D. Parks and R. Mariani. 1993. Altered T cell activaton and development in transgenic mice expressing the HIV-1 nef gene. EMBO J. 12:703-713.

103. Smith, A. J., N. Srinivasakumar, M.-L. Hammarskjold and D. Rekosh. 1993. Requirements for incorporation of Pr160gag-pol from human immunodeficiency virus type 1 into virus-like particles. J. Virol. 67:2266-2275.

104. Smith, D. B. and K. S. Johnson. 1988. Single-step purification of polypeptides expressed in *Excherichia coli* as fusions with glutathione S-transferase. Gene. 67:31-40.

105. Sodroski, J., W. C. Goh, C. Rosen, K. Campbell and W. A. Haseltine. 1986. Role of the HTLV-III/LAV envelope in syncytium formation and cytopathicity. Nature. 322:470-474.

106. Stamnes, M. A., S. L. Rutherford and C. S. Zuker. 1992. Cyclophilins: a new family of proteins involved in intracellular folding. Trends in Cell. Biol. 2:272-276.

107. Steinmann, B., P. Bruckner and A. Superti-Furga. 1991. cyclosporin A slows collagen triple-helix formation in vivo: Indirect evidence for a physiologic role of peptidyl-prolyl cis-trans-isomerase. J. Biol. Chem. 266:1299-1303.

108. Strambio-de-Castillia, C. and E. Hunter. 1992. Mutational analysis of the major homology region of Mason-Pfizer monkey virus by use of saturation mutagenesis. J. Virol. 66:7021-7032.

109. Strebel, K., T. Klimkait, F. Maldarelli and M. A. Martin. 1989. Molecular and biochemical analysis of human immunodeficiency virus type 1 *vpu* protein. J. Virol. 63:3784-3791.

110. Sykes, K., M.-J. Gething and J. Sambrook. 1993. Proline isomerases function during heat shock. Proc. Natl. Acad. Sci. USA. 90:5853-5857.

111. Terai, C., R. Kornbluth, C. Pauza, D. Richman and D. Carson. 1991. Apoptosis as a mechanism of cell death in cultured T lymphoblasts acutely infected with HIV-1. J. Clin. Invest. 87:1710-1715.

112. Thali, M., A. A. Bukovsky, E. Kondo, B. Rosenwirth, C. T. Walsh, J. Sodroski and H. G. Goettlinger. 1994. Specific association of cyclophilin A with human immunodeficiency virus type 1 virions. Submitted.

113. Tristem, M., C. Marshall, A. Karpas and F. Hill. 1992. Evolution of the primate lentiviruses: evidence from *vpx* and *vpr*. EMBO J. 11:3405-3412.

114. Vojtek, A. B., S. M. Hollenberg and J. A. Cooper. 1993. Mammalian Ras interacts directly with the serine/threonine kinase Raf. Cell. 774:205-214.

115. Wainberg, M., A. Dascal, N. Blain, L. Fitz-Gibbon, F. Boulerice, K. Numazaki and M. Tremblay. 1988. The effect of cyclosporine A on infection of susceptible cells by human immunodeficiency virus type 1. Blood. 72:1904-1910.

116. Walsh, C. T., L. D. Zydowsky and F. D. McKeon. 1992. Cyclosporin A, the cyclophilin class of petidylprolyl isomerases, and blockade of T cell signal transduction. J. Biol. Chem. 267:13115-13118.

117. Wang, C.-T. and E. Barklis. 1993. Assembly, processing, and infectivity of human immunodeficiency virus type 1 gag mutants. J. Virol. 67:4264-4273.

118. Wang, T., P. K. Donahoe and A. S. Zervos. 1994. Specific interaction of type I receptors of the TGF-β family with the immunophilin FKBP-12. Science. 265:674-676.

119. Weinhold, K., H. Lyerly, S. Stanley, A. Austin, T. Matthews and D. Bolognesi. 1989. HIV-1 pg120-mediated immune suppression and lymphocyte destruction in the absence of viral infection. J. Immunol. 142:3091-3097.

120. Weiss, R. A. 1989. Defective viruses to blame? Nature. 338:458.

121. Yu, X.-F., M. Matsuda, M. Essex and T.-H. Lee. 1990. Open reading frame *vpr* of simian immunodeficiency virus encodes a virion-associated protein. J. Virol. 64:5688-5693.

122. Zervos, A., J. Gyuris and R. Brent. 1993. Mxi1, a protein that specifically interacts with Max to bind Myc-Max recognition sites. Cell. 72:223-232.

20

LONG-TERM FOLLOW-UP OF HIV POSITIVE ASYMPTOMATIC PATIENTS HAVING RECEIVED CYCLOSPORIN A

Rafaël Levy, Jean-Philippe Jais, Jean-Marc Tourani, Philippe Even, and Jean-Marie Andrieu

Département de Médecine Interne
Hôpital Laennec
Faculté Necker
Paris, France
Département de Biostatistique
Hôpital Necker
Faculté Necker
Paris, France

SUMMARY

The data of the 27 asymptomatic HIV-1 seropositive patients with CD4 + cell count between 300 and 600/µl treated by Cyclosporin A (CSA) (7.5 mg/kg/day) in our institution between october 1985 and 1987 were rewieved in October 1993. Hemoglobin concentration, platelet count, total lymphocytes, CD4$^+$ and CD8$^+$ cell counts and serum core protein p24 antigenemia, as well as creatininemia measured before CSA onset, at CSA cessation and twice a year were recorded as well as clinical signs and CSA toxicities. In October 1993 median duration of CSA treatment was 11 months, median follow-up after CSA cessation was 15 months and median total follow-up was 67 months. Toxicities of CSA were those commonly encountered in other pathologies. Under CSA no patient progressed toward clinical AIDS (1987 definition). The mean CD4$^+$ cell count of the 27 patients remained unchanged (gain of 1 cell/year) under CSA treatment, while it decreased at a rate of 50 cells/year after CSA cessation (p<0,005). On the other hand CSA treatment had no significant impact on the evolution of total lymphocyte count, CD8$^+$ cell counts, and P24 antigenémia.

INTRODUCTION

In 1985, we hypothetized that the potent immunosuppressive drug Cyclosporin A (CSA) could be beneficial for HIV-1 infected subjects not yet profoundly immuno compromised (1). We speculated that CSA, by decreasing CD4 cell activation, - a hallmark of HIV infection, - would decrease HIV replication ; CSA would also down-regulate HIV associated - auto-immune phenomena which were thought to be associated with excessive CD4 cell destruction.

In order to test this hypothesis, between October 1985 and February 1986, CSA was given to 8 patients with AIDS, and 25 without AIDS, of which 10 had less than 300 CD4/µl and 15 were asymptomatic (Centers of Disease Control and Prevention (CDC) stages II or III) with a CD4 cell count between 300 and 600/µl. In patients with AIDS as well as in those with less than 300 CD4/µl, the prognosis of HIV infection did not seem to be modified by CSA treatment (2). On the other hand, none of the 15 patients with CD4 between 300 and 600/µl developed AIDS under CSA treatment; moreover their mean CD4 cell count, after a transient increase (day 10), remained stable over 3-6 months (2,3). At that time, these results, as well as those of a very short-term (2 months) double blinded randomized study sponsored by INSERM (4), were not found positive enough by French AIDS research institution to plan a long term randomized study with CSA.

In october 93 (i.e. 8 years after our first patient began CSA), we decided to evaluate the long-term clinical and biological evolution of all our asymptomatic patients with CD4 cells ranging from 300 to 600/µl who received CSA in our institution.

PATIENTS AND METHODS

A total of 27 asymptomatic patients with CD4 cells ranging between 300 and 600/µl received CSA in our institution from October 21th 1985 to November 25th 1987. This number includes the fifteen patients treated betwen October 1985 and February 86, and 12 other patients treated by CSA betwen March 86 and November 87. All patients gave informed consent.

Details on treatment methods have already been given (2). Briefly, creatinemia, hemoglobin level, platelet count, total lymphocyte count as well as CD4[+] and CD8[+] cells subsets and serum P24 antigenemia were mesured before CSA onset, within the week preeceding CSA cessation as well as at least twice a year during the whole follow-up period. CSA (Sandimune, SANDOZ-FRANCE) was given orally at an initial dosage of 7.5 mg/kg daily. Trough plasma levels of CSA were regularly measured by radio-immunoassay and CSA daily dosage was adjusted to obtain plasma levels ranging from 100 to 300 ng/ml. Dosage was reduced when creatinemia exceeded 140µmol/l. CSA treatment was initially planned for three months. At that time point, patients whose CD4 cell count had decreased under pretherapeutic value were considered as non responders and withdrawn from CSA ; all other patients remained under CSA treatment until appearance of toxicity or their decision to stop the drug.

Statistical analysis: Hemoglobin level, platelet count, creatinininemia, total lympho-cyte count, CD4 and CD8 cell percentages and absolute values and P24 antigenemia were compared at entry and CSA cessation by the Wilcoxon test. Comparison of the evolution of biological parameters measured each 6 month under CSA and after CSA cessation was made by repeated measures analysis of variance (PROC MIXT, SAS, V6)

RESULTS

The characteristics of the 27 patients were as follows: 11 patients were at CDC stage II and 16 at CDC stage III. There were 22 males and 5 females. Routes of contamination were: homosexual sex 19 pts, heterosexual sex 4 pts, and intravenous drug abuse: 4 pts. The mean age of the patients was 37 years (min:23 - max:68).

Table 1. Comparison of biological parameters at the onset and at the end of
Cyclosporin A treatment

	Onset of CSA		End of CSA		
	Mean (± sd)	Median	Mean (± sd)	Median	p*
Lymphocytes/µl	2094 (702)	1825	1491 (687)	1400	0.001
CD4 %	22 (6)	24	28 (10)	27	0.002
CD4 /µl	440 (76)	523	404 (218)	410	0.1
CD8 %	50 (14)	49	50 (11)	48	0.9
CD8 /µl	1052 (487)	945	792 (440)	571	0.02
Hemoglobin (g/dl)	14.7 (1.4)		12 (± 1.6)		0.005
Platelets (x10³/µl)	177 (35)		160 (81)		0.002
Creatinnemia (µml/l)	87.7 (7.4)		168.8 (131.1)		0.005

*p value was determined by the Wilcoxon rank test.

The whole group of patients was evaluated on October 1993. At that time, the median duration of follow-up was 67 months (min:5, max:87, mean:59,5), the median duration of CSA treatment was 11 months (min 2, max 54, mean 14) and the median follow-up after CSA cessation was 45 months (min:2, max:85, mean:45).

Toxicities were those commonly encountered with CSA (paresthesia, gingivitis, hypertension, gastric intolerance, hypertrichosis, asthenia) and have already been described (2). Reasons for CSA cessation were: - no response at 3 months: 7 cases, renal toxicity: 7 cases. hematological toxicity: 4 cases, reactivation of a viral hepatitis: 2 cases, paresthesia: 1 case, hypertension: 1 case, and patient wish: 5 cases.

Under CSA treatment, no patients developed AIDS, while after CSA cessation 18 patients developed AIDS (Opportunistic infection: 9 cases, Kaposi sarcoma: 5 cases, encephalopathy: 2 cases, Non-Hodgkin lymphoma: 1 case).

Overall, under CSA treatment, the total lymphocyte count and its CD8 subset significantly decreased ; in contrast the CD4 cell count remained stable (table 1). At the onset of CSA, p24 antigenemia was detectable in 9 patients and two patients became positive during CSA treatment. The mean value of p24 antigenemia for the entire group increased from 62pg/ml at onset of CSA to 275 pg/ml at CSA cessation (p=0,001). The biological toxicity of CSA treatment was marked (creatinine increased, hemoglobin level and platelet count decreased).

As shown in Figure 1 there was no change in the rate of decrease of the total lymphocyte and CD8 cell counts (absolute value and %) under CSA treatment and after CSA cessation: loss of 20,2 lymphocytes/month under CSA and loss of 10,9 lymphocytes/month after CSA, loss of 9,45 CD8 cell/month and 0,09 CD8 %/month under CSA and loss of 2,85 CD8 cell/month and 0,39 CD8 %/month after CSA (p >0.1). Moreover, there was no change in the rate of increase of p24 antigenemia: increase of 3,89 pg/ml/month under CSA and increase of 2,26 pg/ml/month after CSA cessation (p>0.1). In contrast, there was a highly significant change in the CD4 cell count: gain of 0,8 cell/month and 0,15 CD4 %/month

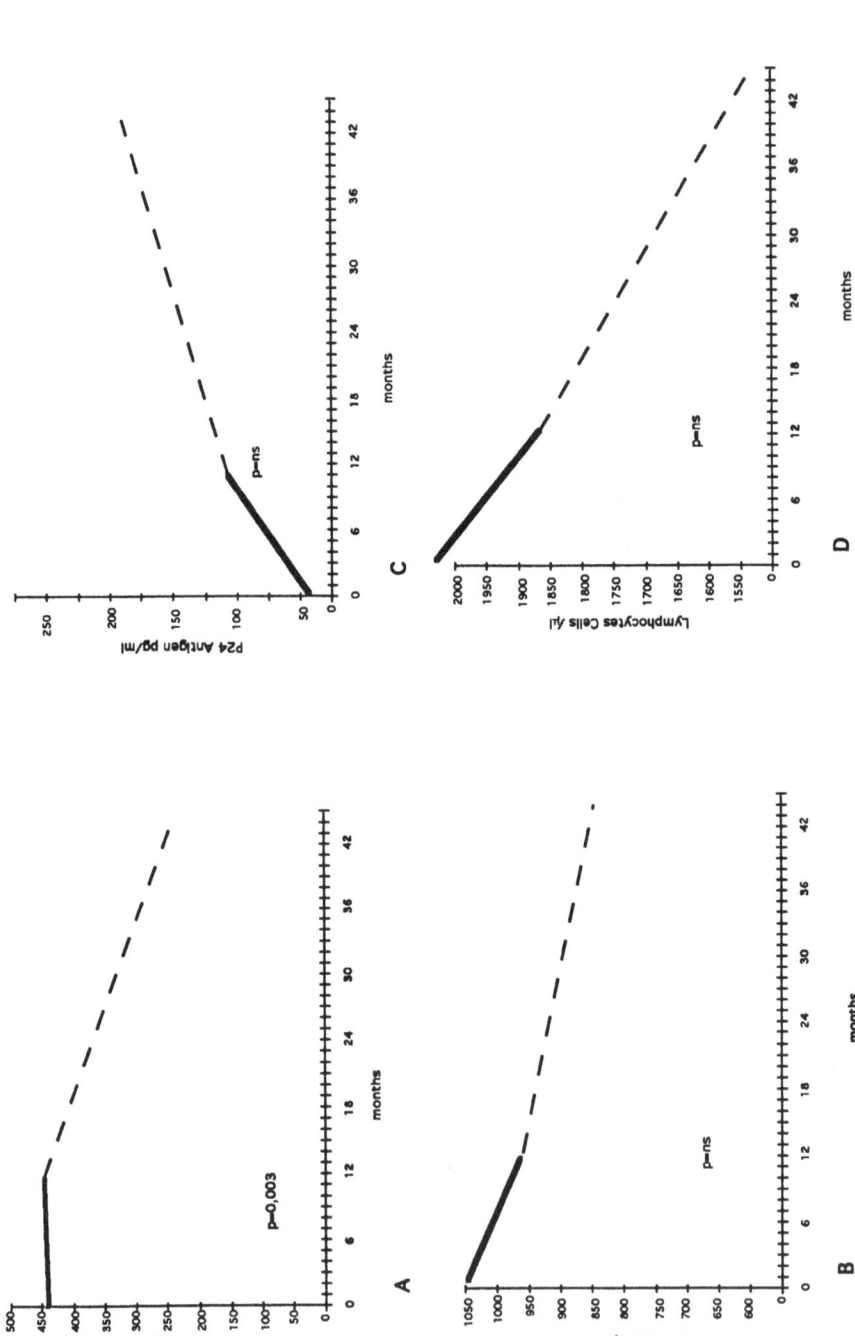

Figure 1. Representation of the calculated slopes of CD4 count (A) CD8 cell count (B), serum P24 antigen level (C), and total lymphocyte count (D). The variation of the slope between the period on CSA (——) and off CSA (···) was calculated by repeated measures analysis of variance ; P: significance of the slope change.

under CSA versus loss of 4,21 cell/month and 0,19 CD4 %/month after CSA cessation (p<0.005 and p<0.001 respectively). Overall the evolution of the total lymphocyte and CD8 cell counts, as well as that of the P24 antigenemia were not significantly affected by CSA treatment ; in contrast the evolution of the CD4$^+$ cell count was profoundly influenced by CSA administration.

DISCUSSION

In this group of 27 patients not yet profoundly immunocompromised, (CD4/µl between 300 and 600) no patient developed AIDS under CSA. On the other hand, the CD4$^+$ cell count remained stable under CSA whereas its rate of decrease returned to around 50 CD4 cells/year after CSA cessation ; interestingly such a rate is that generally observed in untreated or Ziduvudine-treated patients (5). Other biological parameters behave identically whether the patients were on or off CSA. Toxicity of CSA was noticeable but not different from what is observed in other pathologies requiring CSA treatment.

Since the time where in 1985 we formulated the hypothesis that CD4 cell activation could be deleterious in HIV infection by increasing viral replication and by amplifying the immune/auto-immune processes leading to an over destruction of the CD4 cell pool (1), much knowledge has accumulated on these aspects of the pathogenesis of HIV infection (review in 6). - Cellular and humoral markers of immune activation have been demonstrated to be strong predictors of clinical deterioration (7-10) ; - CD4$^+$ cell activation has been recognized as a necessary step preceeding viral replication (11,12); moreover the accelerated CD4 cell apoptosis observed along the course of HIV infection has been shown to result from the chronic HIV-induced CD4 cell activation (13,14).

On the other hand, it has been recently shown in vitro that CSA, by preventing CD4 cell activation was able to inhibit CD4 cell apoptosis as well as viral replication (15,16). Moreover a direct inhibition of HIV replication by CSA (however at extra therapeutic doses) has also been recently demonstrated in vitro (17,18).

A retrospective study of the clinical evolution of kidney transplanted individuals infected by HIV-1 at the time of their transplantation and treated or not by CSA suggested that CSA treatment could slow-down the rate of progression of HIV infection toward AIDS (19).

These various aspects of the viro-immunopathogenesis of HIV infection and the potential role of CSA have been recently summarized (20). Taken to gather, our results and the above-mentionned pieces of information should now allow clicans to design long term double-blinded trials with clinical, virological and immunological end points in order to evaluate the role of CSA in well defined groups of HIV- infected individuals.

REFERENCES

1. Andrieu JM, Even P, Venet A. AIDS and related syndromes as a viral-induced auto-immune disease of the immune system: an anti-MHCII disorder ; therapeutic implications. AIDS Res 1986;2:163-174.
2. Andrieu JM, Even P, Tourani JM et al. Effects of cyclosporin on T-cell subset in human immunodeficiency virus disease. Clin Immunol Immunopathol 1988;46:181-198.13.
3. Andrieu JM, Even P, Tourani JM, Beldjord K, Audroin C. Results of a 2-year exploratory study with cyclosporin A in human immunodeficiency virus infection. Auto-immune aspects of HIV infection (JM Andrieu, JF Bach, P Even Eds). International congress and symposium series N 41, Royal Society of Medicine Services. London New-York 1988.

4. Aboulker JP, Andrieu JM, Gastaud JA et al. Two month double blind placebo controlled trial of cyclosporin in HIV asymptomatic subjects. V international conference on AIDS 1989; p402 (Abst).

5. Concorde Coordinating Committee. Concorde MRC/ANRS randomised double blind controlled trial of immediate and deferred Zidovudine in symptom-free HIV infection. Lancet 1994;343:871-880.

6. Fauci AS. Multifactorial nature of human immunodeficiency virus disease: implications for therapy. Science 1993;262:1011-1018.

7. Malahingam M, Peakman M, Davies ET, Ozniak A, Mac Manus JJ, Vergnani D. T cell activation and disease severity in HIV infection. Clin Exp Immunol 1993;93:337-343.

8. Fahey JL, Taylor JMG, Detels R et al. The prognostic value of cellular and serologic markers in infection with human immunodeficiency virus type 1. N Engl J Med 1990;322:166-172.

9. Lifson AR, Hessol NA, Buchbinder SP, O'Malley PM, Barnhardt L, Segal M, Katz MH, Holmberg SD. Serum β_2-microglobulin and prediction of progression to AIDS in HIV infection. Lancet 1992;339:1436-1440.

10. Simmonds P, Beatson D, Cuthbert RJG et al. Determinants of HIV disease progression; six year longitudinal study in the Edimburgh haemophilia/HIV cohort. Lancet 1991;338:1159-163.

11. Zack JA, Arrigo SJ, Weitsaman Sh, GO AS, Haislip A. Chen ISY. HIV-1 entry into quiescent primary lymphocytes: molecular analysis reveals a labile, latent viral structure. Cell 1990;61:213-222.

12. Bukringsky MI, Stanwick JL, Dempsey MP, Stevenson M. Quiescent T lymphocytes as an inducible virus reservoir for HIV-1 infection. Science 1991;254:423-427.

13. Gougeon ML, Olivier R, Garcia S, Guetard D, Dragic T, Dauguet C, Montagnier L. Mise en évidence d'un processus d'engagement vers la mort cellulaire par apoptose dans les lymphocytes de patients infectés par le VIH. CR Acad Sci Paris 1991;312:529-537.

14. Groux H, Torpier G, Monté D, Mouton Y, Capron A, Ameisen JC. Activation-induced death by apoptosis in CD4+ T cells from human immunodeficiency virus-infected asymptomatic individuals. J Exp Med 1992;175:331-340.

15. Karpas A, Lowdell M, Jacobson SK, Hill F. Inhibition of human immunodeficiency virus and growth of infected T cells by the immunosuppressive drugs cyclosporin A and FK 506. Proc Natl Acad Sci USA 1992;89:8531-8555.

16. Lu W, Salerno-Goncalves R, Yan J, Doré S, Han DS, Andrieu JM. Glucocorticoides rescue CD4+ lymphocytes from activation-induced apoptosis triggered by HIV-1: implication for pathogenesis and therapy. AIDS 1995;9:35-42.

17. Franke EK, Yuan HEH, Luban J. Spenfic incorporation of cyclophilin A into HIV-1 virions. Nature 1994;372:359-362.

18. Thall M, Bukovsky A, Kondo I, Rosewirth B, Walsh C, Sodroski J, Gottlinger HG. Functional association of Cyclophillin A with HIV-1 virions. Nature 1994;372:363-365.

19. Schwarz A, Offerman G, Keller F, Bennhold I, L'Age Stehr J, Krause PH, Mihatsch MJ. The effect of cyclosporin on the progression of human imunodeficiency virus type 1 infection transmitted by transplatnation. Data on four cases and review of the literature. Transplantation 1993;55:95-103.

20. Andrieu JM, Lu W. Viroimmunopathogenesis of HIV disease. Implications for therapy. Immunology today 1995;16:5-7.

21

PROSPECTIVE VIEWS OF HIV PATHOLOGY
Clues for Therapeutic Strategies

Wei Lu and Jean-Marie Andrieu

Laboratorie d'Immunologie des Tumeurs
Hôpital Laènnec
Faculté de Médecine Necker
Université René Descartes–Paris V
Paris, France

INTRODUCTION

The human immunodeficiency virus (HIV) is the causative agent of AIDS. Individuals infected with HIV tolerate an often long, but variable, period of clinical latency characterized by the persistent activation of the multiple components of the immune system as well as by the progressive depletion of the CD4+ T-cell pool. The pathogenic mechanisms governing these processes are complex and composed of overlapping phases where both virological and immunological factors are involved (1-3).

Over the past decade, researchers and clinicians have focused their efforts on attempting to inhibit viral replication using drugs that act on the life cycle of the virus in infected cells. Due to rapid development of drug resistance (4-6), this approach has so far provided transient clinical improvement, and has only slightly delayed clinical progression and death (7). Recent advances in the understanding of the viro-immunopathology of HIV disease open the prospect to alternative therapeutic approaches directed at the pathogenic processes causing the devastation of the immune system.

VIRO-CYTOPATHIC MECHANISMS

HIV-Triggered Apoptosis

HIV infects CD4-positive cells (i.e. T helper lymphocytes and monocytes/macrophages) through a high affinity interaction between the HIV-gp120 env protein and the host CD4 molecules (8,9). In vitro studies demonstrate that HIV strains can differ substantially in their ability to kill CD4+ T-cell lines. Viruses which kill cells by cell-cell fusion are referred as syncytium-inducing (SI) variants while those which provoke single cell death are referred as non-syncytium-inducing (NSI) variants. The major sites in the viral genome

Cell Activation and Apoptosis in HIV Infection
Edited by Jean-Marie Andrieu and Wei Lu, Plenum Press, New York, 1995

responsible for this biological property reside in the VI/V2 or V3 region of the envelope gp120 (10,11) which may also functionally interact with other regions of gp120 (12).

Both types of HIV-triggered cell death occur by apoptosis, an active suicide mechanism which is the principle form of physiological death for lymphocytes (13,14). Several lines of evidence support that HIV replication is a prerequisite for triggering apoptosis in CD4+ T cells (15-19). Although the mechanisms by which apoptosis pathways are activated remain unclear, the env gene product gp120 seems to be required for the induction of apoptosis in infected cells by cell surface CD4 signalling (17,18). The interaction between CD4 molecule and HIV gp120 (C4 domain) appears to play an important role in the single cell-killing process of CD4 lymphocytes (20,21), but not of HIV infected macrophages and microglial cells. The reasons for these differences are so far unidentified. However, HIV-infected macrophages tolerate several functional impairments including alteration of cytokine production (increase in IL-1ß, IL-6, IL-8, and TNF-α production and decrease in IL-12 production) (22,23), alteration of antigen-presenting function (24), and decreased phagocytosis and degradation of micro-organisms (25).

HIV Tropism-Related Cytopathicity

The V3 loop of HIV envelope gp120 has been identified as the primary determinant of the cellular tropism (e.g. the monocyte/macrophage-tropism or the T-cell-line-tropism) at the post-binding level of viral entry (10). Recent evidences indicate that the secondary structure (conformation) of the V3 loop is influenced by the conformation of other regions of HIV envelope gp120 and the overall conformation of gp120 determines the biological properties of the virus (including cytopathicity, cellular tropism, and neutralization) (12,26,27). In addition, regulatory proteins and other host cell factors may be involved in the post-entry processes modulating the kinetics and level of viral replication (10).

The contribution of viral tropism to CD4+ T-cell depletion in AIDS progression was initially suggested by in vitro studies demonstrating that viruses with a T-cell-tropic phenotype (frequently associated with SI and rapidly replicating properties) were recovered with an increased frequency from patients at advanced stages of disease (28). However, the lack of T-cell-line-tropic (SI) isolates in nearly 50% AIDS patients (29,30) indicates that such a property is not a prerequisite for virus-mediated CD4 depletion.

Moreover, infection of severe combined immunodeficiency (SCID) mice grafted with human peripheral blood mononuclear cells (hu-PBMC-SCID mice) with macrophage-tropic/NSI HIV isolates causes the rapid destruction of the grafted CD4+ T cells, whereas in this animal model infection with T-cell-line-tropic/SI isolates causes variable and slower CD4 depletion (31).

On the other hand, we have demonstrated in our laboratory that 66 primary HIV-1 isolates replicate PBMC in a similar fashion regardless of the disease severity of the patients from whom the viruses have been isolated (32); moreover a recent study conducted on a panel of 70 HIV-1 and 12 HIV-2 isolates showed that all HIV isolates could infect and replicate both CD4+ T lymphocytes and primary monocyte-derived macrophages, regardless of the disease severity of the virus donors (33). Furthermore, an in vivo analysis of the V3 loop of the env gp120 revealed that variants of HIV with V3 sequences characteristic of NSI/macrophage-tropic phenotype formed the predominant population in a range of lymphoid and nonlymphoid tissues, irrespective of the severity of disease progression (34). Taken together, these studies, demonstrate the lack of consistent or clear-cut correlation between viral phenotypes and disease progression, and strongly suggest that the role of viral tropism is only marginally involved, if it is, in AIDS pathogenesis.

IMMUNOPATHIC MECHANISMS

Chronic Activation and T-Cell Anergy

The accelerated apoptosis of uninfected T cells (both CD4 and CD8 subsets) from HIV-infected patients when activated in vitro (35-37) does not seem to be correlated with the CD4+ T-cell depletion rate (38). Such an apoptosis could simply be a consequence of the chronic stimulation (or restimulation) (triggered by HIV-related or HIV-unrelated antigens) of the multiple components of the immune system (including monocytes, B lymphocytes, as well as CD4+ and CD8+ T cells) which is hallmark of HIV infection (2,3).

The loss of T-cell proliferative response upon to in vitro recall antigen, alloantigen, and finally mitogen stimulations occurring during the course of the infection (39-41) has been attributed to such an activation (or re-activation) of T-cell compartment causing apoptosis (rather than proliferation) as well as to the selective loss of memory CD4+ T cells (42,43) by virus-induced apoptosis (14-19) and the functional impairment of antigen-presenting cells (44). The T-cell anergy has also been associated with the defective production of IL-12 by infected macrophages which may prevent the Th0-to-Th1 shift in vivo. (3,23).

Cytotoxic T Lymphocytes-Related Immunopathology

The cytotoxic T lymphocytes (CTL) may lyse target cells via a Fas-mediated apoptosis (45,46). HIV-specific CTL response (47,48) is detectable in most seropositive patients with a major HIV-specific CTL expansion during the primary infection (49). Since HIV preferentially replicates in CD4+ T cells as well as macrophages/microglia, and dendritic cells, CTL may destroy these cells when they express or bind viral antigens, which may thus contribute to the development of AIDS (50). This notion is in keeping with a recent study reporting that white pulps of HIV-infected individuals are infiltrated by HIV-specific CTL (51), thereby implicating them in CD4+ T cell destruction in vivo.

Superantigen, Autoimmune Phenomena

A superantigen carried either by HIV or an unrelated microbe has been proposed to bind to the variable (V) region of the TCR β chain in association with binding to the β chain of the class II major histocompatibility complex (MHC) molecules, inducing a massive expansion of the Vβ T cells (2). A recent study has provided evidences that these expanded oligoclonal Vβ T cells are the result of a specific CTL response to HIV and that the intense Vβ expansion observed during primary infection is indeed associated with a rapid progression to AIDS (49). In addition, it has been hypothesized that cross-reactivity between viral proteins and self components such as MHC molecules could induce immunological responses that destroy immune competent cells and damage immunological function such as antigen recognition and cytokine dysmodulation (3). So far no compelling data are however available to confirm such an autoimmune mechanism in vivo.

VIRUS-HOST INTERACTION AND HIV DISEASE

A few weeks after contamination, about 70% of individuals manifest an acute clinical syndrome (52), associated with a burst of infectious viremia (30,53-55), the expansion of CD8+ T cells with a predominant Vβ type (i.e., a HIV-specific CTL response) (49), and a substantial decrease in the CD4+ T-lymphocyte count (resulting from HIV-triggered and CTL-mediated apoptosis). The high level of infectious viremia observed at that time may facilitate virus spread to lymphoid tissues (56,57) as well as to the brain (58). The humoral immune response to HIV (i.e. seroconversion) is then associated with a dramatic decrease in infectious viremia (53,54). At that time, the CD4+ T-cell count may re-increase to some extent, but remains generally lower than before contamination (2). Patients then enter a phase of clinical latency. During this phase, there is an active viral replication in CD4+ T cells and macrophages as well as a progressive disorganization of the follicular dendritic network in the germinal centers (30,56).

The analysis of several cohorts of patients indicates that the rate of progression to AIDS is 0-2% for the first two years after seroconversion and 6 to 8% as of the third year. Thus, 10 years after contamination, about half of the infected individuals have develop AIDS (1). The lymph node architecture at that time is completely disrupted and only vestiges of germinal centers are still observed (30,56). This terminal phase is preceded by the loss of isolate-specific neutralizing antibodies (59) which may be responsible for the tremendous virus spread (through both lymphoid and nonlymphoid tissues) seen in AIDS (2,60).

Although few individuals infected with HIV may develop AIDS during primary infection or shortly (within 12 months) after seroconversion (30,49,61), these rapidly progressing patients often exhibit a broad activation of the immune system with a massive expansion of HIV-specific CTL (predominantly of the Vβ family) (49), an absence of isolate-specific neutralizing antibody response (61), a high level of viremia (30), and a profound decline in CD4+ T-cell count (30,49).

Since the high level of viremia decreases generally after seroconversion (30,53,54), it means that an immune response against HIV is attainable during primary infection. Although there is a temporal association between the anti-HIV CTL activity and the initial control of primary viremia (62), the permanent viral replication and the presence of HIV-specific CTL precursors through the course of HIV disease suggest that CTL alone are not able to eliminate HIV-infected cells in vivo. On the other hand, the fact that the isolate-specific neutralizing antibody activity detectable shortly after seroconversion decreases or disappears in rapidly progressing patients (59,61) while at the same time the infectious virus load increases rapidly (30,59), strongly suggests that the neutralizing antibody response play a primary role in blocking the virus spread in the body.

In this context, the question of how neutralizing antibody production is suppressed arises. One possible explanation is that HIV-specific B cells which are able to process viral antigens, and present their fragments to the class I-restricted CTL may be killed by HIV-specific CTL in the same manner as HBV-presenting B cells are destroyed by anti-HBV CTL (63). This may represent a mechanism of suppression of isolate-specific neutralizing anti-HIV antibody response, a phenomenon that correlates with extensive HIV spread preceding disease progression (30,59,61). Suppression of the highly specific neutralizing antibody response to the evolving HIV variants along the course of infection by the anti-HIV CTL is further rationalized by the fact that anti-HIV CTL have a broader specificity than anti-HIV neutralizing antibodies (64). Consequently, the killing of the B cells highly specific for successive HIV env epitopes by CTL with broad anti-HIV activity may contribute to the establishment of chronic HIV disease as well as eventually to the development of AIDS. While this CTL-mediated B-cell killing mechanism is speculative, the presence of anti-HIV CTL activity, but absence of neutralizing antibodies is clearly demonstrated in the rapidly progressing individuals with HIV infection.

THERAPEUTIC IMPLICATIONS

From a virological view point, HIV replication-induced cell death by apoptosis (13-19) is a major mechanism responsible for CD4+ T-lymphocyte depletion in HIV infection. This direct virus-induced apoptosis is probably the principle component of the acute symptomatic primary infection associated with massive viral replication (30). It is also plausible that the loss of peripheral CD4+ T-cell pool occurring along the course of HIV disease results at least partly from lymphoid organ CD4+ T-cell apoptosis triggered by HIV as well as enhanced by other pathogens (65,66). Moreover, the terminal phase (immunosuppression) of the infection is most likely again dominated by the virus-induced CD4+ T-cell apoptosis as a consequence of the massive viral replication (30).

From an immunological point of view, HIV-specific CTL, by killing virus-expressing cells, may be beneficial in dawn-regulating the viral spread, while at the same time the same CTL would destroy the virus-expressing CD4+ T cells and potentially the virus-presenting B cells or follicular dendritic cells, resulting in the eventual disorganisation of the architecture of lymphoid organs (2,3). This view is in keeping with the fact that the inhibition of CTL activity using anti-activating drugs such as cyclosporin A (CSA) seems to be beneficial in asymptomatic individuals by slowing the rate of disease progression (67-69).

Since HIV-expressing CD4+ T cells (as well as antigen presenting cells) die by apoptosis induced either by viral infection or by anti-HIV CTL via a Fas-mediated mechanism (45,46), the strategy directed at blocking apoptosis by anti-apoptotic drugs might be helpful not only in inhibiting HIV-mediated viropathic effects, but in combating the CTL-mediated immunopathic effects.

In this setting, glucocorticoids (GCC) have recently been discovered in our laboratory to antagonize activation-induced apoptosis in mature human T cells via both HIV-triggered and non-virus-triggered pathways (19). Such an anti-apoptotic action of GCC overbalances the downregulatory effect of GCC on T-cell proliferation, resulting in an overall improvement of CD4+ T-cell survival in patient PBMC. These effects of GCC are prevented by the anti-GCC RU 486 and are not associated with significant suppression of IL-2 receptor expression and IL-2-dependent T-cell blast transformation nor have any impact on viral replication. These findings imply that GCC may have therapeutic potentials in defeating some of the pathogenic processes governing progressive CD4+ T cell destruction in HIV-1 infection. Such a potential has been demonstrated by the one-year results of a glucocorticoid therapy (oral prednisolone 0.5 mg/kg per day for 6 months and 0.3 mg/kg per day thereafter) conducted on 44 asymptomatic patients with CD4+ T-cell count ranging from 200 to 799/µl (median: 438/µl). Not only prednisolone treatment was found to be safe over one year, but a sustained increase in the CD4+ T-cell count (median gain at 1 year: 119 cells/µl) was observed. Moreover, both serum P24 antigen by ELISA and HIV RNA levels by quantitative RT-PCR assay (8,70) coupled with an improved post-PCR detection system (71) remain stable over this period (72).

On the other hand, when looking at the humoral arm of the anti-HIV response, it seems to us probable that the loss of specific neutralizing antibody response is disastrous in favoring viral spread and CD4+ T-cell depletion, and eventually leads to the development of AIDS (59,61). In this setting, strategies aimed at administrating natural (73) or in vitro engineered (74) neutralizing antibodies or at preserving the patient's neutralizing antibody response by biological or pharmacological down-regulation of HIV-specific CTL should be actively developed with the objective of defeating the principal processes proved or suspected to govern the progression to AIDS.

REFERENCES

1. Levy JA. HIV pathogenesis and long-term survival. AIDS 1993; 7:1401-1410.
2. Fauci AS. Multifactorial nature of human immunodeficiency virus disease: Implications for therapy. Science 1994; 262:1011-1018.

3. Andrieu JM, and Lu W. Viro-immunolopathogenesis of HIV disease: Implications for therapy. Immunol Today 1995; 16:5-7.

4. Larder, B.A., G. Darby, D. D. Richman. HIV with reduced sensitivity to zidovudine (AZT) isolated during prolonged therapy. Science 1989; 243:1731-1734.

5. Bucher, CA, Tersmette M, Lange JM, Kellam P, de Guede RE, Mulden JW, Darby G, Goudsmith J, Larder BA. Zidovudine sensitivity of human immunodeficiency viruses from high-risk, symptom-free individuals during therapy. Lancet 1990; 336:585-90.

6. Lu W, and Andrieu JM. Early identification of human immunodeficiency virus-infected asymptomatic subjects susceptible to zidovudine by quantitiative viral coculture and reverse transcription-linked polymerase chain reaction. J Infect Dis 1993; 167:1014-1020.

7. Concorde Coordinating Committee. Concorde MRC/ARNS randomised double blind controlled trial of immediate and deferred zidovudine in symptom-free HIV infection. Lancet; 343:871-880.

8. Dalgleish AG, Beverley PC, Clapham PR, Crawford DH, Greaves MF, and Weiss RA. The CD4 (T4) antigen is an essential component of the receptor for the AIDS retrovirus. Nature 1984; 321:763-767.

9. Klatzmann D, Barre-Sinoussi F, Nugeyre MT, et al. Selective tropism of lymphadenopathy-associated virus (LAV) for helper-inducer T lymphocytes. Science 1984; 225:59-62.

10. Cheng-Mayer C. Biological and molecular features of HIV-1 related to tissue tropism. AIDS 1990; 4 (suppl 1):S49-S56.

11. Sullivan N, Thali M, Ho DD, and Sodroski J. Effect of amino-acid changes in the V1/V2 region of the human immunodeficiency virus type 1 gp120 glycoprotein on subunit association, syncytium formation, and recognition by a neutralizing antibody. J Virol 1993; 67:3674-3679.

12. Freed EO and Martin MA. Evidence for a functional interaction between the V1/V2 and C4 domains of human immunodefiency virus type 1 envelope glycoprotein gp120. J Virol 1994; 68:2503-2512.

13. Gougeon ML, Olivier R, Garcia S, Guetard D, Dragic T, Dougret C, Montanier L. Mise en evidence d'un processus d'engagement vers la mort cellulaire par apoptose dans les lymphocytes de patients infecté par le VIH. CR Acad Sci Paris. 1991; 312:529-537.

14. Gougeon ML, Laurent-Crawford AG, Hovanessian AG, and Montagnier L. Direct and indirect mechanisms mediating apoptosis during HIV infection: contribution to in vivo CD4 T cell depletion. Semin Immunol 1993; 5:187-194.

15. Terai C, Kornbluth RS, Pauza CD, Richman DD, Carson DA. Apoptosis as a mechanism of cell death in cultured T lymphoblasts acutely infected with HIV-1. J Clin Invest 1991; 87:1710-1715.

16. Laurent-Crawford, A. G., Krust B, Muler S, et al. The cytopathic effect of HIV is associated with apoptosis. Virology 1991; 185:829-839.

17. Laurent-crawford AG, Krust B, Riviere Y, Desgranges C, Muller S, Kieny MP, Dauguet C, and Hovanessian AG. Membrane expression of HIV envelope glycoproteins triggers apoptosis in CD4 cells. AIDS Res Hum Retroviruses 1993; 9:761-773.

18. Rey-Cuille MA, Galabru J, Laurent-Crawford A, Krust B, Montagnier L, and Hovanessian AG. HIV-2 EHO isolate has a divergent envolope gen and induces single cell killing by apoptosis. Virology 1994; 202:471-476.

19. Lu W, Salerno-Goncalves R, Yuan J, Sylvie D, Han DS, and Andrieu JM. Glucocorticoids rescue CD4+ T lymphocytes from activation-induced apoptosis triggered by HIV-1: implications for pathogenesis and therapy. AIDS 1995; 9:35-42.

20. Evans LA, Moreau J, Odehouri K, Legg H, Barboza A, Cheng-Mayer C, and Levy JA. Characterization of a noncytopathic HIV-2 strain with unusual effects on CD4 expression. Science 1988; 240:1522-1525.

21. Hoxie JA, Brass LF, Pletcher CH, Haggarty BS, and Hahn BH. Cytopathic variants of an attenuated isolate of human immunodeficiency virus type 2 exhibit increased affinity for CD4. J Virol. 1991; 65:5096-5101.

22. Esser R, von Briesen H, Brugger M, Ceska M, Glienke W, Müller S, Rehm A, Rübsamen-Waigmann H, and Andressen R. Secretory repertoire of HIV-infected human monocytes/macrophages. Pathobiology 1991; 59:219-222.

23. Trinchieri G and Scott P. The role of interleukin 12 in the immune response, disease and therapy. Immunol Today 1994; 15:460-463.

24. Knight SC and Macatonia SE. Effect of HIV on antigen presentation by dendritic cells and macrophages. Res Virol 1991; 142:123-128.

25. Wehle K, Schirmer M, Dünnebacke-Hinz J, Küpper T, and Pfitzer P. Quantitative differences in phagocytosis and degradation of Pneumonystis carinii by alevolar macrophages in AIDS and non-HIV patients in vivo. Cytopathology 1993; 4:231-236.

26. Stamatatos L and Cheng-Mayer C. Evidence that the structural conformation of envelope gp120 affects human immunodefiency virus type 1 infectivity, host range, and syncytium-formating ability. J Virol 1993; 67:5635-5639.

27. Koito A, Harrowe G, Levy JA, and Cheng-Mayer C. Functional role of the V1/V2 region of human immunodefiency virus type 1 envelope glycoprotein gp120 in infection of primary macrophages and soluble CD4 neutralization. J Virol 1994; 68:2253-2259.

28. Fenyo EM, Albert J, and Asjo B. Replicative capacity, cytopathic effect and cell tropism of HIV. AIDS 1989; 3 (suppl 1):S5-S12.

29. Evans LA, McHugh TM, Stites DP, and Levy JA. Differential ability of human immunodeficiency virus isolates to productively infect human cells. J Immunol 1987; 138:3415-3418.

30. Andrieu JM, Levy JP, and Lu W (eds). Workshop on Viral Quantitation in HIV Infection. London: Current Science (AIDS suppl 2), 1993.

31. Mosier DE, Gulizia RJ, Macisaac PD, and Levy JA. Rapid loss of CD4+ T cells in human-PBL-SCID mice by non-cytopathic HIV isolates. Science 1993; 260:689-692.

32. Lu W, and Andrieu JM. Similar replication capacities of primary human immunodeficiency virus type 1 isolates derived from a wide range of clinical sources. J Virol 1992; 66:334-340.

33. Valentin A, Albert J, Fenyo EM, and Asjo B. Dual tropism for macrophages and lymphocytes is a common feature of primary human immunodeficiency virus type 1 and 2 isolates. J Virol 1994; 68:6684-6689.

34. Donaldson YK, Bell JE, Holmes EC, Hughes ES, Brown HK, and Simmonds P. In vivo distribution and cytopathology of variants of human immunodeficiency virus type 1 showing restricted sequence variability in the V3 loop. J Virol 1994; 68:5991-6005.

35. Groux G, Torpier G, Monte D, Mouton Y, Capron A, & Ameisen JC. Activation-induced death by apoptosis in CD4+ T cells from human immunodeficiency virus-induced asymptomatic individuals. J Exp Med 1992; 175:331-334.

36. Meyaard L, Otto SA, Jonker RR, Mijnster MJ, Keet RPM, Miedema F. Programmed death of T cells in HIV-1 infection. Science 1992; 257:217-219.

37. Gougeon ML, Garcia S, Heeney J, et al. Programmed cell death in AIDS-related HIV and SIV infection. AIDS Res Hum Retroviruses 1993; 9:553-563.

38. Meyaard L, Otto S, Keet IPM, Roos MTL, Miedema F. Programmed death of T cells in humanodeficiency virus infection. No correlation with progression to disease. J Clin Invest 1994; 93:982-988.

39. Giorgi JV, Fahey JL, Smith DC, et al. Early effects of HIV on CD4 lymphocytes in vivo. J Immunol 1987; 138:3725-3730.

40. Miedema F, Petit AJ, Terpstra FG, et al. Immunological abnormalities in human immunodeficiency virus (HIV)-infected asymptomatic homosexual men. HIV affects the immune system before CD4+ T helper cell depletion occurs. J Clin Invest 1988; 82:1908-1914.

41. Clerici M, Stocks NI, Zajac RA, et al. Detection of three distinct patterns of T helper cell dysfuction in asymptomatic, human immunodeficiency virus-seropositive patients. Independence of CD4+ cell number and clinical staging. J Clin Invest 1989; 84:1892-1899.

42. Van Noesel CJ, Gruter RA, Terpstra FA, Schellekens PT, Van Lier RA, Miedema F. Functional and phenotypic evidence for a selective loss of memory T cells in asymptomatic human immunodeficiency virus infected men. J Clin Invest 1990; 86:293-299.

43. Schnittman SM, Lane HC, Greenhouse J, Fauci AS. Preferential infection of CD4+ memory T cells by human immunodeficiency virus type 1: Evidence for a role in the selective T-cell functional defects observed in infected individuals. Proc Natl Acad Sci USA 1990; 87:6058-6062.

44. Meyaard L, Schuitemaker H, Miedema F. T-cell dysfunction in HIV infection: anergy due to defective antigen-presenting cell function? Immunol Today 1993; 14:161-164.

45. Cohen JJ, Duke RC, Fadok VA, and Sellins KS. Apoptosis and programmed cell death in immunity. Annu rev Immunol 1992; 10:267-293.

46. Ju ST, Cui H, Panka DJ, Ettinger R, and Marshak-Rothstein A. Participation of target Fas protein in apoptosis pathway induced by CD4+ Th1 and CD8+ cytotoxic T cells. Proc Natl Acad Sci USA 1994; 91:4185-4189.

47. Walker BD and Plata F. Cytotoxic T lymphocytes against HIV. AIDS 1990; 4:177-184.

48. Riviere Y, Tanneau-Salvadori F, Regnault A, Lopez O, Sansonetti P, Guy B, Kieny MP, Fournel JJ, and Montagnier L. Human immunodeficiency virus-specific cytotoxic responses of seropositive individuals: distinct types of effector cells mediate killing of targets expressing gag and env protein. J Virol 1989; 63:2270-2277.

49. Pantaleo G, Demarest JF, Soudeyns H, Graziosi C, Denis F, Adelsberger JW, Borrow P, Saag MS, Shaw GM, Sekaly RP, and Fauci AS. Major expansion of CD8+ T cells with a predominant Vb usage during the primary immune response to HIV. Nature 1994; 370:463-467.

50. Zinkernagel RM, and Hengartner H. T-cell-mediated immunopathology versus direct cytolysis by virus: implications for HIV and AIDS. Immunol Today 1994; 15:262-268.

51. Cheynier, R., Henrichwark, S., Hadida, F., Pelletier E, Oksenhendler E, Autran B, and Wain-Hobson S. Cell 1994; 78:373-378.

52. Tindall B and Cooper DA. Primary HIV infection: host reponses and intervention strategies. AIDS 1991; 5:1-14.

53. Clark SJ, Saag MS, Decker WD, Campbell-Hill S, Roberson JL, Veldkamp PJ, Kappes JC, Hahn BH, and Shaw GM. High titers of cytopathic virus in plasma of patients with symptomatic primary HIV infection. N Engl J Med 1991; 324:954-960.

54. Daar ES, Moudgil T, Meyer RD, and Ho DD. Transient high levels of viremia in patients with primary human immunodeficiency virus type 1 infection. N Engl J Med 1991; 324:961-964.

55. Lu W, Eme D, and Andrieu JM. HIV viraemia and seroconversion. Lancet 1993; 341:113.

56. Pantaleo G, Graziosi C, Demarest JF, et al. HIV infection is active and progressive in lymphoid tissue during the clinically latent stage of disease. Nature 1993; 362:355-358.

57. Embretson J, Zupancic M, Ribas JL, et al. Massive covert infection of helper T lymphocytes and macrophages by HIV during the incubation period of AIDS. Nature 1993; 362;359-362.

58. Price RW, Brew B, Sidtis J, Rosenblum M, Scheck AC, and Cleary P. The brain in AIDS: Central nervous system HIV-1 infection and AIDS dementia complex. Science 1988; 239:586-592.

59. Lu W, Shih JWK, Tourani JM, Eme D, Alter HJ, and Andrieu JM. Lack of isolate-specific neutralizing activity is correlated with an increased viral burden in rapidly progressing HIV-1-infected patients. AIDS 1993; 7 (suppl):S91-S99.

60. Andrieu JM (ed). Viral Quantitation in HIV Infection. Paris: John Libbey Eurotext, 1991.

61. Albert J, Abrahamsson B, Nagy K, et al. Rapid development of isolate-specific neutralizing antibodies after primary HIV-1 infection and consequent emergence of virus variants which resist neutralization by autologous sera. AIDS 1991; 4:107-112.

62. Koup RA, Safrit JT, Cao Y, Andrews CA, McLeod G, Borkowsky W, Farthing C, and Ho DD. Temporal association of cellular immune responses with the initial control of viremia in primary human immunodeficiency virus type 1 syndrome. J Virol 1994; 68:4650-4655.

63. Barnaba V, Franco A, Alberti A, Benvenuto R, and Balsano F. Selective killing of hepatitis B envelope antigen-specific B cells by class I-restricted, exogenous antigen-specific T lymphocytes. Nature 1990; 345:258-260.

64. Chada S, DeJesus CE, Townsend K, Lee WTL, Laube L, Lolly DJ, Chang SMW, and Warner JF. Cross-reactive lysis of human targets infected with prototypic and clinical human immunodeficiency virus type 1 (HIV-1) strain by murine anti-HIV-1 IIIB env-specific cytotoxic T lymphocytes. J Virol 1993; 67:3409-3417.

65. Lu W, Grassi F, Tourani JM, Eme D, Israel-Biet D, and Andrieu JM. High concentration of peripheral blood mononuclear cells harboring infectious virus correlates with rapid progression of human immunodeficiency virus type 1-related disease. J Infect Dis 1993; 168:1165-1168.

66. Lu W, and Israel-Biet D. Virion concentration in bronchoalveolar lavage fluids of HIV infected patients. Lancet 1993; 342:298.

67. Andrieu JM, Bach JF, and Even P (eds). Autoimmune Aspects of HIV Infection. London - New York: Royal Society of Medicine Services, 1988.

68. Andrieu JM, Even P, Venet A. Effects of cyclosporin on T-cell subsets in human immunodeficiency virus disease. Clin Immunol Immunopath 1988; 46:181-98.

69. Levy R, Tourani JM, Jaïs JP, Even P, and Andrieu JM. CD4 cell count of HIV-1 asymptomatic patients remains stable under cyclosporin A. 1994 X Int Conf AIDS I, PB0298 (Abstr).

70. Lu W, and Andrieu JM. Use of the human immunodeficiency virus virion as a universal standard for viral RNA quantitation by reverse transcription-linked polymerase chain reaction. J Infect Dis 1993; 167:1498-1499.

71. Lu W, Han DS, Yan J, Andrieu JM. Multi-target PCR analysis by capillary electrophoresis and laser-induced fluorescence. Nature 1994; 368:269-271.

72. Andrieu JM, Lu W, and Levy R. Sustained increase of the CD4 cell count in asymptomatic HIV-1 seropositive patients treated by prednisolone for one year. J Infect Dis 1995; 171:523-530.

73. Karpus A, Hill F, Youle M, Cullen V, Gray J, Byron N, Howard L, Gilgen D, et al. Effects of passive immunization in patients with the aquired immunodeficiency syndrome-related complex and aquired immunodeficiency syndrome. Proc Natl Acad Sci USA 1988; 85:9234-9237.

74. Burton DR, Pyati J, Koduri R, Sharp SJ, Thornton GB, Parren PWHI, et al. Efficient neutralization of primary isolates of HIV-1 by a recombinant human monoclonal antibody. Science 1994; 266:1024-1027.

INDEX

The manufacturer's authorised representative in the EU is Springer
Nature Customer Service Centre GmbH, Europaplatz 3, 69115 Heidelberg,
Germany. If you have any concerns regarding our products, please
contact ProductSafety@springernature.com

Printed and bound by CPI Group (UK) Ltd, Croydon, CR0 4YY
29/04/2026
02099527-0006